AF822404

Self-Assessment Review in
Gastroenterology
for DM Entrance Exams

Editors

Premashis Kar M.D., DM, PhD., FAMS
Director Professor of Medicine
Head Gastroenterology Division
Department of Medicine
Maulana Azad Medical College and Associated Lok Nayak and G.B. Pant Hospital
University of Delhi
New Delhi - 110002

Hemant Nayak M.D.
Senior Resident, Department of Medicine
Maulana Azad Medical College and Associated Lok Nayak and G.B. Pant Hospital
University of Delhi
New Delhi - 110002

PEEPEE
PUBLISHERS AND DISTRIBUTORS (P) LTD.

Self-Assessment Review in Gastroenterology for DM Entrance Exams

Published by
Pawaninder P. Vij

Peepee Publishers and Distributors (P) Ltd.
Head Office: 160, Shakti Vihar, Pitam Pura, Delhi-110 034 (India)

Correspondence Address:

7/31, First Floor, Ansari Road, Daryaganj
New Delhi-110002 (India)

Ph: 65195868, 23246245, 9811156083

e-mail: peepee160@yahoo.co.in

e-mail: peepee160@rediffmail.com

e-mail: peepee160@gmail.com

www.peepeepub.com

First Edition: 2012

ISBN: 978-81-8445-116-0

Printed at: trident offset works, naraina new delhi

Indian Society of Gastroenterology

FOREWORD

I am pleased to write this foreword for the **Self-Assessment Review in Gastroenterology for DM Entrance Exams** authored by Professor Premashis Kar and Dr. Hemant Nayak. The book contains multiple choice questions in different formats, arranged in individual chapters by topic. The book moreover provides an explanation for each answer at the end of each chapter, with references to standard textbooks in order to assist the reader in identifying the place to obtain more information on a given question. I have read the questions in each chapter and found that they cover a wide spectrum accurately. The questions are designed thoughtfully, and the use of this book in conjunction with the standard gastroenterology textbooks will definitely help those who wish to broaden their knowledge gastroenterology to identify and rectify areas in which their depth of knowledge is insufficient. Professor Kar and the team that contributed to this self-assessment review book ought to be congratulated on the painstaking work that has gone into it. I would recommend it very highly and without reservation to those aspiring for admission to postgraduate training courses in gastroenterology, as well as to those who are already enrolled in training programs in gastroenterology in the country.

B.S. Ramakrishna, MD, DM, PhD, FAMS, FNASc, FNA
President, Indian Society of Gastroenterology

Vellore
14th August 2012

Secretariat: Department of Gastroenterology Moti Lal Medical College, Allahabad-211001, INDIA
Phone: +91-532-2256087, 2256090; Fax: +91-532-2256878
Email: drspmisra@gmail.com; website: http//www.isg.org.in

Preface

The book entitled **"Self-Assessment Review in Gastroenterology for DM Entrance Exams"** is a comprehensive review of gastrointestinal organ system, condition and disorders that has been prepared in conjunction with the Sleisenger Textbook of Gastroenterology. The program is designed for gastroenterologists, hepatologists and physicians with interest in gastroenterology who are involved in day-to-day care of gastrointestinal disorders. The question-answers and the related references would prove helpful for individuals preparing for DM entrance in gastroenterology as well as for practitioners seeking a well rounded clinical update. Efforts were made by all contributors as well as the editors to provide correct answers with reference to various topics covered in the text organ wise. This book is also designed to test the candidates' ability to arrive at a reasonable diagnosis from a set of data and is intended to replicate the day-to-day decision-making faced by all doctors working in gastroenterology. It should be realized that in number of questions there can be more than one answer but weightage is given to the most appropriate answer. The manual has been compiled reflecting the recent trend in the practice of gastroenterology. I believe that this manual of self-assessment in gastroenterology could prove to be an ideal resource for those who seek excellence in the care of gastrointestinal disorders. However there could still be some errors and we would welcome such feedback on controversial answers. Tremendous effort has been put forward by various authors in extensively covering various topics but the manual still needs to be updated every year.

I am grateful to all contributors and colleagues for their commitment to this classic book which has been a labor of love for the field of gastroenterology. The publisher has shown keen interest in the book and we thank for his constant encouragement, co-operation and support.

Premashis Kar

Contributors

Dr. L. Thayumanavan Bhartia, MD, DM
Professor and Head, Department of Gastroenterology
Madurai Medical College and Govt. Rajaji Hospital
Madurai

Dr. Y.K. Chawla, MD, DM
Professor and Head, Department of Hepatology
Postgraduate Institute of Medical Education and Research
Chandigarh

Dr. Ajay Duseja, MD, DM
Add. Professor of Hepatology
Postgraduate Institute of Medical Education and Research
Chandigarh

Dr. A.K. Jain, MD, DM
Professor and Head, Department of Gastroenterology
Institute of Medical Sciences
Varanasi

Dr. Premashis Kar, MD, DM, PhD, FAMS
Director Professor of Medicine
Head Gastroenterology Division
Department of Medicine
Maulana Azad Medical College and Associated Lok Nayak and G.B. Pant Hospital
University of Delhi
New Delhi

Dr. Hemant Nayak, MD
Senior Resident, Department of Medicine
Maulana Azad Medical College and Associated Lok Nayak and G.B. Pant Hospital, University of Delhi
New Delhi

Dr. S.S. Rana, MD, DM
Associate Professor, Department of Gastroenterology
Postgraduate Institute of Medical Education and Research
Chandigarh

Dr. C.S. Reddy, MD, DM
Senior Resident, Department of Hepatology
Postgraduate Institute of Medical Education and Research
Chandigarh

Dr. Rajiv Singla, MD, DNB (Medicine)
Senior Resident, Department of Medicine
Maulana Azad Medical College and Associated Lok Nayak and G.B. Pant Hospital
New Delhi

Dr. J.C. Vij, MD, DM
Senior Consultant
Pushpawati Singhania Research Institute for Liver, Renal and Digestive Diseases
Press Enclave Marg, Sheikh Sarai II
New Delhi

Contents

Chapter 1

Oesophagus

1. The true statement regarding oesophageal anatomy:
A. Length of oesophagus is 30-40 cm
B. It has all the five layers of GIT
C. Mid-oesophagus is supplied by descending aorta
D. Ends after passing through the hiatus in the left crus of diaphragm

2. Dysphagia to normal solid food is always present if esophageal diameter is less than:
A. 1.3 cm
B. 2 cm
C. 2.5 cm
D. 4 cm

3. Postural dysphagia for solids is seen in:
A. Scleroderma
B. Achalasia
C. Diffuse oesophageal spasm
D. None

4. Sitaphobia is seen in:
A. Crohn's disease
B. Viral hepatitis
C. Chronic mesenteric vascular ischemia
D. A + C

5. In achalasia, basic abnormality is:
A. Inhibitory neural degeneration localised to nerve processes
B. Inhibitory neural degeneration localised to nerve cell bodies
C. Excitatory neural degeneration localised to nerve processes
D. Excitatory neural degeneration localised to nerve cell bodies

6. One of the following causes large peristaltic contractions on esophageal manometry:
A. Achalasia
B. Diffuse esophageal spasm
C. Nut cracker esophagus
D. Diabetic neuropathy

7. All are features on esophageal manometry in scleroderma *except:*
A. Abnormal sphincter relaxation of UES
B. Low amplitude peristalsis
C. Hypotensive LES
D. Low amplitude simultaneous onset contractions

8. Candidal esophagitis is best diagnosed by:
A. Endoscopy
B. Endoscopy with plaque smears showing hyphae/yeast
C. Endoscopy with biopsy
D. Endoscopy with culture

9. Severity of radiation esophagitis is increased by all drugs *except:*
A. Doxorubicin
B. Bleomycin
C. Indomethacin
D. Cisplatin

10. The following type of esophageal diverticulum is associated with achalasia:
A. Mid-esophageal
B. Diffuse intramural
C. Zenkers
D. Epiphrenic

11. All are secondary causes of achalasia *except:*
A. Gastric carcinoma
B. African trypanosomiasis
C. Neuropathic intestinal pseudo-obstruction
D. Lymphoma

12. All the following provoke esophageal contractions in DES *except:*
A. Cold water
B. Solid food
C. Edrophonium
D. Ergonovine

13. Most sensitive test for diagnosis of GERD is:
A. Upper GI endoscopy
B. Bernstein test
C. Esophageal biopsy
D. 24 hours ambulatory pH monitoring

14. In the clinical evaluation of chest pain, the symptom that has no significant statistical difference among cardiac and oesophageal causes is:
A. Radiation to left arm
B. Pain lasting several hours
C. Pain awakens at night
D. Provoked by recumbency

15. Most common disorder of esophageal dysmotility:
A. Non-specific dysmotility
B. Nut cracker esophagus
C. Diffuse oesophageal spasm (DES)
D. Achalasia

16. All are causes of odynophagia *except:*
A. Steak-House syndrome
B. Carcinoma esophagus
C. Caustic ingestion
D. Severe GERD

17. The following maneuvers aggravate heart burn *except:*
A. Straining the stool
B. Uplifting of heavy objects
C. Stationary bike riding
D. Running

18. The symptom that does not suggest reflux induced asthma is:
A. Late age of onset
B. Worsening after meals
C. Relieved with bronchodilators
D. Steroid dependent asthma

19. Ora serrata is:
A. Serrations found on buccal mucosa in normal persons
B. Ulcers in the mouth
C. Endoscopic finding of oesophago-gastric junction
D. Variant of geographic tongue

20. All the following types of cells are seen in a normal oesophageal epithelium *except:*
A. Melanocytes
B. Lymphocytes
C. Eosinophils
D. Neutrophils

21. The most common developmental anomaly of esophagus is:
A. Isolated esophageal atresia
B. Esophageal atresia + Distal type of TOF
C. Esophageal stenosis + Distal type of TOF
D. Esophageal stenosis

22. Diet modification is the primary therapeutic approach for:
A. Hiatal hernia
B. Oesophageal rings
C. Dysphagia lustoria
D. Oesophageal webs

23. False statement regarding 'inlet patch':
A. It is a heterotopic gastric mucosa below UES
B. It can secrete acid
C. H. pylori infection can occur
D. No association with adenocarcinoma

24. True statement regarding Schatzki's ring:
A. It represents the proximal border of oesophageal vestibule
B. Contains only mucosa and submucosa
C. This is seen in 40% of patients on routine UGI series
D. Surgery is the most definitive treatment

25. Average normal LES pressure at rest:
A. 10 mm Hg
B. 15 mm Hg
C. 40 mm Hg
D. 30 mm Hg

26. All the following have effect on LES *except:*
A. Truncal vagotomy
B. Fat
C. Peppermint
D. Diazepam

27. The most common neoplasm associated with achalasia:
A. Esophageal squamous cell carcinoma
B. Gastric squamous cell carcinoma
C. Gastric adenocarcinoma
D. Gastric lymphoma

28. Confirmatory test for idiopathic achalasia:
A. Barium swallow
B. Endoscopy with biopsy
C. Barium swallow + videofluoroscopy
D. Oesophageal manometry

29. Test done to differentiate idiopathic achalasia from associated malignancy:
A. Oesophageal manometry
B. Amyl nitrate + barium swallow
C. Barium swallow alone
D. Mecholyl test

30. Barrett's epithelium has all the following histological characters *except:*

A. Absence of goblet cells
B. Lack of intestinal absorptive capacity
C. Presence of villous structure
D. Presence of parietal and chief cells

31. Regarding tLESRs (transient lower oesophageal relaxations), false statement:
A. Occur in patients with normal LES pressure
B. Appear without fixed temporal relation to pharyngeal contractions
C. Persists for shorter duration than swallow induced LESRs
D. Occur physiologically to gastric distension of food/gas

32. Esophageal acid clearance is defined as the duration of time that the oesophageal mucosa remains acidified to a pH less than:
A. 2.5
B. 3
C. 3.5
D. 4

33. Most common predisposing factor for GERD:
A. Scleroderma
B. Pregnancy
C. Nasogastric intubation
D. Obesity

34. If the esophagus endoscopically has confluent erosions of > 50% of the mucosal surface of the last 5 cm of esophageal squamous mucosa, it is graded as.....esophagitis.
A. Grade II
B. Grade III
C. Grade I
D. Grade IV

35. False statement regarding management of Barrett's oesophagus:
A. High grade dysplasia warrants definitive surgical therapy
B. Vigorous anti-secretory therapy is not prescribed in low grade dysplasia
C. Surveillance for low grade dysplasia is every 12 months
D. Surveillance for absent dysplasia is every 18-24 months

36. 'Pseudo-ulcerations' on oesophagogram are seen in esophagitis due to:
A. CMV
B. Candida
C. HSV
D. Pill induced

37. 'Volcano lesions' on oesophagogram are seen in esophagitis due to:
A. CMV
B. Candida
C. HSV
D. Pill induced

38. All are useful in HIV related idiopathic oesophageal ulcers *except:*
A. Sucralfate
B. Dexamethasone
C. Thalidomide
D. Itraconazole

39. Skin condition that is not pre-malignant for oesophageal carcinoma:
A. Epidermolysis bullosa
B. Bullous pemphigoid
C. Cicatricial pemphigoid
D. Tylosis et palmaris

40. The incidence and severity of oesophageal damage increase with radiation doses greater than:
A. 30 Gy
B. 40 Gy
C. 50 Gy
D. 75 Gy

41. Minimum period from exposure of radiation to oesophageal stricture formation is:
A. 3 months
B. 6 months
C. 1 year
D. 2 years

42. Incidence of oesophageal stricture formation following EST:
A. 5%
B. 10%
C. 15%
D. 25%

43. The risk factor for oesophageal squamous cell carcinoma in which endoscopic surveillance is recommended:
A. Partial gastrectomy
B. Chronic stricture
C. Tylosis
D. Plummer-Vinson syndrome

44. Barium swallow finding that excludes resectability in oesophageal carcinoma:
A. Tumor length > 5 cm
B. Apple-core lesion

C. Disruption of oesophageal axis
D. All the above

45. Most common presentation of oesophageal SCC (Squamous cell carcinoma) is in stage:
A. II a
B. II b
C. III
D. IV

46. Ideal palliative modality for circumferential oesophageal carcinoma:
A. Oesophageal dilatation
B. Injection therapy
C. Bipolar electro coagulation
D. Laser

47. Palliative modality of choice for long (>10 cm) tumors of oesophageal carcinoma:
A. Bipolar electro coagulation
B. Laser
C. Photodynamic therapy
D. Endoscopic prosthesis

48. Ideal palliation for short, exophytic, non-circumferential oesophageal carcinoma:
A. Bipolar electro coagulation
B. Laser
C. Photodynamic therapy
D. Endoscopic prosthesis

49. Palliative modality of choice for airway fistulas complicating oesophageal carcinoma:
A. Bipolar electro coagulation
B. Laser
C. Photodynamic therapy
D. Endoscopic prosthesis

50. Most common extrapulmonary site for small cell carcinoma:
A. Hypopharynx
B. Oesophagus
C. Stomach
D. Small intestine

51. Most frequent primary metastasising to oesophagus:
A. Lung
B. Melanoma
C. Thyroid
D. Breast

52. Tracheo-bronchial aspiration unrelated to swallowing occurs with all the following *except:*
A. Pharyngeal paralysis
B. Achalasia
C. Zenker's diverticulum
D. GERD

53. All the foods decrease LES pressure *except:*
A. Onions
B. Carminatives
C. Citrus fruits
D. Sugars

54. All the following drugs decrease LES *except:*
A. Progesterone
B. NSAIDs
C. Adrenergic agonists
D. Adrenergic antagonists

55. All are extra oesophageal manifestations of GERD *except:*
A. Chronic cough
B. Syncope
C. Globus sensation
D. Headache

56. Most common cause of tissue eosinophilia in esophagus:
A. GERD
B. Adenocarcinoma
C. Allergic esophagitis
D. Parasitic infection

57. Treatment of choice in candida esophagitis with granulocytopenia:
A. IV fluconazole
B. IV amphotericin
C. Oral fluconazole
D. A+B

58. Low prevalence of candida esophagitis is seen in:
A. Achalasia
B. Esophageal carcinoma
C. AIDS
D. Post transplant patients

59. Plaque like lesions resembling candida infection are seen with all the following *except:*
A. Swallowed oropharyngeal debris
B. Pill esophagitis
C. CMV infection
D. Aspergillus infection

60. All the following bacterial infections can affect the esophagus without concomitant gastric infection *except:*
A. H. pylori
B. Nocardia

C. Diphtheria
D. Syphilis

61. First line management in GERD during pregnancy:
A. Life style/dietary modification
B. Sucralfate
C. Antacids
D. H_2 receptor antagonists

62. False statement regarding pregnancy and GERD:
A. GERD occurs in less than one-third of pregnant women
B. Resting LES tone decreases in early pregnancy
C. Esophageal motility is altered in late pregnancy
D. Upper GI endoscopy is safe during pregnancy

63. Most common site of esophageal adenocarcinoma:
A. Upper one-third
B. Middle one-third
C. Distal one-third
D. A+B

64. False statement regarding esophageal adenocarcinoma in comparison with squamous cell carcinoma:
A. Around 75% of patients have GERD
B. Fistulas are less common
C. Recurrent laryngeal nerve involvement is less common
D. Extension to adjacent structures is less common

65. Tracheo-oesophageal fistula complicating palliation of esophageal carcinoma by laser treatment is seen in at least:
A. 1%
B. 2%
C. 5%
D. 10%

66. Most common histologic pattern of Barrett's epithelium is:
A. Gastric
B. Small intestinal
C. Colonic
D. A+B

67. One of the following is a wrong statement:
A. Dysphagia is a sensation of sticking or obstruction of passage of food through mouth, pharynx, oesophagus
B. Aphagia signifies complete esophageal obstruction
C. Odynophagia means painful swallowing
D. Globus pharyngeus is lump lodged in throat

68. Phagophobia (fear of swallowing) may occur in all *except:*
A. Rabies
B. Tetanus
C. Hysteria
D. Achalasia

69. Regarding peristaltic contraction pick the correct statement:
A. Primary peristalsis is in response to swallow
B. Deglutitive inhibition is the inhibition that precedes the peristaltic contraction
C. Local distention of esophagus results in secondary peristalsis
D. Tertiary contractions are non-peristaltic and can occur spontaneously
E. All the statements are correct

70. Normal passage of ingested bolus depends on:
A. Size of bolus
B. Luminal diameter
C. Peristaltic contraction
D. Deglutitive inhibition
E. All the above

71. Pick the wrong statement regarding esophagus:
A. Distal esophagus is supplied by left gastric and splenic arteries
B. Venous drainage of distal esophagus is through azygos veins
C. Upper esophagus drains to cervical lymph nodes
D. Distal esophagus drains to celiac and gastric nodes

72. Optical coherence tomography is used to detect:
A. Gastro-esophageal reflux
B. Candidal esophagitis
C. Leiomyoma of esophagus
D. Barrett's esophagus
E. All the above

73. LES pressure is decreased by:
A. Gastrin
B. Motilin
C. VIP
D. Substance P

74. Transfer dysphagia is seen in:
A. Achalasia
B. Carcinoma esophagus
C. Myasthenia gravis
D. Scleroderma

75. One of the following is not a correct combination:
A. Progressive dysphagia lasting weeks to months –carcinoma esophagus

B. Dysphagia to solids and liquids from the very onset–motor dysphagia
C. Episodic dysphagia to solids lasting several years—lower esophageal ring
D. Nasal regurgitation and trachea-bronchial aspiration—pharyngeal paralysis
E. When hoarseness precedes dysphagia primary lesion is in–pharynx

76. Histological definition of low grade reflux esophagitis includes the following criteria *except:*
A. Presence of intraepithelial neutrophils or eosinophils
B. Basal zone> 15% of total thickness
C. Extension of papillae> two-thirds of distance from surface
D. None of the above

77. Hiccups with dysphagia suggest lesion in which part of esophagus?
A. Cervical oesophagus
B. Middle part of esophagus
C. Lower third of oesophagus
D. No such location can be made

78. All the following cause esophageal stricture *except:*
A. Prolonged nasogastric intubation
B. Chronic candidiasis
C. Ingestion of caustic agents
D. Previous radiation therapy
E. Ingestion of pills without water

79. Chest pain with dysphagia occurs in:
A. Leiomyoma of esophagus
B. Schatzki's ring
C. Aberrant subclavian artery
D. Diffuse esophageal spasm
E. All the above

80. Investigation of choice for each condition, match the following:

A. Oropharangeal dysphagia	1. Manometry
B. Carcinoma oesophagus	2. Video fluoroscopy
C. Motor disorders–oesophagus	3. Oesophago gastroscopy
D. GERD	4. 24-hour pH monitoring

81. All are correct regarding carcinoma esophagus *except:*
A. More common in males, most above age 50 years
B. 15% in upper one-third, 45% in middle one-third, 40% in lower one-third
C. More than 75% are squamous cell carcinomas
D. The type of carcinoma can be differentiated radiographically/endoscopically
E. Progressive dysphagia and weight loss are initial symptoms

82. All are premalignant conditions for carcinoma esophagus *except:*
A. Chronic achalasia
B. Corrosive stricture
C. Tylosis palmaris and plantaris
D. Candidiasis
E. Radiation stricture

83. All are premalignant for squamous cell carcinoma *except:*
A. Plummer Vinson syndrome
B. Deficiency of zinc, molybdenum, Vitamin A
C. Cigarette smoking
D. Gastroesophageal reflux disease
E. Excessive alcohol consumption

84. All are correct regarding carcinoma esophagus *except:*
A. Dysphagia occurs when 60% of circumference is infiltrated with cancer
B. Disease spreads to lymph nodes, liver, lung, pleura
C. Tracheo-esophageal fistula develops as disease advances
D. Contrast radiograph's show changes in mucosa and deeper infiltration
E. Oesophagoscopy need not be performed in all the patients

85. Patients with carcinoma esophagus have:
A. Increased incidence of carcinoma lung, head and neck region
B. Endoscopic biopsy success rate is >80% in confirmation
C. More than 5% of patients are alive 5 years after initial diagnosis
D. Results of radiation therapy is less than radical surgery
E. Endoscopic placement of expansive metal stents are useful in tracheobronchial fistula

86. All these statements are correct regarding gastro-esophageal reflux disease *except:*
A. Patients > 40 years with heart burn for 10 years–consider endoscopy to rule out Barrett's esophagus

B. Patients with Barrett's should undergo surveillance every 12-24 months
C. If dysplasia is present patient needs more frequent surveillance
D. High grade dysplasia needs surveillance than oesophagectomy

87. Treatment of choice for malignant trachea esophageal fistula is:
A. Laser ablation
B. Photodynamic therapy
C. Placement of prosthesis
D. Stricture dilatation
E. Chemotherapy

88. All decrease the lower esophageal sphincter pressure *except:*
A. Fatty meal
B. Smoking
C. Substance P
D. Adenosine
E. Nitric oxide donor, i.e., nitrates

89. All cause lower esophageal sphincter contraction *except:*
A. M_2 receptor agonist
B. Alpha adrenergic agonist
C. Gastrin
D. Vasoactive intestinal peptide (VIP)
E. Prostaglandin F_2 Alpha

90. All aggravate heart burn *except:*
A. CCK
B. Secretin
C. Dopamine
D. Metoclopramide
E. Nicotine

91. Odynophagia is characteristic of all *except:*
A. Monilial esophagitis
B. Barrett's ulcer
C. Carcinoma with periesophageal involvement
D. Achalasia
E. Caustic injury

92. Most frequent esophageal cause of chest pain is:
A. Reflux oesophagitis
B. Carcinoma oesophagus
C. Diffuse oesophageal spasm
D. Oesophageal ulcers
E. Herpes esophagitis

93. Water brash is:
A. Effortless appearance of gastric or esophageal contents in mouth
B. Because of incompetence of upper and lower esophageal sphincter
C. Associated with achalasia or diverticulum
D. Salivary hypersecretion, which occurs in response to peptic esophagitis
E. All the above

94. Investigation of choice for detection and analysis of oral and pharyngeal functions is:
A. Oesophagoscopy
B. Videofluoroscopy
C. Manometers
D. 24-hour pH monitoring

95. Esophageal peristalsis is best studied in:
A. Recumbent position
B. Upright position
C. Right lateral position
D. Left lateral position

96. Esophageal motility disorders are useful to study all *except:*
A. Diffuse esophageal spasm
B. Carcinoma esophagus
C. Achalasia
D. Scleroderma

97. Oropharyngeal paralysis causes all *except:*
A. Dysphagia
B. Nasal regurgitation
C. Chest pain
D. Tracheobronchial aspiration
E. All the above

98. All these conditions cause oropharyngeal dysphagia *except:*
A. Myasthenia gravis
B. Polymyositis
C. Cerebrovascular accident
D. Fibrosis in cricopharyngeus
E. None of the above

99. Globus pharyngeus is:
A. Difficulty in swallowing
B. More common in men
C. Barium studies and manometry are abnormal
D. Treatment is pharyngomyotomy
E. Associated with GERD

100. Achalasia shows all these features *except:*
A. LES does not relax with swallowing
B. Abnormal contractions in esophagus body
C. Loss of inhibitory neurons containing VIP and nitric oxide synthetase

D. Manometry can differentiate the primary from secondary achalasia
E. Dysphagia, chest pain, regurgitation are main symptoms

101. Secondary achalasia can be caused by:
A. Gastric carcinoma infiltrating esophagus
B. Lymphoma
C. Chagas' disease
D. Chronic intestinal pseudo-obstruction
E. All the above

102. Achalasia shows all these features *except:*
A. Dysphagia
B. Chest pain
C. Gastro-esophageal reflux
D. Regurgitation
E. All the above

103. All are shown in achalasia *except:*
A. Dysphagia for solids and liquids
B. Symptoms worsened by emotional stress
C. Valsalva manoeuver aids the passage of bolus into stomach
D. Chest pain is more in classical achalasia than vigorous achalasia
E. Associated carcinoma has severe weight loss and down-hill course

104. Manometric findings in achalasia will show:
A. Absence of gastric air bubble
B. Tubular mediastinal mass beside aorta
C. Air fluid level in mediastinum in upright position
D. Sigmoid esophagus on barium swallow
E. Presence of peristalsis in lower esophagus

105. Monomeric findings in achalasia are all *except:*
A. Basal LES pressure normal or elevated
B. Swallow induced relaxation is reduced
C. CCK paradoxically causes contraction of LES because of absence of the neurally transmitted inhibitory effect
D. All the above are correct

106. All are used in treatment of achalasia *except:*
A. Nitroglycerin 0.3 - 0.6 mg sublingual
B. Isosorbide dinitrate 2.5-5 mg sublingually before meals
C. Botulinum toxin injection at LES blocking cholinergic excitatory nerves
D. Esophageal stenting
E. Balloon dilatation to reduce LES pressure by tearing muscle fibers

107. Scleroderma shows all these changes by manometry:
A. Reduced amplitude of contractions that are simultaneous or peristaltic in onset
B. Reduced LES pressure
C. Normal sphincter relaxation
D. All are correct

108. Diffuse esophageal spasm shows all these changes *except:*
A. Large amplitude, long duration, repetitive multiple simultaneous, spontaneous contractions
B. Patchy neural degeneration localized to nerve process
C. Chest pain and dysphagia occur at rest, swallowing or emotional stress
D. Barium X-ray will show classical features
E. Nitroglycerine, nifedipine, isosorbide dinitrate are helpful

109. Simultaneous esophageal contractions are seen in:
A. Collagen vascular disease, diabetic neuropathy
B. Reflux esophagitis, irradiation esophagitis
C. Esophageal obstruction
D. All the above
E. None of the above

110. Gastrointestinal contents will reflux when:
A. Gastric volume is increased
B. Intra-gastric pressure is increased
C. When gastric contents are located near the gastro-esophageal junction
D. All the above

111. All cause decreased LES pressure *except:*
A. Pregnancy
B. Scleroderma
C. Intestinal pseudo-obstruction syndrome
D. Antacids
E. Aminophylline

112. Incidence of peptic stricture in patients with reflux esophagitis is:
A. 1%
B. 3%
C. 5%
D. 10%
E. 12%

113. GERD can cause all *except:*
A. Heart burn
B. Aspiration pneumonia
C. Squamous cell carcinoma

D. Chronic asthma
E. Peptic stricture

114. Investigations useful in diagnosis of GERD are all *except:*
A. 99m Tc sulfur colloid scan
B. 24-hour pH esophageal recording
C. Barium swallow
D. Bernstein test
E. Mucosal biopsy

115. Simultaneous onset contractions (> 10% of wet swallows) with intermittent normal peristalsis on oesophageal manometry is characteristic of:
A. Diffuse esophageal spasm
B. Nut cracker esophagus
C. Achalasia
D. Scleroderma

116. Bernstein test is useful in diagnosis of:
A. Barrett's esophagus and adenocarcinoma
B. Candidiasis, viral or bacterial infection of esophagus
C. Reflux esophagitis, which is not obvious endoscopically
D. Achalasia can be diagnosed
E. Scleroderma affecting the esophagus be diagnosed

117. All are used for treatment of GERD *except:*
A. Stop smoking
B. Weight reduction
C. Avoid fatty foods
D. Sleeping with foot end of the bed raised
E. Avoid lot of fluids with food

118. All are used in treatment of GERD *except:*
A. Avoiding smooth muscle relaxants
B. Mild to moderate cases respond to H_2 receptor blockers and prokinetics
C. Proton pump blockers (Omeprazole 20-40 mg)
D. Fundoplication
E. Oesophagectomy and esophagogastric anastomosis

119. Metaclopramide has all these effects *except:*
A. Increased LES pressure
B. Increased gastric emptying
C. Increased esophageal clearance
D. Extrapyramidal effects
E. Has action on small intestine and colon

120. Surveillance for GERD includes all *except:*
A. Endoscopic surveillance every 1-2 years in patients without dysplasia
B. Low grade dysplasia
C. High grade dysplasia
D. All are correct

121. Most useful in alkaline esophagitis is:
A. Omeprazole
B. Sucralfate
C. Cholestyramine
D. Aluminium hydroxide
E. Cisapride

122. Esophagitis in immunocompromised patients is because of all *except:*
A. HSV esophagitis
B. CMV esophagitis
C. Candidiasis
D. Varicella-zoster esophagitis
E. Reflux esophagitis

123. Patients with herpetic esophagitis present with all these features *except:*
A. Acute onset of chest pain, odynophagia, dysphagia
B. Nausea, vomiting, fever, chills, leucocytosis are present
C. Herpetic vesicles of nose and lips provide clues to the diagnosis
D. Barium swallow can adequately distinguish from other lesions
E. Endoscopy shows small discrete, punched out superficial ulceration

124. Mucosal cells taken from biopsy samples of HSV ulcers show:
A. Ballooning degeneration
B. Ground glass changes in nuclei with eosinophilia intranuclear inclusions
C. Giant cell formation
D. All the above

125. Necrotizing esophagitis is caused by:
A. HSV esophagitis
B. Varicella zoster esophagitis
C. CMV esophagitis
D. Candida esophagitis
E. All show these changes

126. Match the following:

A. Vesicles and small superficial ulcers	(1) CMV esophagitis
B. Vesicles, confluent ulcers	(2) HSV esophagitis
C. Serpiginous ulcers initially	(3) Varicella-zoster esophagitis
D. Curdy white precipitates	(4) Candidal esophagitis

127. CMV esophagitis show all these features *except:*
A. Occurs in immunocompromised patients
B. Can cause giant ulcers in distal esophagus
C. Diagnosis is by endoscopy and mucosal brushings
D. Intranuclear, cytoplasmic inclusions in fibroblast and endothelial cells in biopsy
E. Immunohistology with monoclonal antibodies to CMV is helpful for diagnosis

128. Treatment of choice for CMV esophagitis is:
A. Acyclovir 800 mg twice daily orally
B. Ganciclovir 5 mg/kg every 12 h IV
C. Foscarnet 60 mg/kg every 8 hours IV
D. Local steroid injections

129. Esophagitis in AIDS is caused by:
A. Cryptosporidium
B. Pneumocystis carinii
C. Mycobacterium tuberculosis
D. All the above

130. Esophageal bullous lesions are seen with:
A. Dystrophic epidermolysis bullosa
B. Cicatricial pemphigoid
C. Stevens-Johnson syndrome
D. Toxic epidermolysis bullosa
E. All the above

131. All these conditions involving oesophagus respond to steroids *except:*
A. Graft-versus-host disease
B. Behcet's disease
C. Eosinophilic enteritis
D. Crohn's disease
E. Erosive lichen planus

132. Match the following:
A. Zenker's diverticulum
B. Mid oesophageal diverticulum
C. Epiphrenic diverticulum
D. Diffuse intramural diverticulosis
(1) Traction from old adhesions
(2) Posterior hypopharyngeal wall weakness
(3) Associated with achalasia
(4) Dilatation of deep esophageal glands

133. Zenker's diverticulum shows all these features *except:*
A. Causes halitosis and regurgitation of saliva
B. Can cause dysphagia or complete obstruction
C. Endoscopy, NG tube placement can cause perforation
D. Treated by cricopharyngeal myotomy with or without diverticulectomy
E. All are correct

134. Plummer Vinson's syndrome shows all these features *except:*
A. Common in middle aged women
B. Iron deficiency anemia
C. Causes intermittent dysphagia to solids
D. No malignant potential
E. Symptomatic hypo pharyngeal webs

135. Schatzki's ring shows all these features *except:*
A. Weblike constriction located in squamo columnar junction
B. Produces dysphagia when diameter is less than 13 mm
C. Muscular ring with dysphagia only to solids and is intermittent
D. Asymptomatic rings are seen in 10% patients
E. Symptomatic rings are treated by dilatation

136. All these conditions causing dysphagia respond to rubber dilators *except:*
A. Peptic, corrosive stricture
B. Achalasia, diffuse esophageal spasm
C. Schatzki ring
D. Muscular ring (lower esophageal contractile ring)

137. Sliding hiatus hernia is:
A. GE junction and fundus of stomach slide upwards
B. Incidence decreases with age
C. Small hernias by themselves produce symptoms
D. Not associated with reflux esophagitis
E. All are correct

138. Sliding hiatus hernia results from:
A. Weakening of anchors of GE junction to diaphragm
B. Longitudinal contraction of esophagus
C. Increased intra-abdominal pressure
D. All the above

139. Para-esophageal hernia shows all these *except:*
A. Stomach herniates beside GE junction through esophageal hiatus
B. May become incarcerated and strangulated
C. Leads to acute chest pain, dysphagia and mediastinal mass
D. Herniated gastric pouch cause dysphagia, gastritis, chronic blood loss
E. Surgical therapy is required for all

140. One of this does not cause esophageal perforation
A. Instrumentation of esophagus or external trauma
B. Forceful vomiting or retching
C. Corrosive esophagitis, ulcers
D. Reflux esophagitis
E. Esophageal carcinoma

141. Esophageal perforation presents with all these *except:*
A. Severe retrosternal chest pain
B. Palpable subcutaneous emphysema
C. Mediastinal crackling sounds on auscultation
D. Massive hematemesis
E. Pneumothorax

142. Spontaneous rupture of esophagus mimics all *except:*
A. Myocardial infarction
B. Pancreatitis
C. Acid peptic disease
D. Rupture of abdominal viscus
E. All

143. Confirmation of spontaneous rupture of esophagus is by:
A. Chest X-ray PA view
B. CT scan of chest
C. Gastrograffin swallows
D. Barium contrast
E. Endoscopic US

144. Mallory Weiss syndrome shows all these features *except:*
A. Tear usally involves gastric mucosa near GE junction
B. Severe GI bleed may be the presenting symptom
C. Most patients need surgery
D. Response to vasopressin or embolisation is good
E. All are correct

Explanation

1. **Ans. (C)** Esophagus is a 10 inch structure. Serosa is not present. It enters the abdomen through right crus of diaphragm.

   (Sleisenger, 9th edition, P-665)

2. **Ans. (A)** Dysphagia to solid food is usually present of esophageal diameter is less than 13 mm. It is corrected by dilating with mercury dilator to a diameter 13 mm.

   (Sleisenger, 9th edition, P-674)

3. **Ans. (D)** Postural dysphagia is seen in conditions of oropharyngial causes of dysphagia for example– Zenker's diverticulum, cricopharyngeal bar (etc).

   (Sleisenger, 9th edition, Pp-679-681)

4. **Ans. (C)** Sitophobia–fear for intake of food it usually seen in chronic mesenteric ischemia.

   (Sleisenger, 9th edition, P-2104)

5. **Ans. (B)** In achalasia, the basic abnormality is due to inhibitory neural degeneration localized to nerve cell bodies.

   (Sleisenger, 9th edition, Pp-691-692)

6. **Ans. (C)** In nutcracker oesophagus the amplitude of esophageal body contraction is more than 180 cm Hg.

   (Sleisenger, 9th edition, P-699)

7. **Ans. (D)** In scleroderma, upper esophageal sphincter (UES), characteristically spared.

   (Sleisenger, 9th edition, P-693)

8. **Ans. (B)** Candida esophagitis best diagnosed by endoscopy and brushing the lesion to demonstrate hyphae of yeast.

   (Sleisenger, 9th edition, P-741)

9. **Ans. (C)** Vinca alkaloids, bleomycin, donorubicin, cisplation all are implicated in increasing severity of radiation injury.

   (Sleisenger, 9th edition, P-738)

10. **Ans. (D)** Epiphrenic diverticular is associated with achalasia.

    (Sleisenger, 9th edition, P-693)

11. **Ans. (C)** Neuropathic idiopathic intestinal pseudo-obstruction is not associated with symptoms of achalasia.

    (Sleisenger, 9th edition, Pp-692-693)

12. **Ans. (D)** Cold water, solid food and edrophonium all provokes symptoms in distal esophageal spasm.

    (Sleisenger, 9th edition, P-692)

13. **Ans. (D)** 24 hours ambulatory PH monitoring is the most sensitive test for diagnosis of GERD.

    (Sleisenger, 9th edition, Pp-717-718)

14. **Ans. (A)** The symptoms of radiation to left arm are a non-specific finding in differentiation cardiac from non-cardiac chest pain.

    (Sleisenger, 9th edition, P-693)

15. **Ans. (A)** Non-specific dysmotility is the most common form of oesophageal motility disorder.

    (Sleisenger, 9th edition, P-686)

16. **Ans. (A)** In steak-house syndrome, characteristic sensation of food bolus impaction but not odynodysphagia.

    (Sleisenger, 9th edition, P-694)

17. **Ans. (A)** Straining leads to move LES relaxation leading to aggravation of reflux esophagitis.

    (Sleisenger, 9th edition, P-708)

18. **Ans. (C)** Reflux induced asthma relieved by PPI therapy.

    (Sleisenger, 9th edition, P-714)

19. **Ans. (C)** Ora serrata characteristically simulate endoscopic finding of Z-like line in oesophago gastric junction.

    (Sleisenger, 9th edition, P-681)

20. **Ans. (D)** No neutrophil found in normal oesophagus.

    (Sleisenger, 9th edition, P-425)

21. **Ans. (B)** Most common type–development a normally of esophagus is – esophageal atresia and distal type tracheo-oesophageal fistula.

    (Sleisenger, 9th edition, P-668)

22. **Ans. (C)** Diet modification is primary therapeutic approach for dysphagia lustoria.

    (Sleisenger, 9th edition, P-672)

23. **Ans. (D)** In inlet patch, there is no risk of adenocarcinoma, since there is no evidence of metaplasia.

(Sleisenger, 9th edition, P-675)

24. **Ans. (C)** Schatzki ring found in approximately 10% of general population located in the LES and contains only mucosa and submucosa.

(Sleisenger, 9th edition, P-674)

25. **Ans. (B)** Normal LES pressure is 10-30 mm of Hg.

(Sleisenger, 9th edition, P-683)

26. **Ans. (B)** Truncal vagotomy has no effect on LES.

(Sleisenger, 9th edition, P-882)

27. **Ans. (C)** Tumor infiltration especially carcinoma in gastric fundus is the most common malignant cause of achalasia.

(Sleisenger, 9th edition, P-693)

28. **Ans. (D)** Esophageal manometry is the confirmatory test for achalasia.

(Sleisenger, 9th edition, P-699)

29. **Ans. (B)** Differentiation between idiopathic achalasia from mechanical achalasia by amyl nitrate test.

(Sleisenger, 9th edition, P-693)

30. **Ans. (D)** No parietal and chief cells in the Barrett's epithelium (only intestinal metaplastic cell).

(Sleisenger, 9th edition, P-727)

31. **Ans. (B)** Transient lower esophageal sphincter relaxation (TLER), most episodes occur in relation to swallowing.

(Sleisenger, 9th edition, P-709)

32. **Ans. (D)** Esophageal acid clearance is said to be detective when esophageal PH remain less than 4.

(Sleisenger, 9th edition, P-718)

33. **Ans. (B)** In pregnancy 70% of cases, associated with some amount of reflux episodes.

(Sleisenger, 9th edition, P-710)

34. **Ans. (B)** According to Savary-Miller classification non-circumferential erosion, classified as grade-III injury.

(Sleisenger, 9th edition, P-716)

35. **Ans. (B)** Anti-secretory therapy prescribed even in low grade dysplasia of Barrett's esophagus.

(Sleisenger, 9th edition, P-730)

36. **Ans. (B)** Pseudoulceration on upper G.I. endoscopy seen in candida oesophagitis.

(Sleisenger, 9th edition, P-741)

37. Volcano lesion on upper GI endoscopy seen in HSV esophagitis.

(Sleisenger, 9th edition, Pp-741-742)

38. **Ans. (D)** Itraconazole is not effective in idiopathic esophageal ulceration in HIV patient.

(Sleisenger, 9th edition, P-643)

39. **Ans. (D)** Tylosis is a premalignant risk factor for esophageal carcinoma.

(Sleisenger, 9th edition, Pp-748-749)

40. **Ans. (C)** Incidence and severity of esophageal injury increases with radiation dose greater than 50 GY.

(Sleisenger, 9th edition, P-640)

41. **Ans. (B)** Abnormal peristalsis reported 1-3 months following treatment completion whereas most strictures developed in 4-8 months following treatment completion of radiotherapy.

(Sleisenger, 9th edition, P-640)

42. **Ans. (C)** Average 15% of cases developed esophageal strictures following endoscopic sclerotherapy.

(Sleisenger, 9th edition, P-39)

43. **Ans. (B)** Endoscopic surveillance for chronic stricture patient to role out evolution into squamous cell carcinoma.

(Sleisenger, 9th edition, P-75)

44. **Ans. (C)** Barium swallow finding if suggestive of disruption of esophageal axis excludes possibility of resection.

(Sleisenger, 9th edition, P-753)

45. **Ans. (A)** Most commonly esophageal cancer present in stage-IIa.

(Sleisenger, 9th edition, P-758)

46. **Ans. (A)** Ideal palliative modality for circumferential esophageal carcinoma is dilation with self expandable metallic stent.

(Sleisenger, 9th edition, P-766)

47. **Ans. (D)** Self-expanding metal stents used as a palliation for long tumors of esophagus.

(Sleisenger, 9th edition, P-766)

48. **Ans. (A)** Bipolar electrocoagulation is adequate palliation for short, exophytic non-circumferential esophageal carcinoma.

(Sleisenger, 9th edition, P-764)

49. **Ans. (D)** Self-expandable metallic stents (SEMS) is the best form of palliation in patients with esophagus

respiratory fistula with success rate of 70%-100% in relieving dysphasia.

(Sleisenger, 9th edition, P-767)

50. **Ans. (A)** Most common site of squamous cell carcinoma is upper aerodigestive tract.

(Sleisenger, 9th edition, P-758)

51. **Ans. (B)** Metastatic carcinoma to esophagus is unusual, with melanoma and breast cancer the two cancers most frequently metastatic to the esophagus.

(Sleisenger, 9th edition, P-768)

52. **Ans. (D)** In gastroesophageal reflux disease (GERD), micro aspiration due to relaxation of LES and not related to swallowing.

(Sleisenger, 9th edition, Pp-720-722)

53. **Ans. (D)** Carbohydrate food not effect on relaxation of lower esophageal sphincter.

(Sleisenger, 9th edition, P-708)

54. **Ans. (B)** NSAIDs has no effect on lower esophageal sphincter (LES) pressure. Progesterone, â-agonist and á-antagonist causes LES relaxation.

(Sleisenger, 9th edition, P-708)

55. **Ans. (B)** Syncope is not an extra esophageal manifestation of GERD.

(Sleisenger, 9th edition, Pp-714-715)

56. **Ans. (A)** GERD is the most common cause of tissue eosinophilia in esophagus.

(Sleisenger, 9th edition, P-716)

57. **Ans. (C)** Oral fluconazole is the treatment of choice for candida esophagitis.

(Sleisenger, 9th edition, P-742)

58. **Ans. (B)** Esophageal candidiasis seen in achalasia, scleroderma, diabetes mellitus, adrenal insufficiency, alcoholism immunosuppressed state and in motility disorders.

(Sleisenger, 9th edition, P-741)

59. **Ans. (D)** Plague like lesion resembling esophageal candidiasis, seen in CMV esophagitis, pill esophagitis and swallowed pharyngeal debris.

(Sleisenger, 9th edition, Pp-741-742)

60. **Ans. (A)** H. pylori can affect stomach with feature of pangastritis and lower the chance of reflux esophagitis.

(Sleisenger, 9th edition, P-862)

61. **Ans. (A)** First line management of GERD during pregnancy is lifestyle modification and avoid drugs which relaxes lower esophageal sphincter (LES).

(Sleisenger, 9th edition, P-721)

62. **Ans. (A)** GERD occurs in upto 70% of pregnant patient which is more common in 1st trimester due to relaxing effect of estrogen and progesterone on lower esophageal sphincter (LES).

(Sleisenger, 9th edition, P-715)

63. **Ans. (C)** Distal on third is the most common risk factor esophageal adenocarcinoma and usually develops from Barrett's esophagus.

(Sleisenger, 9th edition, P-745)

64. **Ans. (D)** Extension into adjacent structure also common and equal in case of esophageal adenocarcinoma in comparison of esophageal squamous cell carcinoma.

(Sleisenger, 9th edition, P-752)

65. **Ans. (C)** 5% of cases developed tracheo-oesophagus fistula as a complication to laser therapy.

(Sleisenger, 9th edition, P-765)

66. **Ans. (B)** Most common histologic pattern of Barrett's epithelium is specialized intestinal metaplastic cells followed by gastric cardiac type cell.

(Sleisenger, 9th edition, P-727)

67. **Ans. (B)** Aphagia indicates absence of swallowing may be due to mechanical causes or due to mortality disorders.

(Sleisenger, 9th edition, P-716)

68. **Ans. (D)** Phagophobia not seen in achalasia.

(Sleisenger, 9th edition, P-699)

69. **Ans. (E)** The esophagus does not show spontaneous contractions. Primary peristalsis initiated with swallowing secondary peristalsis initiated in response to focal esophageal dilation.

(Sleienger, 9th edition, P-681)

70. **Ans. (E)** Normal passage of ingested bolus depends on site of bolus, luminal diameter, peristaltic contraction and deglutitive inhibition.

(Sleisenger, 9th edition, P-681)

71. **Ans. (C)** Venous drainage of distal esophagus through portal vein and midoesophagus through azygous vein.

(Sleisenger, 9th edition, P-667)

72. **Ans. (C)** Optic coherence tomography is used to detect leiomyoma of esophagus.

(Sleisenger, 9th edition, Pp-754-755)

73. **Ans. (C)** VIP, no decreases LES pressure, whereas gastrin, motilin and substance-pancreases LES pressure.

(Sleisenger, 9th edition, P-788)

74. **Ans. (B)** Transfer dysphagia seen in esophageal carcinoma.

(Sleisenger, 9th edition, P-766)

75. **Ans. (B)** In case of motor dysphagia to liquid occurs first, later on it involves the solid dysphagia also.

(Sleisenger, 9th edition, P-669)

76. **Ans. (C)** Low grade esophagitis characterized by presence of intra epithelial neutrophils and eosinophil with involvement of 715% of basal fine thickness.

(Sleisenger, 9th edition, Pp-738-739)

77. **Ans. (C)** Hiccups originated from irritation of diaphragm, so hiccough and dysphagia may suggest disease pathology from lower esophagus.

(Sleisenger, 9th edition, P-679)

78. **Ans. (A)** Chronic candidiasis rarely leads to esophageal stricture.

(Sleisenger, 9th edition, P-742)

79. **Ans. (D)** Chest pain with dysphagia occurs in distal esophageal spasm.

(Sleisenger, 9th edition, P-690)

80. **Ans.**

A. Oropharyangeal dysphagia–video fluoroscopy
B. Carcinoma of oesophagus–oesophageal gastroscopy
C. Motor disorder–oesophageal manometry
D. GERD–24-hour PH monitoring

Oropharyangeal dysphagia best demonstrated by video fluoroscopy. GERD is best diagnosed by 24-hour oesophageal PH measurement.

(Sleisenger, 9th edition, Pp-689-693)

81. **Ans. (D)** Type of esophageal carcinoma (Histological type can't be differentiated by radiologically. Worldwide squamous cell carcinoma is the most common variety and middle third is the most common site.

(Sleisenger, 9th edition, P-896)

82. **Ans. (D)** Candidiasis (esophageal) is a very rare etiology of esophageal stricture and esophageal malignancy.

(Sleisenger, 9th edition, Pp-747-748)

83. **Ans. (D)** GERD and Barrett's esophagus are the premalignant condition for esophageal adenocarcinoma not squamous cell carcinoma.

(Sleisenger, 9th edition, P-748)

84. **Ans. (E)** Oesophagoscopy should be done in all patients for histological diagnosis of type of esophageal carcinoma. Management is different from different histology.

(Sleisenger, 9th edition, P-756)

85. **Ans. (C)** The 5-year survival rate for esophageal carcinoma is around 15%-20%.

(Sleisenger, 9th edition, P-745)

86. **Ans. (D)** High grade dysplasia of Barrett's esophagus. Patient should be offered surgical or endoscopic therapy. Low grade dysplasia due to low rate of progression of cancer invasive therapy generally not recommended however frequent surveillance recommended.

(Sleisenger, 9th edition, P-731)

87. **Ans. (C)** Treatment of choice for malignant tracheo-esophageal fistula is self expanding metallic stents.

(Sleisenger, 9th edition, P-765)

88. **Ans. (C)** Substance P increases LES pressure. Rest all decreases LES pressure.

(Sleisenger, 9th edition, P-708)

89. **Ans. (D)** VIP causes LES relaxation thereby decreases LES pressure.

(Sleisenger, 9th edition, P-708)

90. **Ans. (D)** Metoclopramide and other prokinetic drugs are used for treatment of GERD.

(Sleisenger, 9th edition, P-708)

91. **Ans. (D)** Caustic ingestion, pill induced injury, infectious esophagitis, severe reflux esophagitis and esophageal carcinoma are the causes of odynophagia.

(Sleisenger, 9th edition, P-176)

92. **Ans. (C)** Most frequent esophageal causes of chest pain is reflux esophagitis.

(Sleisenger, 9th edition, P-177)

93. **Ans. (C)** Water brash type sensation occurs in achalasia or diverticulum.

(Sleisenger, 9th edition, P-175)

94. **Ans. (B)** Video fluoroscopy is the investigation of choice for detection and analysis of oral pharyngeal secretion.

(Sleisenger, 9th edition, P-694)

95. **Ans. (A)** Esophageal peristalsis is best evaluated by manometry done in upright position.

(Sleisenger, 9th edition, P-695)

96. **Ans. (B)** Diffuse esophageal spasm. Achalasia and scleroderma all are motility disorder and esophageal manometry is most useful for their diagnosis and management.

(Sleisenger, 9th edition, P-699)

97. **Ans. (E)** Oropharyngeal paralysis causes dysphasia nasal regurgitation, tracheobronchial aspiration on and chest pain.

(Sleisenger, 9th edition, Pp-679-681)

98. **Ans. (E)** Myasthenia, stroke, parkinsonism, cerebral palsy etc are important causes of oropharyngeal dysphagia.

(Sleisenger, 9th edition, P-687)

99. **Ans. (E)** Globus pharyngeus is a feeling of a lump or tightness in the throat unrelated to swallowing. It may be associated with gastroesophageal reflux disease.

(Sleisenger, 9th edition, P-177)

100. **Ans. (B)** Esophageal body aperistalsis with failure of LES relaxation on swallowing are the definite nonmonetary criteria for achalasia.

(Sleisenger, 9th edition, P-699)

101. **Ans. (E)** Secondary achalasia can be caused by gastric adenocarcinoma, infiltrating esophageal metastatic tumor, Chaga's disease.

(Sleisenger, 9th edition, P-693)

102. **Ans. (E)** Dysphagia is the most common symptoms of achalasia. However chest pain, GERD can occur in achalasia.

(Sleisenger, 9th edition, P-692)

103. **Ans. (D)** Chest pain is more common in spastic achalasia than classic achalasia.

(Sleisenger, 9th edition, P-691)

104. **Ans. (E)** Esophageal body aperistalsis is the characteristic finding in esophageal manometry.

(Sleisenger, 9th edition, P-699)

105. **Ans. (D)** Basal LES pressure usually elevated in achalasia with lack of LES relaxation on swallowing. CCK paradoxically increases LES pressure.

(Sleisenger, 9th edition, P-699)

106. **Ans. (D)** Esophageal stenting is used for mechanical dysphagia. Pharmacologic therapy (Smooth muscle relaxants), Botulinum toxin and endoscopic balloon dilation are used for treatment.

(Sleisenger, 9th edition, P-701)

107. **Ans. (A)** In scleroderma due to fibrosis, there is failure of LES relaxation; LES pressure may be normal or increased. There is also reduced amplitude of contraction of lower part of oesophagus.

(Sleisenger, 9th edition, Pp-686-688)

108. **Ans. (D)** Barium swallow may be normal in distal esophageal spasm. However on oesophageal manometry LES is normal, but contraction force velocity (CFV>8 cm/second).

(Sleisenger, 9th edition, P-699)

109. **Ans. (D)** Simultaneous esophageal contraction seen in reflux esophagitis, esophageal obstruction and connective tissue disorder.

(Sleisenger, 9th edition, P-697)

110. **Ans. (D)** Gastroesophageal reflex occur when there is increase in abdominal pressure 1, increasing transient lower esophageal sphincter relaxation (t-LER).

(Sleisenger, 9th edition, Pp-708-709)

111. **Ans. (D)** Antacids increases LES pressure, so, GERD is less common.

(Sleisenger, 9th edition, P-708)

112. **Ans. (D)** Incidence of stricture in reflux esophagitis is 6%-12%.

(Sleisenger, 9th edition, P-726)

113. **Ans. (C)** GERD leads to Barrett's esophagus lead to adenocarcinoma not squamous cell carcinoma.

(Sleisenger, 9th edition, Pp-714-715)

114. **Ans. (A)** Colloid sulfur scan (99 Technetium) is not used for diagnosis of GERD).

(Sleisenger, 9th edition, Pp-716-718)

115. **Ans. (A)** Simultaneous onset contraction with intermittent normal peristalsis on esophageal manometry is characteristic of diffuse esophageal spasm.

(Sleisenger, 9th edition, P-699)

116. **Ans. (C)** Bernstein useful for diagnosis of reflux esophagitis.

(Sleisenger, 9th edition, Pp-716-719)

117. **Ans. (D)** Sleeping with head end elevated is a recommended therapy for treatment of GERD.

(Sleisenger, 9th edition, Pp-722-726)

118. **Ans. (E)** Oesophagectomy is not indicated in uncomplicated GERD, rather it indicated when associated with Barrett's esophagus with severe dysplasia and adenocarcinoma.

(Sleisenger, 9th edition, Pp-722-726)

119. **Ans. (E)** Metoclopramide no action on small intestine and colon.

(Sleisenger, 9th edition, P-714)

120. Ans. (D) Endoscopic surveillance indicated in Barrett's esophagus, high grade dysplasia and low grade dysplasia.

(Sleisenger, 9th edition, Pp-732-733)

121. Ans. (B) Most useful in alkaline esophagitis is symptomatic treatment. Sucralfate is the best option among the option provided. No role of gluco-corticoids and prophylactic antibiotics.

(Sleisenger, 9th edition, P-592)

122. Ans. (E) Reflux esophagitis occur in normal person with relaxed LES.

(Sleisenger, 9th edition, P-708)

123. Ans. (D) Barium swallow cannot adequately distinguish between HSV esophagitis from CMV esophagitis. About 20% of cases of HSV esophagitis oropharynx involved.

(Sleisenger, 9th edition, Pp-742-743)

124. Ans. (D) HSV esophagitis on histology characteristically demonstrate multinucleate giant cell, ballooning degeneration, ground glass intra nuclear cowdry type-A inclusion body.

(Sleisenger, 9th edition, P-742)

125. Ans. (A) Varicella faster esophagitis produces necrotizing esophagitis.

(Sleisenger, 9th edition, P-743)

126. Ans.

A. Vesicle and small superficial ulcer–HSV oesophagitis

B. Vesicles with confluent ulcer–Varicella zoster esophagitis

C. Serpiginous ulcer–CMV esophagitis

D. Curdy white precipitates–Candidal esophagitis

(Sleisenger, 9th edition, Pp-741-743)

127. Ans. (D) In CMV esophagitis there is intra-cytoplasmic inclusion cowl's eye inclusion body. Diagnosis is by endoscopy and biopsy of mucosal brushings. Diagnosis is confirmed by immuno-histology with monoclonal antibodies to CMV.

(Sleisenger, 9th edition, Pp-524-526)

128. Ans. (B) Treatment of choice for CMV esophagitis is ganciclovir. Alternatively cidofovir and foscarnet can be used. Steroid has no role.

(Sleisenger, 9th edition, Pp-527-530)

129. Ans. (D) Esophagitis in AIDS is caused by all of the above mentioned.

(Sleisenger, 9th edition, Pp-526-529)

130. Ans. (E) Esophageal bullous lesion can be seen in TEN, SJ syndrome, Epidermolysis bullosa.

(Sleisenger, 9th edition, P-526)

131. Ans. (D) Crohn's disease involving esophagus is rare and more likely responds to anti-TNF therapy and rarely surgery is required.

(Sleisenger, 9th edition, Pp-1968-1970)

132. Ans.

A. Zenker's diverticulum–Posterior hypopharyngeal weakness

B. Midoesophageal diverticular–Traction from old adhesion

C. Epiphrenic diverticulum–Associated with achalasia

D. Diffuse intramural diverticulosis–Dilation of deep esophageal glands

(Sleisenger, 9th edition, Pp-371-375)

133. Ans. (E) Zenker's diverticulum causes halitosis and regurgitation of saliva endoscopy and NG tube placement cause perforation. Cricopharyngeal myotomy with or without diverticulocity is the treatment of choice.

(Sleisenger, 9th edition, Pp-371-372)

134. Ans. (D) The risk of squamous cell carcinoma increased in Plummer Vinson syndrome.

(Sleisenger, 9th edition, P-748)

135. Ans. (C) Schatzki ring is B-ring located in squamo-columnar 2 junctions is a mucosal ring and not muscular ring. It is found in 7-12% of patients. It is usually asymptomatic. Rarely produces intermittent dysphagia.

(Sleisenger, 9th edition, Pp-672-673)

136. Ans. (B) In case of peptic or corrosive stricture, dysphagia responds to metallic dilator.

(Sleisenger, 9th edition, P-726)

137. Ans. (A) Sliding hernia occurs when gastroeso-phageal junction and some portions of the stomach are displaced above the diaphragm. Most small sliding hernias are asymptomatic. Large sliding hernias are associated with gastroesophageal reflux.

(Sleisenger, 9th edition, Pp-379-381)

138. Ans. (D) Sliding hernia occurs due to displacement of GE junction and stomach into thoracic cavity. It occurs due to increase in abdominal pressure, weakness of diaphragm support.

(Sleisenger, 9th edition, Pp-379-381)

139. Ans. (A) In paraoesophageal hernia, although stomach herniates through esophageal hiatus but GE junction not displaced.

(Sleisenger, 9th edition, P-379)

140. Ans. (D) Reflux esophagitis rarely causes esophageal perforation.

(Sleisenger, 9th edition, P-98)

141. Ans. (D) Massive hematemesis is rare in esophageal perforation. Severe chest pain, subcutaneous emphysema, pneumothorax can occur.

(Sleisenger, 9th edition, P-524)

142. Ans. (D) Spontaneous perforation of esophagus may mimic MI, pancreatitis APD etc.

(Sleisenger, 9th edition, P-742)

143. Ans. (C) Confirmation of spontaneous rupture of esophagus confirmed by esophageal contrast study using gastrograffin.

(Sleisenger, 9th edition, P-741)

144. Ans. (C) Treatment for Mallory-Weiss tear is supportive because of self-limited nature of bleed. Surgery rarely required 10% of cases may present with massive hematemesis.

(Sleisenger, 9th edition, P-740)

Chapter 2

Stomach and Duodenum

1. **Peptic ulcers are labeled refractory after treatment for a minimum of:**
A. 4-6 weeks B. 8-12 weeks
C. 3-6 months D. 1 year

2. **One of the following is not an important factor for refractory ulcers:**
A. Persisting H. pylori B. Dense fibrosis
C. Irritable gut D. Giant ulcers

3. **Drug of choice for patients who continue to take NSAIDs in peptic ulcer:**
A. Omeprazole B. Famotidine
C. Sucralfate D. Misoprostol

4. **During maintenance of anti-secretory therapy, the highest risk for recurrences appear between:**
A. 2-3 months B. 3-6 months
C. 6-9 months D. < 2 years

5. **Least frequent ulcer complication is:**
A. Gastric outlet obstruction
B. Hemorrhage
C. Perforation
D. Penetration

6. **In saline load test for gastric outlet obstruction, the quantity of gastric aspirate which excludes significant obstruction is:**
A. < 200 ml B. 200-300 ml
C. 300-400 ml D. 400 ml

7. **The finding which indicates gastric retention include all *except:***
A. Succussion splash more than 4 hours after eating
B. Gastric residual volume less than 200 ml on fasting
C. More than 50% barium retention at 4 hours
D. Scintigraphic fractional emptying rate of less than 10% min for liquids and less than 0.5% min for solids

8. **Cell of origin of gastrinomas is:**
A. Ectoderm B. Endoderm
C. Mesoderm D. Neuroectoderm

9. **All are features of sporadic gastrinomas *except:***
A. They are usually solitary
B. More than 60% are malignant
C. Occur in both duodenum as well as in pancreas
D. Metastasize to lymph nodes and liver

10. **The level of serum gastrin at which metastasis is suspected in ZE syndrome is:**
A. >500 pg/ml B. >1000 pg/ml
C. >1500 pg/ml D. >450,000 pg/ml

11. **Most frequently performed elective surgery for peptic ulcer worldwide:**
A. Proximal gastric vagotomy
B. Vagotomy + antrectomy
C. Selective gastric vagotomy
D. Vagotomy + hydroplasty

12. **Type of peptic ulcer associated with highest recurrence rate following proximal gastric vagotomy is:**
A. Post-pyloric ulcer B. Pre-pyloric ulcer
C. Intra-pyloric ulcer D. Post-bulbar ulcer

13. **Nissen closure is for:**
A. Duodenal stump after Billroth II
B. Billroth I
C. Roux-en-y anastomosis
D. None

14. **Surgical procedure for type IV gastric ulcers at cardia is:**
A. Pouchet procedure
B. Ulcer excision
C. Kelling-Madlener procedure
D. Roux-en-y oesophageogastrojejunostomy

15. **Factors predicting mortality for inhospital bleeding duodenal ulcer include all *except:***
A. Age >60 years
B. NSAID abuse
C. Blood transfusions >5 units
D. Co-existing medical illness

16. **Lowest recurrence and highest complication rate for peptic ulcer surgery is seen with:**
A. Gastric resection
B. Vagotomy + GJ
C. Highly selective vagotomy
D. Vagotomy + Antrectomy

17. **All are vasomotor symptoms of early dumping syndrome *except:***
A. Palpitations B. Diarrhoea
C. Dizziness D. Sweating

18. **All cause erosive/hemorrhagic gastritis *except:***
A. H. pylori
B. Reactive gastropathy
C. Lymphocytic gastritis
D. Radiation

19. **Snake skin/Mosaic appearance of stomach on endoscopy is typical of:**
A. Prolapse gastropathy
B. Congestive gastropathy
C. Reactive gastropathy
D. Hypertrophic gastropathy

20. **Type of gastritis associated with vigorous running:**
A. Hemorrhagic B. Non-erosive
C. Distinctive D. None

21. **Feveolar hyperplasia on gastric biopsy is seen all the following *except:***
A. Post gastrectomy stoma
B. Menetrier's disease
C. Chronic superficial gastritis
D. Hyperplastic polyps

22. **Phlegmonous gastritis is most frequently caused by:**
A. Radiation
B. Alcohol
C. Group-Á hemolytic streptococci
D. Clostridium Welchii

23. **Fungal disease most commonly affecting stomach is:**
A. Histoplasmosis B. Candida
C. Aspergillosis D. Mucormycosis

24. **The most frequent site affected in gastric Crohn's is:**
A. Fundus B. Antrum
C. Pylorus D. Body

25. **All are causes of gastric granulomas *except:***
A. Allergic granulomatosis
B. Whipple's disease
C. Chronic Granulomatous disease
D. Pseudolymphoma

26. **In children Menetrier's disease is caused by:**
A. CMV B. Tuberculosis
C. Autoimmune D. H. pylori

27. **Risk factor for gastric cancer for which surveillance is not indicated:**
A. Adenoma
B. FAP
C. Intestinal metaplasia
D. High grade dysplasia

28. **All the following are definitive risk factors for gastric carcinoma *except:***
A. Intestinal metaplasia
B. H. pylori infection
C. Lynch II syndrome
D. Menetrier's disease

29. **Most common genetic abnormality seen in gastric adenocarcinoma:**
A. Ras-oncogene mutation
B. P53 allelic loss
C. DNA aneuploidy
D. Erb-B2 oncogene amplification

30. **Surveillance for gastric carcinoma is warranted for the following paraneoplastic syndrome:**
A. Lesar-Trelat sign
B. Dermatomyositis
C. Trousseau's syndrome
D. Microangiopathic hemolytic anemia

31. **Most common presentation of early gastric cancer:**
A. Peptic ulcer symptoms
B. Anorexia
C. Abdominal pain
D. Early satiety

32. **Most common presentation of advanced gastric cancer is:**
A. Weight loss
B. Abdominal pain
C. Nausea and vomiting
D. Anorexia

33. **All of the following are radiological signs of benign gastric ulcers *except:***
A. Radiating mucosal folds
B. Distorted areae gastricae
C. Ulcer crater projecting outside the gastric lumen
D. Smooth surrounding mucosal odema

34. **Most sensitive and specific technique(s) for diagnosis of gastric carcinoma:**
A. Double contrast radiography
B. Endoscopy + Biopsy
C. EUS
D. Endoscopy + Biopsy + Cytology

35. **According to JRSGC, the morphological classification of EGC, an excavated lesion involving mucosa and submucosa belongs to:**
A. Type I B. Type II
C. Type III D. Type IV

36. **Type IV lesions of Bormann morphological classification for advanced gastric cancer (AGC) refers to:**
A. Polypoid masses projecting into the lumen
B. Ulcerated masses/fungating lesions
C. Both ulcerations with infiltration
D. Linitis plastica

37. **Differential diagnosis for multiple polyps or masses in the stomach during endoscopy include all *except:***
A. Hyperplastic polyps B. Metastases
C. Fundic gland polyps D. Lymphoma

38. **On endoscopy, flat superficial lesions of stomach are seen in:**
A. EGC (Early gastric cancer)
B. Linitis plastica
C. Kaposi's sarcoma
D. Smooth muscle tumor

39. **On endoscopy all the following lesions can appear as masses with ulceration in the stomach *except:***
A. Smooth muscle tumor
B. Metastases
C. Gastric carcinoid
D. Peptic ulcer disease

40. **Endoscopic ultrasound (EUS) is most sensitive in detecting all the following features in carcinoma of stomach *except:***
A. Lymph node involvement
B. Liver involvement
C. Overall staging accuracy
D. Depth of invasion

41. **Early gastric carcinoma (ECG) has 5 years survival rate of:**
A. 40% B. 60%
C. 90% D. 98%

42. **Poor prognostic factor in carcinoma stomach is:**
A. Upper third tumors
B. Early TNM stage
C. Age of the patient
D. Nodal involvement in ECG

43. **One of the following factors in carcinoma stomach indicates poor prognosis *except:***
A. Degree of differentiation
B. Stromal fibrosis
C. Age and gender
D. Aneuploid tumors

44. **Which of the following surgical option for gastric carcinoma has highest mortality rate?**
A. Curative resection
B. Anastomotic leak
C. Palliative resection
D. None

45. **One of the following chemotherapy regimens affect survival in gastric carcinoma:**
A. 5FU+ Doxorubicin + Mitomycin
B. 5FU + Doxorubicin + Cisplatin
C. Etopiside + Doxorubicin + Cisplatin
D. None

46. **All are EUS features of gastric lymphoma *except:***
A. Hyperechoic infiltration
B. Localised non-homogenous polypoid matrix
C. Gastric wall thickening with ulcers
D. Multiple hypoechoic mass lesions

47. **One of the following staging system is not associated with gastric lymphoma:**
A. Ann Arbor
B. Bormann
C. Musshoff
D. Black ledge

48. **One of the following is not a poor prognostic feature of gastric lymphoma:**
A. MALT features
B. Associated HIV infection
C. Tumors > 10 cm site
D. T-cell tumors

49. **Poor prognostic indicator of gastric lymphomas is:**
A. Tumors <10 cm
B. Diffuse or large cell type
C. Presentation with acute abdomen
D. Musshoff stage II E1

50. **For the following stage of gastric lymphoma surgery is the first line treatment:**
A. IE B. IE1
C. IE2 D. MALT lymphoma

51. **CARNEY's triad includes all *except:***
A. Extra adrenal paragangilloma
B. Smooth muscle/Stromal tumor of stomach
C. Gastric carcinoid
D. Pulmonary chondroma

52. **Best and the most commonly used predictor of malignancy in gastric stromal tumor is:**
A. Size > 10 cm
B. Presence of necrosis
C. High nuclear atypia
D. Mitotic index > 10/HPF

53. **Pre-malignant gastric polyps are:**
A. Peutz-Jeghers polyps
B. Adenoma
C. Hyperplastic polyps
D. Fundic gland polyps

54. **Most common site of hyperplastic polyps of stomach is:**
A. Body B. Fundus
C. Pylorus D. Antrum

55. **Most common cause of death in ZE syndrome is:**
A. Complications of ulcer disease
B. Malignant tumor invasion
C. Malabsorption
D. Other comorbid illness

56. **Gastric acid hypersecretion with normal gastrin levels are seen in all *except:***
A. Non-gastrinoma islet cell tumors
B. Pancreatic carcinomas
C. Gastrinoma related to MEN-1
D. Ampullary carcinoma

57. **'Extended' highly selective vagotomy includes:**
A. Division of right and left gastroepiploic bundles
B. Division of crow's foot
C. Division of criminal nerve (grassis nerve)
D. Preservation of celiac and hepatic branches

58. **Risk factors for mortality in peptic ulcer perforation include all *except:***
A. Advance age
B. Duration >24 hours
C. NSAID use
D. Corticosteroid use

59. **'Minigastrin' is:**
A. G14 B. G17
C. G10 D. G20

60. **Most common cause of acute gastric dilatation is:**
A. Diabetes
B. Carcinoma stomach
C. Idiopathic
D. Peptic ulcer

61. **Gastric polyps in FAP are of following type:**
A. Adenomas B. Hyperplastic
C. Fundic gland D. Hamartomas

62. **In a post operative stomach all the following histological features can be seen *except:***
A. Foveolar hyperplasia
B. Reactive gastropathy
C. Moderate-severe inflammation
D. Stromal erythema

63. **All the following veins drain the stomach *except:***
A. Splenic vein
B. Gastroduodenal vein
C. Short gastric vein
D. Right gastroepiploic vein

64. **One of the following is not a function of gastric juice:**
A. Facilitation of duodenal calcium absorption
B. Killing ingested micro-organisms
C. Initiation of dietary triglyceride hydrolysis
D. Facilitation of duodenal iron absorption

65. **Precursors of parietal cells in oxyntic gland:**
A. Surface mucous cells
B. Mucous neck cells
C. D-cells
D. ECL-like cells

66. **H+K+ ATPase is predominantly located in:**
A. Cytoplasm
B. Apical membrane
C. Protrudes into the lumen
D. Baso lateral membrane

67. **Hyperpepsinogenema I is an indicator of all *except:***
A. H. pylori infection
B. NSAID usage
C. Increased parietal cell mass
D. Refractory ulcer

68. **Most common initial clinical presentation of ZE syndrome is:**
A. Single DU in D1
B. Multiple DUs in D1
C. Single DU in D2
D. Multiple in D1+D2

69. **All are effects of ZE syndrome on small intestine *except:***
A. Denuded villi
B. Infiltration of lamina propria with polymorphs and eosinophils
C. Multiple superficial mucosal erosions
D. Brunner's gland hypoplasia

70. **False statement regarding gastrectomy and carcinoma stomach:**
A. Carcinoma develops after 15 years
B. There is a 50-70% increased risk after 15-25 years

C. Commonly occurs at anastomotic site
D. Surveillance is indicated for detection

71. **All are dietary risk factors for gastric adenocarcinoma *except:***
A. High intake of fruits and vegetables
B. High intake of salted and pickled food
C. High intake of preserved foods
D. High intake of alcohol

72. **One of the following is a possible risk factors for carcinoma stomach:**
A. Hyperplastic polyps
B. Fundic gland polyps
C. Benign gastric ulcers
D. Hamartomas

73. **All the following surgeries can cause dumping syndrome *except:***
A. Highly selective vagotomy
B. Nissen fundoplication
C. Ramsted's operation
D. Pyloroplasty

74. **Urease of H. pylori is not essential for:**
A. Adherence
B. Colonisation
C. Tissue injury
D. All the above

75. **Congenital anomaly causing dumping syndrome:**
A. Gastric duplication
B. Gastric atresia
C. Microgastria
D. Malrotation of gut

76. **Gastric mucous gel thickness is not decreased by:**
A. Gastric distention
B. Pepsin
C. NSAIDs
D. N-Acetyl cysteine

77. **False statement regarding serology of H. pylori:**
A. It is used as an epidemiological tool
B. Can differentiate between active and remote infection
C. There is a high correlation between antibody titers and histological gastritis
D. ELISA is the most common method used for detection

78. **Gastric lipase is secreted by:**
A. Parietal cells
B. ECL cells
C. Chief cells
D. Surface mucous cells

79. **Pepsinogen secretion is increased by each of the following *except:***
A. Somatostatin
B. Gastrin
C. Histamine
D. Vagal stimulation

80. **The gastric acid secretory pump located on the apical surface of the parietal cell uses:**
A. Na+,K+-ATPase
B. H+,K+-ATPase
C. Tyrosine kinase
D. Carbonic anhydrase

81. **Which of the following statement regarding the regulation of gastric acid secretion is the most accurate?**
A. Basal gastric acid secretion exhibits a circadian variation; the highest secretion occurs in the early morning and the lowest secretion occurs at night
B. The cephalic phase of acid secretion is mediated primarily by vasoactive intestinal polypeptide containing vagal fibers
C. The gastric phase of acid secretion consists of two components: a physical component (i.e. distention of the stomach) and a chemical component
D. The primary stimulatory factors involved in the intestinal phase of acid secretion include distention and fat

82. **All the following statements regarding the cellular basis for the regulation of gastric acid secretion are true *except:***
A. Parietal cells express cell surface receptors for gastrin, acetylcholine, histamine and somatostatin
B. Transforming growth factor directly inhibits parietal cell activity by epidermal growth factors receptor occupancy
C. Occupancy of the muscarinic receptor on parietal cells leads to stimulation of acid secretion by activation of the adenylate cyclase signaling pathway
D. Stimulation of parietal cells leads to morphologic transformation, rapid changes in H+, K+-ATPase location and opening of ion channels

83. **Which is not member of the epidermal growth factor family of growth factors?**
A. Betacellulin
B. TGF-α
C. TGF-β
D. Amphiregulin

84. The gastric source of histamine is:
A. Parietal cells
B. G cells
C. ECL cells
D. D cells

85. The arterial blood supply to the stomach is derived from all of the following *except:*
A. Right hepatic artery
B. Common hepatic artery
C. Superior mesenteric artery
D. Left gastric artery

86. Each of the following statements regarding carcinoid tumors of the stomach is true *except:*
A. The stomach is the most common site for the development of carcinoid tumors
B. Gastric carcinoid tumors are usually discovered incidentally
C. Gastric carcinoid tumors typically synthesize serotonin
D. A gastric carcinoid tumor occurs more frequently in patients with atrophic gastritis and pernicious anemia

87. Which of the following characteristics describes the lymphoid follicles that accompany infection with Helicobacter pylori?
A. They are common in non-infected individuals
B. They may precede the development of mucosa associated lymphoid tissue (MALT) lymphoma
C. They are rare in childre
D. Their presence does not correlate with H. pylori antibody titer

88. A 38-year-old man is referred to you for the evaluation of abdominal pain and duodenal ulcer that has failed to heal after an 8-week regimen of full-dose H_2 blockers. Serology and antral biopsy confirm that his Helicobacter pylori status is negative. The patient denies cigarette smoking and the ingestion of non steroidal anti-inflammatory drugs (NSAIDs). Each of the following statement regarding his condition is true *except:*
A. The majority of duodenal ulcers that fail to heal after 8 weeks of therapy are associated with Zollinger-Ellison syndrome
B. A careful history regarding the patient's compliance with the anti-ulcer medication must be performed before recommending further diagnostic evaluation or therapy
C. The likelihood that NSAID ingestion (inadvertent of surreptitious) is contributing to the persistence of this patient's ulcer may be as high as 40% of higher
D. Gastric acid hypersecretion may be a contributing factor in this clinical picture

89. After performing a complete evaluation of the patient presented in the pervious question, including medication history, esophagogastroduodenoscopy biopsy specimens, salicylate screen and serum gastric and gastric acid analyses. You fail to identify or explain the refractory ulcer. Each of the following statements regarding therapy for this patient are true *except:*
A. There is a 50% to 60% chance of this ulcer healing with an additional 8 weeks of H_2-receptor antagonists
B. Maintenance therapy with full-dose or half-dose H_2 blockers yields a 1-year symptomatic recurrence rate of less than 20%
C. Virtually all refractory ulcer can be healed with omeprazole (40 mg/day) or its equivalent
D. Omeprazole at 20 mg/day appears to be less effective in maintaining ulcer remission than is the dose of 40 mg/day

90. All of the following statements regarding cyclooxygenase (COX) isoenzymes are true *except:*
A. The expression of COX is the rate-limiting catalytic step in the production of prostaglandins from membrane-esterified arachidonic acid
B. COX-1 is expressed in a constitutive manner and plays a house keeping role in macrophages, leukocytes, fibroblasts and endothelial cells
C. COX-2 is the inducible form of the enzyme, which is up-regulated in areas of inflammation
D. The expression of COX-2 is regulated by physiologic stimuli and leads to the synthesis of thromboxane A2, PG12 and PGE2

91. The relative incidence of gastric ulcers resulting from the use of non-steroidal anti-inflammatory drugs can be significantly reduced by all of the following *except:*
A. Standard-dose H_2-receptor antagonists
B. Non-acetylated salicylates
C. Misoprostol
D. Co-therapy with a proton pump inhibitor

92. Select the best answer regarding non-steroidal anti-inflammatory drug (NSAID) related gastroduodenal mucosal injury.
A. There is no difference among NSAIDs in their likelihood to cause mucosal injury

B. The potency and duration of cyclooxygnease-2 inhibition by an NSAID correlates with the risk of the development of ulcers and the risk of ensuing complications
C. Nonacetylated NSAIDs may be associated with a decreased incidence of mucosal injury compared to acetylated compounds
D. Nonacetylated NSAIDs are associated with less gastrointestinal toxicity because of the relative selectivity of these agents for the different cylooxygenase isoenzymes

93. **All of the following statements regarding the effects of truncal vagotomy on gastric motility are true *except:***
A. Receptive relaxation of the stomach is enhanced
B. Gastric accommodation is impaired
C. Antral contractile force and frequency are reduced
D. The fed motor pattern is typically of shorter duration compared with that of normal subjects

94. **Truncal vagotomy in the treatment of duodenal ulcer achieves which of the following results?**
A. Reduces basal acid output by 50% and maximal acid output by 25%
B. Reduces acid secretion by decreasing the influence of acetylcholine on G cells
C. Reduces the sensitivity of the parietal cell to gastric and histamine
D. Enhances proximal gastric non-phasic motor activity

95. **What is the best surgical procedure for a perforated anterior ulcer associated with an acutely bleeding 'kissing' duodenal ulcer along the posterior wall?**
A. Closure of perforation
B. Closure of perforation, suture ligature of the ulcer bed and proximal gastric vagotomy
C. Total gastrectomy and closure of perforation
D. Proximal gastric vagotomy

96. **Which form of anemia most commonly occurs in postgastrectomy patients?**
A. Iron deficiency
B. Vitamin B_{12} deficiency
C. Folate deficiency
D. Hemolytic anemia

97. **Non-surgical management of peptic ulcer perforation includes each of the following *except:***
A. Nasogastirc suction
B. Intravenous H_2-receptor antagonists
C. Antibiotics
D. Octreotide

98. **True statements regarding nausea and vomiting during pregnancy include all of the following *except:***
A. Nausea and vomiting during pregnancy are more common in nonsmokers
B. They are more common in primigravida
C. They are more common in those who have taken oral contraceptives
D. They are more common in women with less than a tenth-grade education
E. They are more common in obese women

99. **Which statement about hyperemesis gravidarum is true?**
A. Hyperemesis gravidarum typically begins in the second trimester
B. The incidence is increased with nulliparity and younger age
C. Serum human chronic gonadotropin level correlate with the degree of symptoms
D. Nearly one-third of the women with nausea and vomiting during the first trimester of pregnancy will develop hyperemesis gravidarum

100. **The metabolic consequences of severe nausea and vomiting include each of the following *except:***
A. Hypochloremic metabolic alkalosis
B. Normal anion gap metabolic acidosis
C. Hyponatremia
D. Hypokalemia

101. **Which of the following statements regarding the passage of a nasogastric tube is the most appropriate?**
A. A nasogastric tube for occult blood in the nasogastric aspirate
B. It allows testing for occult blood in the nasogastric aspirate
C. It allows treatment of upper gastrointestinal bleeding by ice water lavage
D. Passage of a nasogastric tube is contraindicated if the patient has liver disease with possible bleeding varices

102. **The most important step in the resuscitation of this patient is to:**
A. Obtain a complete history from the patient's wife
B. Send a blood specimen to the blood bank for typing and cross matching, so that a transfusion can be performed immediately

C. Replete the intravascular volume with intravenous saline to prevent the consequences of shock
D. Determine the hematocrit to assess the severity of his blood loss and perform urgent endoscopy to determine the etiology of bleeding

103. After this patient has been adequately resuscitated and is hemodynamically stable, upper endoscopy should be performed:
A. Urgently to allow for possible therapeutic endoscopy
B. Urgently, because findings of diagnostic endoscopy favorably affect the survival of patients with upper gastrointestinal bleeding
C. Only if the bleeding fails to stop spontaneously
D. Only if medical therapy (i.e. H_2 receptor antagonists fails to control bleeding)

104. A 57-year-old man with a long history of alcoholism presents with an upper gastrointestinal hemorrhage from isolated gastric varices in the fundus. No other endoscopic abnormalities are noted. The levels of serum amino transferees, bilirubin and albumin are normal as is the prothrombin time. Treatment of this patient should include:
A. Repeat sclerotherapy until variceal obliteration is achieved
B. Portosystemic shunt surgery
C. Medical therapy with a β blocker, because sclerotherapy in the gastric mucosa is associated with a high complication rate
D. Angiography to assess splenic vein patency

105. All of the following statement regarding arteriovenous malformations (AVMs) in the upper gastrointestinal tract are true *except:*
A. Estrogen-progesterone therapy decreases blood transfusion requirement in some patients
B. Rebleeding is rare after endoscopic coagulation therapy in hereditary hemorrhagic telangiectasi
C. AVMs have been reported in association with aortic valve disease
D. AVMs are a common cause of upper gastrointestinal bleeding in patients with chronic renal failure

106. Patients presenting with upper gastrointestinal bleeding in whom upper endoscopy reveals a clean ulcer base:
A. Have a 0% to 3% risk of re-bleeding
B. Account for 75% to 80% of patients with significant upper gastrointestinal hemorrhage (i.e. requiring >2 U of red blood cells) when the endoscopy is performed within 24 hours of the initial bleed
C. Have a risk of re-bleeding comparable to patients with falt pigmented spots in the ulcer base
D. Are unlikely to have bled from the ulcer even though the rest of the upper endoscopic evaluation revealed no abnormalities

107. All of the following statements concerning optimal therapeutic endoscopic technique in the setting of acute upper gastrointestinal hemorrhage are correct *except:*
A. Use of a therapeutic endoscope with two suction channels is advantageous
B. For electrocoagulation or heater probe treatment firm tamponade is indicated for artery coaptation in bleeding ulcers
C. Follow-up endoscopy is necessary within 24 hours of the initial treatment
D. Arterial compression likely contributes to the mechanism of action of epinephrine injection

108. Although there are some conflicting studies, the thermal techniques of multipolar electrocoagulation and heater probe are generally considered:
A. Superior to injection techniques for obtaining hemostasis in bleeding ulcers
B. Superior to the Nd: YAG laser because they are portable, less expensive and require less technical support
C. Superior to medical management in the subgroup of ulcer patients with minor stigmata
D. Frequently complicated by perforation when more than 20 seconds of electrocoagulation or more than 90 joules are used per ulcer

109. Lesions other than bleeding ulcers that have been reported to benefit from epinephrine injection or thermal therapy include all of the following *except:*
A. Gastric varices
B. Dieulafoy lesion
C. Gastric tumors
D. Mallory-Weiss tears
E. Upper gastrointestinal angiodysplasia

110. Which of the following statements about the pathogenesis of non-ulcer dyspepsia is not true?
A. Altered vagal function may occur with non-ulcer dyspepsia
B. Duodenogastric reflux is more common in patients who have non-ucler dyspepsia than in relative subjects

C. Postprandial antral hypomolitiy and disorganized patterns of intestinal motility are not specific findings in non-ulcer dyspepsia
D. Helicobacter pylori gastritis occurs in about 30% to 60% of patients with non-ucler dyspepsia

111. Which statement regarding dyspepsia is incorrect?
A. The most common symptom cluster in patients with dyspepsia is categorized as ulcer-like
B. Upper endoscopy identifies structural abnormalities in about 75% of patients with dyspeptic symptoms
C. Of the patient with non-ulcer dyspepsia, at least some of them have concurrent syndrome
D. An extended functional workup, including the evaluation of gastric emptying, identifies abnormalities in about 50% of new patients with dyspepsia who have normal findings on upper endoscopy

112. Which of the following statements regarding percutaneous endoscopic gastrostomy tubes is false?
A. Post procedural infections are most commonly caused by staphylococcus aureus and β-hemolytic streptococci
B. Antibiotics must be given for a 48-hour period to reduce the risk of infection
C. Peritoneal dialysis is an absolute contraindication to percutaneous endoscopic gastrostomy tube placement
D. Neoplastic seeding to the skin from oropharyngeal and esophageal cancers can occur

113. Which of the following statements concerning the prevention of recurrent variceal hemorrhage is true?
A. Treatment to prevent re-bleeding includes sclerotherapy, rubber band ligation, transjugular intrahepatic portosystemic shunt (TIPS), surgical shunts and pharmacologic therapy including propranolol and isosorbide mononitrate
B. Prophylactic portacaval shunt surgery prevents re-bleeding and improves survival
C. β-adrenergic antagonists are beneficial in treating grade I varices
D. Mortality is better correlated with variceal size than with a patient's child-pugh score

114. Which of the following statements regarding a dieulafoy lesion is true?
A. This lesion typically occurs in the proximal stomach, along the lesser curvature
B. The mean age for presentation of this disorder is the third decade of life
C. Optimal surgical treatment of this disorder involves oversewing of the lesion
D. Acid reduction therapy (e.g. H_2-receptor antagonists) decreases the risk of recurrent hemorrhage

115. Endoscopic evaluation reveals an anastomotic ulcer in patient who has undergone antrectomy and gastrojunostomy in the past. Which of the following test results suggest the presence of retained antral tissue?
A. A positive response on a secretin stimulation test, which is a provocative test for gastrinoma
B. Normal acid secretion from the gastric remnant
C. An abnormal increase in the serum gastric level in response to meal ingestion
D. An increased basal serum gastrin level

116. All of the following statements regarding pernicious anemia are true *except:*
A. Malabsorption of cobalamin is a characteristic feature of pernicious anemia
B. Pernicious anemia is caused by an absence of or a reduction in the number of chief cells
C. Pernicious anemia causes megaloblastic anemia
D. Absent or dysfunctional terminal ileal absorption leads to pernicious anemia

117. Each of the following conditions can cause hypergastrinemia *except:*
A. Renal failure
B. Diabetes insipidus
C. Rheumatoid arthritis
D. Pheochromocytoma

118. All of the following statements regarding the pathogenesis of diarrhoea in patients with Zollinger-Ellison syndrome are true *except:*
A. Hypergastrinemia leads to colonic hypersecretion of fluid and electrolytes
B. Acid hypersecretion leads to extreme acidification of the duodenum, resulting in inactivation of pancreatic enzymes and concomitant steatorrhea
C. Extreme acidification of the small intestine can lead to mild disruption of enterocyte integrity, resulting in mild malabsorption
D. Gastric hypersecretion can lead to significant volume overload of the small intestine

119. The following statements regarding multiple endocrine neoplasia (MEN) type I syndrome are true *except:*

A. Twenty five percent of patients with gastrinoma have MEN I syndrome
B. Pancreatic tumors are the most common gastrinoma have MEN I syndrome
C. MEN I is an autosomal dominant genetic disorder there is a genetic defect in the long arm of chromosome II
D. Patients with MEN I syndrome and gastrinoma may develop gastric carcinoid tumors

120. All of the following are currently considered valid therapeutic options for the initial treatment of Zollinger-Ellison syndrome *except:*
A. Surgical resection of the gastrin-producing tumor
B. H+K+-ATPase inhibitors
C. Total gastrectomy
D. Combination chemotherapy with streptozoein, 5-fluorouracil and doxorubicin

121. Which of the following is not associated with an increased risk of the development of gastric adenocarcinoma?
A. Common variable immunodeficiency
B. Billroth II gastrectomy and gastrojejunostomy
C. Chronic atrophic gastritis
D. Long term proton pump inhibitor therapy
E. Lynch syndrome II

122. Which statement regarding the epidemiology of gastric cancer is not true?
A. Gastric cancer is directly correlated with the seroprevalence of Helicobacter pylori
B. It is equally common in men and women
C. Incidence and morality rates are higher in groups with lower socio-economic status
D. First generation emigrants have incidence rates similar to those in their country of origin
E. High risk areas frequently have high nitrate levels in the water

123. The prognosis of gastric cancer is worsened by each of the following *except:*
A. Diffuse-type histology
B. Penetration beyond the muscularis propria
C. Lymph node metastases
D. Location in the proximal stomach
E. Elevation of the carcinoembryonic antigen level

124. Which of the following statements regarding the preoperative staging of gastric cancer is not true?
A. Endoscopic ultrasonography is most accurate T and N-stage cancer
B. Computed tomography is best to rule out distant metastases
C. Laparoscopy can be of value to exclude occult peritoneal involvement.
D. Enlarged celiac nodes render the lesion incurable
E. Endoscopic ultrasonography can be used to evaluate the extent of both proximal and distal tumors

125. Which of the following statements regarding surgery for gastric cancer is incorrect?
A. Surgical resection should provide 5 cm tumor-free margins
B. Perigastric and regional nodes should be removed
C. Most patients with metastatic disease should have a palliative resection
D. Routine splenectomy is unnecessary
E. Adjuvant chemotherapy is of unproven benefit and potential harm

126. Which of the following statements regarding gastric lymphoma is not true?
A. It can be cured with radiotherapy alone
B. Most gastric lymphomas are T-cell in origin
C. Endoscopic ultrasonography is highly accurate in staging
D. Patients with stages II, III and IV disease should receive chemotherapy
E. Subtotal gastrectomy may be adequate treatment and avoids the morbidity of esophagojejunostomy

127. Which of the following statements regarding gastric lymphoma is not true?
A. It is often associated with Helicobacter pylori infection
B. It is associated with a relatively favorable prognosis if the lymphoma is derived from mucosa associated lymphoid tissue (MALT)
C. It is not a tumor for which surgical resection is recommended
D. It may regress after treatment with antibiotics
E. Diffuse large B cell lymphoma makes up the largest subgroup

128. The most common type of gastric polyp is:
A. Hyperplastic
B. Adenomatous
C. Fundic gland
D. Juvenile
E. Carcinoid

129. A 65-year-old man underwent subtotal gastrectomy for advanced gastric adenocarcinoma. A Bormann type III lesion was resected from the proximal third of his stomach. He was noted to have 15 of 17 positive para-aortic lymph nodes. The depth of invasion was to the muscularis

propria. Which of the following statements regarding his prognosis is not correct?

A. The most important predictors of prognosis include the depth of tumor invasion and the extent of lymph node metastasis
B. The histologic degree of tumor differentiation is independently predictive of prognosis
C. Increased p53 expression in cancers is associated with a reduced 5-year survival rate
D. Cancers involving the proximal stomach tend to have a worse prognosis than distal lesions

130. **Which statement regarding the association between Helicobacter pylori infection and gastric malignancy is false?**

A. H. pylori has been linked to both mucosa-associated lymphoid tissue lymphoma and gastric carcinoma
B. In patients infected with H. pylori, epidemiologic studies suggest an inverse association between duodenal ulcer and gastric cancer
C. H. pylori has been linked to the intestinal type but not the diffuse type of gastric adenocarcinoma
D. H. pylori infection alone is probably not sufficient to cause gastric cancer

131. **A 55-year-old man presents with a new onset of epigastric pain. He reports mild postprandial nausea but denies vomiting, weight loss, gastrointestinal bleeding and use of non-steroidal anti-inflammatory drugs. What is the most appropriate diagnostic study for this patient?**

A. Upper gastrointestinal tract radiologic examination
B. Upper endoscopy
C. Non-invasive test for Helicobacter pylori
D. Trial with a proton pump inhibitor and follow-up in 4 weeks

132. **A 51-year-old woman is referred to you for the evaluation of a recent upper gastrointestinal hemorrhage from peptic ulcer disease. She brings record indicating that a local physician performed endoscopy and gastric biopsies. Review of these studies reveals that a duodenal ulcer was documented and that Helicobacter pylori was discovered in the gastric biopsy specimens. Each of the following statements regarding H. pylori is correct *except:***

A. H. pylori are gram negative, microaerophilic, flagellated, urease-producing rod, which is found in the gastric antrum in over 50% of patients with peptic ulcer disease
B. This organism appears to play an important role in the pathogenesis of peptic ulcer disease
C. Eradication of this organism with the appropriate antibiotic regimen will lead to ulcer healing; however, it will not alter the recurrence rate of duodenal ulcers
D. Examination at 1 month or more after cessation of therapy is necessary to verify the eradication of H. pylori

Explanation

1. **Ans. (B)** 90% peptic ulcer heal with conventional therapy. A gastric ulcer that fails to heal after 12 weeks and a duodenal ulcer that does not heal after 8 weeks of therapy should be considered as refractory.

   (Harrison, 17th edition, P-1868)

2. **Ans. (C)** The factors important for refractory ulcers are:
   - Size: 7 cm.
   - H. pylori infection.
   - Cigarette smoking.
   - Compliance to treatment.
   - NSAIDs abuse.

   (Harrison, 17th edition, P-1869)

3. **Ans. (A)** The treatment of choice for NSAIDs related mucosal injury is proton pump inhibitor.

   (Harrison, 17th edition, P-1864)

4. **Ans. (B)** The highest risk for recurrence appears between 3-6 months.

   (Harrison, 17th edition, P-1870)

5. **Ans. (A)** Gastric outlet obstruction is the least common ulcer related complication occurring in 1-2% of patients.

   (Sleisenger, 9th edition, Pp-868-869)

6. **Ans. (A)** A gastric aspirate volume of >300 ml 4 hours after a meal or greater than 200 ml after an overnight fast is evidence of delayed gastric emptying.

   (Sleisenger, 9th edition, Pp-868-869)

7. **Ans. (B)** A gastric aspirate volume of greater than 300 ml 4 hours after meal or greater than 200 ml after an overnight fast in case of delayed gastric emptying.

   (Sleisenger, 9th edition, Pp-868-869)

8. **Ans. (B)** Gastrinoma is a neuroendocrine tumor that secretes gastrin.

   (Harrision, 17th edition, P-2354)

9. **Ans. (C)** Most gastrinoma (50-70%) are present in the duodenum followed by (20-40%) and other intra-abdominal site.

   (Sleisenger, 9th edition, Pp-498-503)

10. **Ans. (C)** The level of gastrin at which metastasis is suspected >1500 pg/ml.

    (Sleisenger, 9th edition, Pp-498-503)

11. **Ans. (A)** Surgical treatment is designed to decrease gastric acid secretion. Procedures performed:
    1. Vagotomy.
    2. Highly selective vagotomy.
    3. Vagotomy with antrectomy.

    Highly selective vagotomy is one of the elective surgery. It is also known as parietal cell or super selective or proximal vagotomy.

    (Sleisenger, 9th edition, P-894)

12. **Ans. (B)** Highly selective vagotomy is procedure of choice in elective surgery except in situation where ulcer recurrence rates are high.

    (Harrsion, 17th edition, P-1866)

13. **Ans. (A)** Nissen closure is done for duodenal stump after billroth II procedure (Linkkinghub.clasvier.com).

    (Sleisenger, 9th edition, Pp-882-883)

14. **Ans. (D)** Ulcer located near the esophageal gastric junction may require a more radial approach, a subtotal gastrectomy with esophagaus gastrojejunostomy.

    (Sleisenger, 9th edition, Pp-882-883)

15. **Ans. (B)** (a) Age > 65 years (b) shock (c) Hb level (d) multiple transfusion (e) illness (f) comorbid condition (g) fresh bleeding in emergency.

    (Sleisenger, 8th edition, P-1122)

16. **Ans. (D)** The procedure that provides lowest recurrence rate (17%) but high complication rate in vagotomy in combination with antrectomy.

    (Harrison, 17th edition, P-1867)

17. **Ans. (B)** Diarrhoea is a G.I. symptom.

    (Sleisenger, 9th edition, Pp-853-854)

18. **Ans. (A)** Lymphocytic gastritis is characteristically histologically by intense infiltration of surface epithelium with lymphocytes. No specific symptoms suggest lymphocytic gastritis.

    (Sleisenger, 9th edition, Pp-853-854)

19. **Ans. (B)** Snake skin or mosaic appearance on U.G.I.E. is characteristics of portal gastropathy (congestive gastropathy).

(Sleisenger, 9th edition, P-306)

20. **Ans. (A)** Hemorrhagic gastritis possible associated with running vigorous.

(Sleisenger, 9th edition, P-856)

21. **Ans. (C)** Chronic superficial gastritis faveola hyperplasia is seen in Menetrie's disease, Hyperplastic polyps, Postgastrectomy stomach, Gastric gland, Hyperplasia, Hypertrophic hypersensitivity gastropathy.

(Robbin Path, 7th edition, P-820)

22. **Ans. (C)** Bacterial infection of the stomach phlegmonous gastritis is rare, potentially life threatening disorder characterized by mark and diffuse acute, inflammatory infiltrates of the entire gastric wall, accompanied by necrosis organisms includes streptococcus, stephylococcus, E. coli, protein and hemophilus.

(Harrison, 17th edition, P-1870)

23. **Ans. (D)** Mucormycosis–fungal disease–most commonly affects stomach.

(Sleisenger, 9th edition, P-851)

24. **Ans. (B)** Antrum: Most frequent site affected in gastric Crohn's is Antrum.

(Sleisenger, 9th edition, P-853)

25. **Ans. (D)** Gastric granulomas occur in – Crohn's disease, Wegener's granulomatosis, whipple's disease, eosinophilic gastritis, chronic granulomas disease, sarcoidosis (benign inflammatory condition a/w chronic gastric ulcer and mimicking gastric carcinoma or malignant lymphoma).

(Sleisenger, 9th edition, Pp-852-853)

26. **Ans. (A)** Large gastric folds can be caused by: CMV, Histoplasma, Syphilis.

(Harrison, 17th edition, P-1871)

27. **Ans. (C)** In Western countries endoscopic surveillance done for patients with (1) Low to moderate grade dysplasia (2) Adenoma (3) History of FAP.

(Sleisenger, 8th edition, P-1149)

28. **Ans. (D)** Definite risk factors for gastric adenopathy (1) FAP (2) Adenoma (3) Dysplasia (4) H. pylori (5) Chronic atrophic gastritis (6) HNPCC (7) Post gastrectomy (8) 1st degree relative with gastric cancer. Menetrie's disease possible risk factor (not definite).

(Sleisenger, 8th edition, P-1149)

29. **Ans. (C)** Most common genetic abnormality seen in gastric adenocarcinoma is DNA an aneuploidy seen in 60-75% of cases. P53 deletion is next with 60-70% cases.

(Sleisenger, 9th edition, P-893)

30. **Ans. (C)** Trousseau's syndrome, other para neoplastic syndrome a/w gastric adenocarcinoma – Neuropathy, Nephrotic syndrome, DIC.

(Harrison, 17th edition, P-1150)

31. **Ans. (A)** Most common presentation of early gastric cancer is peptic ulcer symptoms. They produce symptoms mainly after penetrating muscularis propria.

(Harrison, 17th edition, P-1150)

32. **Ans. (A)** Weight loss is the most common symptom of advanced gastric adenocarcinoma seen in 62% of patients abdnominal pain is second most common symptom (52%) patient.

(Harrison, 17th edition, P-1150)

33. **Ans. (B)** *Radiological sign Benign ulcer:* (1) Symmetric with smooth margins (2) Hampton's line + radiolucent band between ulcer and lumen (3) Symmetric radiating mucosal folds (4) Smooth surrounding mucosal edema. *Malignant:* (1) Asymmetric ulcer (2) An ulcer with a mass (3) Presence of irregular fold (4) Nodularity (5) Loss of gastric distensibility.

(Sleisenger, 8th edition, P-1154)

34. **Ans. (D)** Most sensitive and specific technique for diagnosing gastric carcinoma is a combination of endoscopy guided biopsy and it cytological analysis 6 to 8 biopsies from base and edges must be taken from non healing ulcer.

(Sleisenger, 8th edition, P-1151)

35. **Ans. (C)** Type III, Type O: Superficial, Flat tumor with or without minimal elevation or depression, Type I poly tumor Type II a-elevated, b-flat, c-depressed, type III excavated.

(Gastrointestinal Oncology, 6th edition, P-360)

36. **Ans. (D)** Linitis plastica, Type 1-Polypoid, Type 2- Fungated, Type 3 - Ulcerated, Type 4- Infiltration.

(GI Oncology, 6th edition, P-360)

37. **Ans. (B)** The following disorder can present as multiple polyps or masses: Hyperplastic polyps, Fundic gland polyp, Lymphoma, Gastric carcinoma.

(Sleisenger, 9th edition, Pp-858-859)

38. Ans. (A) Early gastric cancer endoscopic appearance may be flat.

(Sleisenger, 9th edition, P-901)

39. Ans. (C) Gastric carcinoid.

(Sleisenger, 9th edition, Pp-478-479)

40. Ans. (B) EUS uses high transducer and allow visualizing of 5 layers of gastric wall and thus is the best modality to determine depth of invasion. Diagnostic accuracy of EUS for lymph nodes is 50 to 80% and is comparable to CT scan. However CT scan is must better modality for detection of liver metastasis.

(Harrison, 17th edition, P-1152)

41. Ans. (C) EGC has 5 years survival rate of greater than 90% in Japan and of 88% in Western countries.

(Sleisenger, 8th edition, P-1154)

42. Ans. (A) Upper third tumor – Upper third tumors spread more frequently in a spleen and pancreatic tail and require more aggressive surgical approach.

(GI Oncology, 6th edition, Pp-384-386)

43. Ans. (D) Aneuploid tumor: Poorly differentiated tumors have worse prognosis. Elderly and males have more progression as young and females.

(Harrison, 17th edition, P-1154)

44. Ans. (B) Possibly: Anastomotic leak has highest mortality rate.

(Sleisenger, 9th edition, P-883)

45. Ans. (D) Survival benefit is seen with following regimes: (1) Epirubicin + Cisplatin + 5 Fu (ECA), (2) Epirubicin + LV+S-Fu (ECF) (3) Epirubicin + folate + 5-Fu + Etoposide.

(Harrison, 17th edition, P-1157)

46. Ans. (A) Hyperechoic infiltration. Not seen in gastric lymphoma.

(Sleisenger, 9th edition, P-450)

47. Ans. (B) Bormann following stating systems are used for gastric lymphoma.

- Ann arbor.
- TNM staging.
- Lugano staging.
- Mushoff staging.
- Black ledge staging.
- Bormann staging used for gastric adenocarcinoma staging B-cell.

(Sleisenger, 9th edition, Pp-448-453)

48. Ans. (A) MALT features.

- Maltoma has better prognosis than diffuse B-cell lymphoma of stomach and other uncommon tumors.
- Stage 1: Maltoma regresses with antibiotic therapy for H. pylori.

(Sleisenger, 9th edition, Pp-449-453)

49. Ans. (C) Acute abdominal symptom.

- Gastric lymphoma generally presents as: Epigastric pain, Dyspepsia, Large tumors may present with features of obstruction and thus may present as acute obstruction.

(Sleisenger, 8th edition, Pp-570-572)

50. Ans. (A) Surgery was thought to be curative if tumor was limited to submucosa. Debulking of tumor has led to modest improvement in survival in stage I-II.

(Sleisenger, 9th edition, P-846)

51. Ans. (C) Carney's triad.

- Extra adrenal paraganglioma.
- Smooth muscle/stromal tumor of stomach.
- Pulmonary chondroma (www.gist support.org)
- Extremely rare syndrome (30 cases reported).
- Mainly females (80% case), present in teenage group.

(Sleisenger, 9th edition, Pp-473-474)

52. Ans. (D) Most useful clinical predictor of outcome in GIST in mitotic index of tumor those with necrotic rate > 2 per 10 HPA have much higher risk for recurrence and metastasis. Tumor size > 5 cm are also at higher risk of metastasis.

(Sleisenger, 9th edition, Pp-467-468)

53. Ans. (B) Majority of gastric polyps that undergo malignant transformation are adenoma. It has been documented that approximately 11% of gastric adenomas develop carcinoma in stiu within 4 years of follow-up.

(Sleisenger, 8th edition, P-847)

54. Ans. (D) Hyperplastic polyps are a type of benign stomach polyps.

- They occur singly in antrum or in multiply at the more distal regions of stomach.
- They are a/w chronic gastritis caused by H. pylori

(www.essortment.com)

55. Ans. (B) Most common cause of death in ZE syndrome is malignant tumor invasiveness.

(Sleisenger, 8th edition, P-639)

56. **Ans. (C)** Gastrinoma is a/w more badly elevated fasting serum gastric level combined with gastric acid hypersecretion.

(Sleisenger, 8th edition, P-785)

57. **Ans. (A)** Extended highly selective vagotomy includes–division of right and left gastroepiploic bundles.

(Sleisenger, 9th edition, P-883)

58. **Ans. (C)** Risk factors for morality:

- Advanced age.
- Shock.
- Perforation > 12 hours.
- Major medical illness.

(Sleisenger, 8th edition, Pp-1129-1130)

59. **Ans. (A)** G-14-3 Active forms of gastrins are:

- Big gastrin–G-34 (Contains 34 amino acids).
- Little gastrin–G-17 (Contains 14 amino acids).
- Mini gastrin–G-14 (Contains 14 amino acids).

(Sleisenger, 9th edition, P-821)

60. **Ans. (D)** Peptic ulcer disease.

(Sleisenger, 9th edition, Pp-862-865)

61. **Ans. (C)** Gastric polyps occur in 30-100% of FAP patients but most polyps in stomach are non-neoplastic fundic gland polyps.

(Sleisenger, 8th edition, P-2199)

62. **Ans. (C)** All except moderate to severe inflammation can occur in postoperative stomach.

(Sleisenger, 9th edition, P-896)

63. **Ans. (B)**

- R and L gastric vein drain lesser curvature of stomach.
- R and L gastroepiploic veins drain in aspect and protion of greater curvature of stomach.
- R gastroepiploic veins becomes gastrocolic vein.
- L gastroepiploic veins becomes splenic vein which later receives short gastric veins draining the fundus. There no gastroduodenal veins.

(Sleisenger, 8th edition, P-677)

64. **Ans. (A)** Gastric secretion helps in draining fundus duodenal iron absorption, suppress ingested microorganisms gastric lipase causes early hydrolysis of dietary triglyceride.

(Sleisenger, 8th edition, P-716)

65. **Ans. (B)** Surface mucous cells are cytoprotective mucosal neck cell function as stem cell precursor for surface mucous, parietal chief and endocrine cell.

(Sleisenger, 8th edition, P-679)

66. **Ans. (A)** When HCL secretion is stimulated, tubular membranes which are prominent in cytoplasma or resting cells diminish along with increase in apical canalicular membrane with fuse with each other. Proton pump are translocated from tubulovesicular to secretory canaliculas.

(Sleisenger, 8th edition, P-716)

67. **Ans. (B)** Pepsinogen I is elevated in 50% of patients with duodenal ulcers, reflect the increase gastric secretory mass.

(Harrison, 17th edition, P-1868)

68. **Ans. (A)** Most common clinical presentation of ZE syndrome is single DU in D1 (duodenal bulb).

(Sleisenger, 8th edition, P-633;
Harrison, 17th edition, P-1868)

69. **Ans. (D)** Brunner is gland hypoplasia–Not occur ZE syndrome.

(Sleisenger, 9th edition, Pp-498-502)

70. **Ans. (D)** Cost effectiveness of endoscopic surveillance for gastric cancer is postgastrectomy patients has not been focus.

(Sleisenger, 8th edition, P-806)

71. **Ans. (A)** Decline in gastric cancer rate coincides with widespread use of refrigeration concomitant increase intake of fresh fruits and vegetables and decrease intake of pickles and slated food. Highly preserved food increases gastric cancer rate.

(Sleisenger, 8th edition, P-834)

72. **Ans. (D)** Peutz-Jeghers syndrome (Hamartomas) is a probable risk factor for gastric carcinoma.

(Sleisenger, 8th edition, P-1149, Table 52-5)

73. **Ans. (C)** Dumping syndrome occurs:

- Vagotomy.
- Drainage procedure (Bilroth procedures and pyloroplasty).
- Nissen's fundoplication.

(Sleisenger, 9th edition, P-882)

74. **Ans. (B)** Urease is not essential for colonization because in urease-ve H. pylori have been cultured from patients with duodenal ulcer disease and have been used to successfully infect experimental animals.

(Sleisenger, 8th edition, P-734)

75. Ans. (C) Possibly microgastria.

(Sleisenger, 9th edition, P-896)

76. Ans. (A) Gastric gel thickness not decreased by gastric dilation.

(Sleisenger, 9th edition, Pp-884-885)

77. Ans. (B) Test for IgA/IgM Abs is unreliable. Chronic H. pylori infection elicit IgG antibody which can be measured by Elisa.

(Sleisenger, 8th edition, P-739)

78. Ans. (C)

- Chief cells: Pepsin and lipase.
- Parietal cell: Acid.
- ECL cells: Histamine.

(Sleisenger, 9th edition, Pp-817-819)

79. Ans. (A) Pepsinogen secretion is evoked by the same stimulants that increase gastric acid secretion.

(Sleisenger, 9th edition, Pp-822-825)

80. Ans. (B) When parietal cells are activated, H^+, K^{+-} ATPase is translocated from vesicular membranes within the cells to the canalicular membranes at the apical cell surface, where it actively pumps hydrogen ions in exchange for potassium.

(Sleisenger, 9th edition, Pp-823-824)

81. Ans. (C) Basal gastric acid secretion is highest at night and lowest in the early morning. Cholinergic vagal fibers are primarily responsible for the cephalic phase of gastric acid secretion. The primary stimulatory factors involved in the intestinal phase include distention, proteins, and products of protein digestion.

(Sleisenger, 9th edition, P-827)

82. Ans. (C) Occupancy of muscarinic receptors on parietal cells results in phospholipase C activation, which leads to the hydrolysis of phosphatidylinositol bisphosphate to diacylglycerol (DAG) and inositol triphosphate (IP3) IP3 promotes an increase in cytosolic calcium, and DAG leads to the translocation of protein kinase C. These events in turn lead to the stimulation of parietal cell secretory activity.

(Sleisenger, 9th edition, P-822)

83. Ans. (C) Transforming growth factor-á, amphiregulin, betacelulim, heparin-binding epidermal growth factor (EGF) and neuregulins are members of the EGF family.

(Sleisenger, 9th edition, P-823)

84. Ans. (C) Enterochromaffin-like (ECL) cells of the gastric mucosa release histamine by the action of the gastrin.

(Sleisenger, 9th edition, P-821)

85. Ans. (A) Most of the stomach is supplied by branches of the celiac artery (i.e. splenic, left gastric, and common hepatic arteries). The right, middle and left hepatic arteries supply the liver and biliary tree.

(Sleisenger, 9th edition, P-775)

86. Ans. (A) Only 2% to 3% of carcinoid tumors are found in the stomach. Carcinoid tumors are most commonly found in the appendix (47%), ileum (28%) and rectum (17%).

(Sleisenger, 9th edition, Pp-475-477)

87. Ans. (B) Mucosa-associated lymphoid tissue lymphoma is strongly associated with helicobacter pylori infection and may be preceded by the development of lymphoid follicles. Lymphoid follicles are rare in normal gastric mucosa except in children and correlate with H. pylori density and antibody titers. Lymphoid follicles decrease in number with antibiotic therapy.

(Sleisenger, 9th edition, Pp-445-447)

88. Ans. (A) Zollinger-Ellison syndrome is a rare cause of refractory peptic ulcer disease. Poor compliance with medical therapy and the ingestion of non-steroidal anti-inflammatory drugs are important factors to exclude in patients with no evidence of Helicobacter pylori. Gastric acid hypersecretion may contribute to the failure of standard medical therapies in a subset of patients with peptic ulcer disease.

(Sleisenger, 9th edition, Pp-499-503)

89. Ans. (A) Fifty percent to 70% of ulcer recurrences are asymptomatic in patients on maintenance therapy with H_2 blockers.

(Sleisenger, 9th edition, Pp-503-505)

90. Ans. (D) COX-1 expression occurs in response to physiologic stimuli and leads to the synthesis of thromboxane A_2, PG_{I2} and PGE_2.

(Sleisenger, 9th edition, P-543)

91. Ans. (A) Switching to nonacetylated salicylates or reducing the analgesic dose, avoiding concomitant corticosteroid use and co-therapy with misoprostol or a proton pump inhibitor have all been demonstrated to reduce the incidence of non-steroidal anti-inflammatory.

(Sleisenger, 9th edition, Pp-872-874)

92. Ans. (C) There are differences in the ability of non-steroidal anti-inflammatory drugs (NSAIDs) to selectively block COX-1 and COX-2; the newer selective agents are associated with less gastrointestinal toxicity. The potency and duration of COX-1 inhibition is related to duodenal ulcer development. Non-acetylated NSAIDs do not significantly inhibit COX activity.

(Sleisenger, 9th edition, P-862)

93. **Ans. (A)** After truncal vagotomy, both the receptive relaxation and accommodation reflexes are blunted in response to a meal, resulting in accelerated liquid emptying. Vagal denervation of the antrum reduces the force and frequency of contractions during the fasted and fed states. Conversely, reflex inhibition of antral contractions elicited by food passing into the small intestine is also impaired. Truncal vagotomy shortens the duration of fed motor activity after a meal.

(Sleisenger, 9th edition, Pp-882-884)

94. **Ans. (C)** In addition to decreasing the sensitivity of parietal cells to gastrin and histamine, truncal vagotomy reduces basal acid output by 85% and maximal acid output by 50%, decreases the influence of acetylcholine on parietal cells and abolishes proximal gastric non-phasic motor activity.

(Sleisenger, 9th edition, Pp-882-883)

95. **Ans. (B)** When perforation of an anterior duodenal bulb ulcer is associated with a bleeding posterior "kissing" ulcer it is necessary to perform a definitive surgical procedure.

(Sleisenger, 9th edition, P-882)

96. **Ans. (A)** Iron deficiency is a common cause of anemia in postgastrectomy patients. This condition is related to reduced postoperative acid secretion and a decreased ability to dissociate ferric iron from food. Folate and Vitamin B_{12} deficiencies can also develop in these patients, but these deficiencies are much less common.

(Sleisenger, 9th edition, P-912)

97. **Ans. (D)** Poor surgical candidates and patients with a negative result from a gastrografin swallow can be managed conservatively if there are no sign of generalized peritonitis. There is no evidence suggesting that octreotide is of any benefit in the management of these cases.

(Sleisenger, 9th edition, Pp-883-884)

98. **Ans. (C)** Prior use of oral contraceptives does not alter the incidence of nausea and vomiting during pregnancy. However, nausea during the first trimester of pregnancy is more common in non-smokers, primigravidas obese women and women with lower levels of education.

(Sleisenger, 9th edition, P-628)

99. **Ans. (B)** Hyperemesis gravidarum usually starts at 4 weeks of gestation and resolves by the end of the first trimester. Although serum human chorionic gonadotropin levels are increased in patients with hyperemesis gravidarum, these levels do not correlate with the severity of symptoms. One percent to 5% of women with pregnancy-associated nausea and vomiting develop hyperemesis gravidarum, which is characterized by volume depletion and electrolyte abnormalities.

(Sleisenger, 9th edition, P-628)

100. **Ans. (B)** Unlike the other metabolic abnormalities listed, acidosis is not a consequence of vomiting.

(Sleisenger, 9th edition, P-628)

101. **Ans. (A)** In patient with an obvious upper gastrointestinal source of bleeding (indicated by a history of hematemesis, a nasogastric tube allows the assessment of ongoing acute hemorrhage.

(Sleisenger, 9th edition, P-878)

102. **Ans. (C)** Maintenance of tissue perfusion with adequate intravascular volume is more important than replacement of blood cells in the initial management.

(Sleisenger, 9th edition, P-878)

103. **Ans. (A)** Urgent endoscopy is warranted in patients with continued bleeding. Diagnostic endoscopy alone has not been shown to significantly alter the outcome of actively bleeding patients.

(Sleisenger, 9th edition, Pp-878-879)

104. **Ans. (D)** Pancreatitis can be complicated by splenic vein thrombosis, which can be successfully managed by splenectomy.

(Sleisenger, 9th edition, Pp-315-316)

105. **Ans. (B)** Angiodysplasias cause 5% to 7% of upper gastrointestinal hemorrhages. High rates of re-bleeding occur after endoscopic therapy for gastro-intestinal angiodysplasia because most patients will have multiple lesions. Especially those with hereditary hemorrhagic telangiectasia.

(Sleisenger, 9th edition, P-628)

106. **Ans. (A)** Most studies have shown that patients with a clean ulcer base at endoscopy have a 0% to 3% risk of re-bleeding. The identification of a visible vessel or adherent clot at endoscopy is associated with a significantly increased risk of ulcer re-bleeding. Visible vessels are identified in 20% to 50% of endoscopies performed with 6 to 24 hours of hospital admission. Other stigmata, such as the flat pigmented spot or white clot, confer a lower risk of re-bleeding.

(Sleisenger, 9th edition, P-309)

107. **Ans. (C)** In general, prompt follow-up endoscopy in patients with hemorrhage from peptic ulcer disease is reserved for those with recurrent bleeding.

(Sleisenger, 9th edition, Pp-290-292)

108. **Ans. (B)** Thermal methods have been reported to be superior, inferior, and equal to injection techniques for bleeding ulcer; in general, their efficacy rates are comparable. The ulcer patients who seem to benefit most from therapeutic endoscopy, in term of need for surgery, transfusion requirements and length of hospitalization are those with major stigmata (e.g. arterial spurting, visible vessels). The joules per tamponade station vary from 60 to 150 and a mean of 40 seconds of electrocoagulation per ulcer has been used safely.

(Sleisenger, 9th edition, Pp-291-292)

109. **Ans. (A)** Gastric varices have not been shown to benefit from epinephrine injection or thermal therapy.

(Sleisenger, 9th edition, Pp-1510-1512)

110. **Ans. (B)** Duodenogastric reflux is not more common in patients with non-ucler dyspepsia than in control subjects.

(Sleisenger, 9th edition, P-184)

111. **Ans. (B)** Upper endoscopy identifies structural disease in about 50% of previously unevaluated dyspeptic patients. An extended functional work-up can identify abnormalities in about 50% of the remaining patients.

(Sleisenger, 9th edition, Pp-183-186)

112. **Ans. (B)** A single intravenous dose of antibiotics can be given periprocedurely to decrease the risk of infection with staphylococcus aureus and â-Adrenergic antagonists have a beneficial effect for large (i.e. grade II or III) varices only. The Child-Pugh score correlates better with mortality than with variceal size.

(Sleisenger, 9th edition, P-654)

113. **Ans. (A)** Prophylactic shunt surgery reduces re-bleeding rates (vs. sclerotherapy) but does not improve long-term morality in patients with cirrhosis. β-Adrenergic antagonists have a beneficial effect for large (i.e., grade II or III) varices only. The Child-Pugh score correlates better with mortality than with variceal size.

(Sleisenger, 9th edition, Pp-1490-1498)

114. **Ans. (A)** A dieulafoy lesion is a condition in which a histologically normal artery running within the submucosa fails to reduce in caliber near the mucosal surface thus causing pressure erosion of the overlying epithelium and possible rupture and hemorrhage. The optimal surgical treatment is a wide wedge resection. Endoscopic coagulation is often successful and precludes the need for surgical management.

(Sleisenger, 9th edition, Pp-593-595)

115. **Ans. (D)** In patients with retained antrum syndrome, little or no gastrin is released after a meal, although the basal gastrin level is increased. Unlike the results in patients with gastrinoma, secretin stimulation tests in patients with retained antrum syndrome do not produce significant increases in the serum gastrin concentration. Acid secretion in these individuals is significantly elevated.

(Sleisenger, 9th edition, Pp-880-885)

116. **Ans. (B)** Pernicious anemia is caused by circulating factors or parietal cell antibodies that lead to a decrease in cobalamin absorption in the terminal ileum and consequent megaloblastic anemia.

(Sleisenger, 9th edition, Pp-837-838)

117. **Ans. (B)** In addition to gastrinomas, the differential diagnosis of hypergastrinemia includes hypochlorhydria or achlorhydria, retained gastric antrum, antral G-cell hyperplasia, renal insufficiency, massive small bowel resection, gastric outlet obstruction, rheumatoid arthritis, vitiligo, diabetes mellitus and pheochromocytoma.

(Sleisenger, 9th edition, P-503)

118. **Ans. (A)** Hypergastrinemia may lead to active gastric and small bowel secretion, but it does not cause colonic hypersecretion.

(Sleisenger, 9th edition, P-501)

119. **Ans. (B)** The most common clinical manifestation of multiple endocrine neoplasia (MEN) type I is hypercalcemia secondary to hyperparathyroidism.

(Sleisenger, 9th edition, P-502)

120. **Ans. (C)** With the advent of potent anti-secretory agents, there is no need to perform a gastrectomy for the initial treatment of gastrinoma. This procedure is currently used only in rear patient with unresectable gastrinomas who have not responded to medical therapy, or in individuals who are unable to take oral medications. Chemotherapy is used only for unresectable metastatic gastrinoma.

(Sleisenger, 9th edition, Pp-503-504)

121. **Ans. (D)** Patients with common variable hypogammaglobulinema are at an increased risk for gastric cancer. Because of exposure of the stomach to bile in the setting of hypochlorhydria and hypergastrinemia, patients with Billroth II gastrojejunostomy have increased cancer risk. Atrophic gastritis

has a similar premalignant potential. Long term proton pump inhibitor therapy can produce enterochromaffin-like cell hyperplasia and carcinoid tumors in rats but not in humans. Lynch syndrome II is a also known as the cancer family syndrome, a genetic with a propensity for gastrointestinal and other tumors.

(Sleisenger, 9th edition, P-889)

122. **Ans. (B)** Mens have upto a 2-fold risk for the development of gastric cancer compared with women in some population. Gastric cancer compared with women in some populations. Gastric cancer is associated with Helicobacter pylori seropositivity and with lower socio-economic status; it is likely that these two factors are at least partially related to each other because H. pylori infection is more common in lower socio-economic group. Gastric cancer affects first generation emigrants at rates comparable to those in their countries of origin. Gastric cancer is more common in areas where there are high nitrate levels in the water, such as Columbia.

(Sleisenger, 9th edition, Pp-888-893)

123. **Ans. (C)** Tumor markers have been studied as prognostic markers for gastric cancer; however, they are not predictive of survival. Depth of invasion and nodal involvement predict outcome. Proximal tumors tend to have a worse prognosis, possibly because they are frequently advanced at the time of diagnosis.

(Sleisenger, 9th edition, Pp-902-903)

124. **Ans. (D)** Computed tomography is required to exclude distant metastatic disease, particularly to the liver. Endoscopic ultrasonography is very accurate for TNM staging and for the evaluation of tumor extent, but cannot determine whether lymph node enlargement is the result of tumor involvement or inflammation. Enlarged nodes should be biopsied prior to precluding a curative resection. Laparoscopy is used in some centers prior to resection for cure to investigate for peritoneal lesions that may have been missed by preparative radiographic studies.

(Sleisenger, 9th edition, Pp-900-902)

125. **Ans. (C)** Palliative resection is most appropriate in patients undergoing resection when preoperative staging has failed to predict unresectability and survival is expected beyond a few months.

(Sleisenger, 9th edition, Pp-902-904)

126. **Ans. (B)** Gastric lymphomas arise from mucosa-associated lymphoid tissue and are B cell in origin.

(Sleisenger, 9th edition, Pp-445-447)

127. **Ans. (C)** Surgical therapy may be beneficial for patients with gastric lymphoma, but its central role in management is being challenged by advances is chemotherapy and radiotherapy. The diffuse variant is the most common subtype in the stomach. Mucosa-associated lymphoid tissue lymphomas have a relatively good prognosis and have been reported to regress with therapy to eradicate Helicobacter pylori infection.

(Sleisenger, 9th edition, Pp-447-451)

128. **Ans. (A)** Benign hyperplastic polyps constitute about 80% of all gastric polyps. They are unusually less than 2 cm in diameter; sessile and often multiple.

(Sleisenger, 9th edition, Pp-889-890)

129. **Ans. (B)** The most important predictors of prognosis in patients with gastric adenocarcinoma include depth of invasion and the distribution of lymph node metastasis. The degree of histologic differentiation of the tumor is not an independent predictor of prognosis. Proximal tumors tend to have a worse prognosis than more distal lesions. Increased P53 expression in cancers is associated with a reduced 5-year survival rate.

(Sleisenger, 9th edition, P-902)

130. **Ans. (C)** Infection with Helicobacter pylori has been linked to both histologic variants of gastric adenocarcinoma–the intestinal type and the diffuse type.

(Sleisenger, 9th edition, P-895)

131. **Ans. (B)** The onset of dyspeptic symptoms in patients older than 45 to 50 or the presence of "Warning sign" such as dysphagia, nausea, vomiting, bleeding, weight loss or a family history of gastric cancer support the need for early diagnostic evaluation with endoscopy.

(Sleisenger, 9th edition, P-899)

132. **Ans. (C)** The eradication of Helicobacter pylori leads to both ulcer healing and decreased recurrence rates. The documentation of H. pylori eradication is absolutely necessary only in patients with complicated peptic ulcer disease, mucosa-associated lymphoid tissue, lymphoid tissue and after the resection of early gastric cancer.

(Sleisenger, 9th edition, Pp-841-843)

Chapter 3

Small Intestine

1. **Barium small intestine radiography may display thickening of the valvulae conniventes in each of the following small intestine diseases *except:***
   A. Lymphoma
   B. Amyloidosis
   C. Whipple disease
   D. Celiac sprue

2. **Each of the following statements about abetalipoproteinemia is true *except:***
   A. The plasma cholesterol concentration is typically low
   B. There is a positive association with acanthocytosis
   C. Enterocytes appear normal under light microscopy
   D. It exhibits autosomal recessive inheritance

3. **Intraepithelial lymphocytes are predominantly:**
   A. B-lymphoblasts B. NK-cell
   C. CD4 T cells D. CD8 T cells

4. **Which of the following statements regarding secretory IgA is true?**
   A. It facilitates cell-mediated opsonization of infectious organisms
   B. It is protective only when the mucosal barrier is intact
   C. It is protective as a result of its ability to activate complement
   D. It prevents the adherence of bacteria to epithelial cells

5. **The major mucosal defense system against parasitic infection includes each of the following *except:***
   A. Eosinophils B. IgD
   C. IgE D. Mast cells

6. **Histamine secretion by mast cells can be triggered by each of the following *except:***
   A. Gastrin
   B. Vasoactive intestinal polypeptide
   C. Substance P
   D. Somatostatin

7. **The following statement regarding selective IgA deficiency are true *except*:**
   A. Most patients with selective IgA deficiency are asymptomatic
   B. Selective IgA deficiency is associated with celiac disease and pernicious anemia
   C. IgA deficiency is the most common primary immune deficiency
   D. Jejunal biopsy specimens are usually histologically abnormal

8. **A predisposition to the development of diarrheal illness from Giardia lamblia infection exists with each of the following immuno deficiency syndromes:**
   A. X-line or Bruton hypogammaglobulinemia
   B. Severe combined immunodeficiency syndrome
   C. Common variable hypogammaglobulinemia

9. **In intestinal epithelia the rate limiting barrier restricting the passive movement of hydrophobic solutes through the paracellular space is:**
   A. The plasma membrane
   B. The tight junctions
   C. The intestinal mucus
   D. The basement membrane

10. **All of the following statements about tight junctions are true *except:***
   A. The permeability of tight junctions decreases moving distally from the duodenum to the ileum
   B. Water small molecules with molecular weights less than 300 D and electrolytes are unable to pass through the tight junctions
   C. Tight junctions in the villous regions are less permeable than those in the small intestine crypts
   D. The intestinal epithelial cell cytoskeleton is connected directly to the tight junctions

11. **Gap junctions:**
   A. Behave as conduits to allow the direct passage of ions and small molecules between the cytoplasms of adjacent cells
   B. Are located on the apical membrane of cells
   C. Consist of homologous proteins that are identical in the epithelia of different organs
   D. Are also known as desmosomes

12. **All of the following statements concerning chloride channels are true *except:***
   A. There are at least three different choloride channels in intestinal epithelial cells
   B. The most important channel in the intestine is the calcium-activated chloride channel
   C. cAMP-activated chloride channels are defective in cystic fibrosis
   D. Calcium-calmodulin is an important intracellular regulator of one type of chloride channel

13. **Hereditary angioedema (CI esterase inhibitor deficiency):**
   A. Can be effectively treated with anabolic steroids
   B. Is characterized by recurrent, pitting edema of the extremities
   C. Commonly presents in association with pruritus
   D. Commonly presents with associated leukocytosis

14. **Intestinal lymphangiectasia is typically associated with:**
   A. A rash resembling dermatitis herpetiformis
   B. Skin test anergy
   C. Pruritus
   D. Decreased $á_1$ antitrypsin level is stool

15. **All of the following statements regarding travelers diarrhea are true *except:***
   A. Most cases of travelers' diarrhea are caused by enterotoxigenic Escherichia coli
   B. The treatment of choice for adults is trimethoprimsulfamethoxazole
   C. Antibiotics decrease the duration of illness as well as the number of stools per day
   D. Bismuth subsalicylate is an effective prophylaxis for travelers' diarrhea

16. **All of the following statements regarding food-borne illness are true *except:***
   A. Shigella species are the most common causes of food-borne illness in the United States
   B. The ingestion of fried rice contaminated with Bacillus cereus produces an emetic illness
   C. Botulinum toxin produces an illness characterized by nausea, vomiting and mild abdominal pain
   D. Food poisoning caused by a staphylococcal toxin typically occurs 6 to 24 hours after ingestion of the affected food

17. **The vibrionaceae are a family of bacteria whose members include Vibrio, Aeromonas, and Plesiomonas species, members of this family all of the following statements are true *except:***
   A. Decreased gastric acid is associated with an increased risk of acquiring vibrio cholerae infection
   B. The use of oral rehydration formula in the treatment of vibrio cholerae infection relies on small intestine glucose-sodium cotransport mechanism to induce sodium and water absorption
   C. Vibrio parahemolyticans found in fresh water

18. **Which of the following studies would best confirm the diagnosis of tropical sprue?**
   A. Upper gastrointestinal endoscopy with small intestine biopsy
   B. Colonoscopy with biopsy of the terminal ileum
   C. A dedicated small intestine barium radiographic series
   D. A 72 hours stool collection for quantitative fecal fat determination
   E. Stool cultures

19. **Anemia in patients with tropical sprue is secondary to:**
   A. Pseudosplenectomy
   B. Sickling of erythrocytes
   C. Malabsorption resulting in Vitamin B_{12} and folate deficiencies
   D. Chronic disease
   E. Loss of appetite

20. **Clinical manifestations of ascariasis lumbricodies can include all the following *except:***
   A. Pulmonary hypersensitivity reactions
   B. Intestinal obstruction
   C. Common bile duct obstruction
   D. Granulomatous hepatic inflammation

21. **All of the following intestinal nematodes can be associated with pulmonary hypersensitivity reactions *except:***
   A. Trichuris trichiura
   B. Necator americanus
   C. Ascaris lumbricoids
   D. Strongyloides stercoralis

22. **All of the following statements regarding hookwork infections are true *except:***
   A. Iron deficiency is a hallmark of chronic disease
   B. Abdominal pain is common
   C. Direct fecal examination for ova is inadequate to detect significant infections
   D. Eosinophilia is common

23. **The epithelial lining of the intestinal mucosa includes each of the following *except:***

A. Enterocytes
B. B-lymphocytes
C. Paneth cells
D. Enteroendocrine cells
E. Goblet cells

24. **Congenital atresia of the small intestine:**
A. Is associated with an overall mortality of 80%
B. Most often occurs in the distal ileum
C. Is rarely associated with other birth defects
D. When involving the duodenum, is associated with Down syndrome

25. **Malrotation of the midgut is associated with all of the following complications *except:***
A. Duodenal obstruction
B. Acute intestinal ischemia
C. Hirschsprung disease
D. Small intestine arteriovenous malformations

26. **A 7-month-old boy presents with "currant jelly" stools and a palpable midabdominal mass. His parents report intermittent irritability and crying over the past few days. After the initiation of intravenous hydration and surgical evaluation, the next most useful step would be:**
A. Computed tomography of the abdomen
B. Barium enema radiography
C. Scintigraphy, i.e., a Meckel scan
D. Exploratory laparotomy

27. **Which of the following statements regarding Meckel diverticula is true?**
A. They result from ectopic evagination of the primitive appendix
B. They most commonly present with gastrointestinal obstruction in adults
C. They are usually located in the distal jejunum
D. They may be falsely diagnosed by a sodium pertechnetate technetium-99-m radionuclide scan in patients with Crohn's disease

28. **Congenital lymphangiectasia typically presents with each of the following *except:***
A. Diarrhea secondary to an opportunistic infection
B. Asymmetric edema of the extremities
C. Steatorrhea
D. Hypoalbuminemia and lymphocytopenia

29. **Volvulus of the small intestine is:**
A. Most common in adolescents
B. More common than colonic volvulus
C. Often associated with an underlying anatomic defect
D. Often treated medically with conservative measures

30. **Which statement regarding plicae criculares is true?**
A. They are important for generating coordinated perostaltic movement
B. They consist of invaginations of the mucosa, submucosa and muscularis propria
C. They enhance the surface area and absorptive function of the small intestine
D. They are most prominent in the ileum

31. **Which of the following neurotransmitter candidates is thought to play a role in the descending relaxation component of intestinal peristalsis?**
A. Substance P
B. Vasoactive intestinal polypeptide
C. Acetylcholine
D. Somatostatin

32. **Which of the following neurotransmitter candidates is thought to play a role in the ascending contraction component of intestinal peristalsis?**
A. Vasoactive intestinal polypeptide
B. Substance P
C. Norepinephrine
D. Calcitonin gene-related peptide

33. **All of the following are risk factors for the development of small bowel lymphoma *except:***
A. X-linked or Bruton hypogammaglobulinemia
B. Celiac sprue
C. Human immunodeficiency virus
D. Intestinal lymphangiectasia

34. **An infant with congenital chloride diarrhea can benefit from treatment with:**
A. NaCI supplementation
B. Omeprazole
C. Glucose supplementation
D. Cimetidine

35. **Each of the following statements regarding abetalipoproteinemia is true *except:***
A. Abetalipoproteinemia is an autosomal recessive disease characterized by the absence of apolipoprotein B (apo B) and apo B containing lipoproteins in the plasma of affected subjects
B. Symptoms of malabsorption and failure to thrive are characteristic of this disease
C. Plasma lipid and lipoprotein profiles of patients with abetalipoproteinemia include hypocholesterolemia, low triglyceride levels and virtually non detectable chylomicrons, very-low-density lipoproteins, low-density lipoproteins and apo B

D. mRNA for apo B and apo B protein are absent in the intestinal mucosa and liver of affected subjects

36. **A 22-year-old Asian student presents with complaints of intermittent abdominal pain, cramps, nausea, flatulence and diarrhea. He has had these symptoms for several years. He describes his stools as bulky, frothy and watery. He denies weight loss, blood in the stools, fever or chills. He has no significant medical history. He recently spent 2 weeks in India visiting relatives. Finding on physical examination and results of laboratory tests are normal. The most likely cause of this patient's discomfort is:**
A. Lactose intolerance
B. Inflammatory bowel disease
C. Sprue
D. Amebiasis

37. **The diagnostic test of choice would be:**
A. Serum analysis of antiendomysial antibody
B. Lactulose breath test
C. Stool culture
D. Quantitative fecal fat test

38. **Small bowel biopsy specimens reveal infiltration of the lamina propria by Periodic Acid-Schiff (PAS) positive macrophages containing gram-positive non-acid-fast bacilli, accompanied by lymphatic dilation. This man's illness is caused by:**
A. Mycobacterium avium complex
B. Giardia lamblia
C. Tropheryma whippelii
D. Mycosplasma species

39. **Which of the following statements about the treatment of this disease is true?**
A. Treatment with antibiotics results in gradual improvement; full clinical recovery can take up to 1 year
B. Small bowel biopsy to document the absence of bacilli is recommended prior to discontinuing therapy at 1 year
C. Relapse is uncommon
D. Yearly surveillance with endoscopy is recommended

40. **The most common skin disorders associated with celiac disease is:**
A. Dermatitis herpetiformis
B. Dermatomyositis
C. Polyarteritis nodosa
D. The result of niacin deficiency

41. **All of the following statements regarding this condition are true *except:***
A. Atopic eczema may respond to treatment of the underlying disease
B. Skin biopsy specimen will reveal IgA at the dermopeidermal junction in areas not affected by blisters
C. No specific treatment for the skin disorder is warranted if the underlying problem is treated
D. This patient has a high likelihood of being HLA-DQ2 positive

42. **This patient is at increased risk for all of the following *except:***
A. Lactose and sucrose intolerance
B. Small bowel lymphoma
C. Adrenal insufficiency
D. Hyposplenism

43. **All of the following statements regarding the histology of the small intestine in celia sprue are true *except*:**
A. There is a loss of villous architecture with a reduction in the ratio of villous height to crypt dept
B. There is a decrease in the total thickness of the mucosa because of crypt atrophy
C. Mitotic activity is no longer confined to the base of the crypt
D. The cell migration time from the base of the crypt to the villous tip is shortened

44. **A woman with celiac sprue confirmed by biopsy has been compliant with her recommended diet. Her most recent laboratory studies reveal hypoalbuminemia, possibly complication she developed:**
A. Gluten in the diet
B. Small bowel lymphoma
C. Pancreatic insufficiency
D. Achlorhydria

45. **Gluten shock is best treated with:**
A. Immune globulin
B. Systemic corticosteroids
C. Somatostatin
D. Antibiotics

46. **Patients with extensive ileal resections have an increased incidence of:**
A. Cholesterol gallstones
B. Pigment gallstones
C. Both
D. Neither

47. Which of the following patients with Crohn's disease would not be predisposed to the formation of calcium oxalate renal stones?

A. A patient who has had more than 100 cm of terminal ileum resected
B. A patient who has had less than 100 cm of terminal ileum resected
C. A patient with an ileostomy who has had a total colectomy
D. A patient with extensive terminal ileum disease who has not had any resections

48. Which of the following is not a mechanism by which neutrophils contribute to epithelial destruction in inflammatory bowel disease?

A. Release of granule-bound proteases
B. Increased IgG secretion
C. Production of superoxide and other reactive oxygen species
D. Breakdown of the tight junction during migration of neutrophils across the epithelium into the lumen

49. Crohn's disease involving the terminal ileum and right colon is diagnosed in a 28-year-old woman. Olsalazine is started. Within 1 week, profound watery diarrhea develops without constitutional symptoms. How should this case be managed?

A. Prescribe steroids
B. Measure serum gastrin and vasoactive intestinal polypeptide levels
C. Stop olsalazine and start mesalamine
D. Perform enteroscopy

50. The most common presenting symptoms of Crohn's disease are diarrhea and:

A. Bleeding
B. Abdominal pain
C. Perianal disease
D. Arthritis

51. Which of the following conditions is not included in the differential diagnosis of terminal ilea ulcerations?

A. Crohn's disease
B. Behcet syndrome
C. Histoplasmosis
D. Whipple disease
E. Non-steroidal anti-inflammatory drug-induced ulcerations

52. Which of the following statements regarding the outcome of patient with irritable bowel syndrome is true?

A. Most persons with irritable bowel syndrome are free of symptoms after 5 years
B. Female patients with a long history of diarrhea and a good initial response to treatment are most likely to achieve long-term improvement
C. Patients who receive education regarding the roles of psychologic stress and precipitating factors require fewer physician visits for management of their disorder
D. Persons with irritable bowel syndrome have higher mortality rates than do unaffected persons

53. Which of the following statements regarding tropical sprue is correct?

A. Involvement of the ileum and deficiency of vitamin B_{12} are rare in tropical sprue
B. Tropical sprue is thought to be due to bacterial overgrowth

54. The following persons are at increased risk for gastrointestinal tuberculosis *except*:

A. Persons from endemic areas
B. Persons infected with human immunodeficiency virus
C. Person with a history of alcohol abuse
D. Persons who have splenectomy

55. What is the most frequent site of gastrointestinal tuberculosis infection?

A. Stomach
B. Duodenum
C. Jejunum
D. Terminal ileum and cecum

56. Which of the following mycotic infection of the small intestine affects immunocompetent as well as immunocompromised persons?

A. Histoplasmosis
B. Aspergillosis
C. Candidiasis
D. Mucormycosis

57. All of the following statements concerning gastrointestinal hemorrhage in immuno compromised persons are correct *except*:

A. Viral ulceration represents the most common causes of gastrointestinal hemorrhage in patients following bone marrow transplantation
B. Non-healing peptic-appearing ulcer in the stomach and duodenum may be caused by cytomegalovirus infection
C. Herps simplex virus infection commonly presents endoscopically with large intestinal nodules

D. Graft-versus-host disease is a common cause of hemorrhage in the bone marrow transplant patients

58. The most common cause of occult gastrointestinal hemorrhage in the western world is:
A. Acid-peptic disease
B. Colonic neoplasms
C. Vascular malformations
D. Hookworm infection

59. All of the following statements regarding giardiasis are correct *except*:
A. Giardiasis is major cause of acute diarrhea in patients with acquired immunodeficiency syndrome
B. In the United States, giardia lamblia is the leading infectious agent identified in waterborne outbreaks of diarrhea
C. Treatment is indicated if cysts or trophozoites are identified in stool specimens from symptomatic patients
D. Recommended therapies include quinacrine of metronidazole for 5 to 10 days

60. All of the following statements regarding diarrhea are true *except*:
A. The mean frequency of stools with diarrhea resulting from colonic disease is greater than that resulting from small intestine disease
B. Stool volumes are generally smaller with colonic causes of diarrhea compared with small intestine diseases resulting in diarrhea
C. Stool frequencies are more regular with small intestine disease that cause diarrhea than with colonic causes of diarrhea
D. Colonic disease that causes diarrhea commonly result in positive tests for fecal occult blood

61. The most prevalent intestinal helminth is:
A. Ascaris lumbricoides
B. Strongyloides stercoralis
C. Enterobias vermicularis
D. Clonorchis sinensis

62. The clinical triad associated with visceral larva migrans infection includes each of the following *except*:
A. Eosinophilia
B. Hepatomegaly
C. Pleuritis
D. Hypergammaglobulinemia

63. A 54-year-old man with degenerative joint disease presents with iron deficiency anemia and hemocultpositive stools. He has been an oral indomethacin 25 mg twice daily for 12 months. Colonoscopy and upper endoscopy have failed to define the cause of his blood loss. Small intestine enteroscopy demonstrated several 0.3 to 0.6 cm shallow ulcers distal to the ligament of Treitz. Which of the following statement regarding this disorder is true?
A. Almost 25% of patients taking non-steroidal anti-inflammatory drugs (NSAIDs) have evidence of increased intestinal permeability or inflammation
B. Non-specific small intestine ulcers are found in 50% of patients who were prescribed NSAIDs during the 6 months prior to death

64. Each of the following medications is associated with intestinal ischemia *except*:
A. Cocaine
B. Oral contracepatives
C. Angiotensin-converting enzyme (ACE) inhibitors
D. Ergotamine
E. Dopamine

65. All of the following statements regarding hemorrhage from aortoenteric fistulas are true *except*:
A. They almost always involve the third portion of duodenum
B. The classic presentation is a 'herald' bleed
C. Aortography is often helpful in making the correct diagnosis
D. With a Dacron graft, the fistula usually arises from the proximal part of the graft

66. A 5-year-old infant presents with increasing abdominal girth. Occasional vomiting and decreased activity. The infant was born 6 weeks prematurely, but has been taking formula until the day prior to presentation. The pediatrician notes bloods in the infant's stool. Abdominal radiographs reveal pneumatosis intestinalis. The child is admitted for management of necrotizing enterocolitis (NEC). Which of the following statements is most accurate?
A. Prematurity is a risk factor for the development of NEC
B. Intestinal penumatosis is largely caused by aerophagia
C. Breastfeeding places infants at an increased risk for NEC
D. The transverse colon is most commonly involved in NEC

67. **All of the following statements regarding radiation enteritis are true *except*:**
   A. It is often seen with total radiation doses of 40 Gy
   B. It commonly present with diarrhea as the only symptom
   C. It may present with nausea and vomiting
   D. Barium radiographic studies are often non-diagnostic

68. **A 21-year-old woman presents to the emergency department with a 3-day history of upper abdominal cramping and vomiting. She has recently returned from New Guinea, where she worked for 2 years in the peace corps. On examination, the patient is afebrile but appears dehydrated. Abdominal examination reveals absent bowel sounds, diffuse abdominal tenderness with guarding, and a papable segment of bowel in the periumbilical region. Rectal examination is negative for masses or tenderness, but reveals maroon-colored stool that is guaiac-positive. A pelvic examination reveals nothing abnormal. Routine laboratory evaluation, including a serum pregnancy test is negative except for evident leukocytosis white blood cell count of 17000 cell/mm^3. Abdominal radiographs reveals multiple air-fluid levels with a thickened jejunal wall. The patient undergoes a laparotomy and is found to have patchy, plum-colored bacilli are observed in the microscopic sections:**
   A. Clostridium perfringens is most likely etiologic agent for the jejunal inflammation
   B. Stool cultures are not helpful in the diagnosis of this infection
   C. Infections with this organism rarely respond to antibiotics
   D. Surgical management should include wide resection of any involved segments of intestine

69. **A 26-year-old woman presents to her local physician for an evaluation of peripheral edema. The patient denies having any other symptoms and reportedly has a normal medical history. The laboratory evaluation is remarkable for a serum albumin level of 2.8 g/dl, with normal liver chemistries (aspirate aminotransferase, alkaline, phosphatase, prothrombin time) and normal results from renal function tests and urinalysis. All of the following studies are indicated:**
   A. Measure the serum angiotensin-converting enzyme level
   B. Echocardiography
   C. Small intestine biopsy
   D. Analyze stool for α-antitrypsin concentration

70. **A 28-year-old man is referred for the evaluation of recurrent epistaxis and a family history of recurrent gastrointestinal hemorrhage in one sibling. You tender a tentative diagnosis after noting abnormal vascular ectasias on his lips. Which of the following statement is most accurate?**
   A. The most likely is Peutz-Jeghers syndrome
   B. The disease is likely to be autosomal recessive
   C. Connective tissue disorders are often associated with this disease
   D. Lower gastrointestinal hemorrhage is more common than upper gastrointestinal bleeding in this disease

71. **A 43-year-old homosexual mart with pneumocystis carinii pneumonia is referred for the evaluation of persistent guaiac-positive stools that began with a single episode of melena 10 days ago. Of the following disease process is most likely to account for gastrointestinal blood loss?**
   A. Diverticulitis
   B. Kaposi sarcoma
   C. Infection with giardia lamblia
   D. Infection with isospora belli I

72. **All of the following statements concerning pneumatosis intestinalis are true *except*:**
   A. It is defined as gas-filled cysts in the wall of the small intestine and colon
   B. A linear pattern of gas accumulation may be associated with intestinal ischemia
   C. Cystic-like pneumatosis intestinalis may be seen in scleroderma
   D. Pneumoperitoneum may occur as a result of this disorder
   E. It represents a severe form of enteritis and is usually fatal

73. **Ischemic injury to the gastrointestinal tract is likely tract is likely to be mediated by all of the following *except*:**
   A. Free radicals generated by xanthine oxidase
   B. Superoxide dismutase
   C. Proteases
   D. Bacteria and toxins

74. **All of the following are thought to modulate gastrointestinal blood flow *except*:**
A. Adenosine and oxygen
B. Parasympathetic nervous system
C. Arteriolar and precapillary sphincters
D. Hormones

75. **Which of the following statements regarding primary small intestine tumor is most accurate?**
A. Most small intestine tumors will eventually become symptomatic
B. Small intestine tumors account for approximately 10% of all gastrointestinal malignancies
C. Japanese immigrants to Hawaii acquire the same risk of the development of small intestine tumors as that found in the Hawaiian white population
D. Small intestine tumors are more common in Asia than in other parts of the world

76. **Which of the following statement regarding the treatment of carcinoid syndrome with octreotide is correct?**
A. Octreotide improves symptoms in 90% of patients with carcinoid syndrome
B. Octreotide reduces plasma serotonin levels in patients with carcinoid syndrome
C. Octreotide increases the urinary excretion of 5-hydroxyindoleacetic acid (5 HIAA in patient with carcinoid syndrome
D. Octreotide decreases tumor bulk but does affect mortality rates

77. **Each of the following statements regarding the genetic and environmental etiologies of celiac sprue is true *except*:**
A. Ten percent to 15% of first-degree relatives of patients with celiac sprue also have the disease
B. The prevalence of prior infection with adenovirus serotype 12 is higher in patients with celiac sprue compared with healthy controls
C. There is significant amino acid homology between A-gliadin and a cell wall protein of non-pathogenic anaerobes
D. Worldwide, HLA-DR and HLA-DQ antigens have the strongest association with celiac sprue

78. **Of which statements regarding adynamic ileus, which is the most accurate?**
A. Bowel ischemia may result from decreased arterial blood flow secondary to increased intraluminal pressure in adynamic ileus
B. The initial presentation of adynamic ileus typically includes focal pain and borborygmi
C. The etiology of adynamic ileus often relates to metabolic abnormalities of infection
D. The observation of multiple air fluid levels on up-right abdominal radiographs differentiates adynamic ileus from mechanical intestinal obstruction

79. **All of the following statements concerning small intestine motor dysfunction is scleroderma are true *except*:**
A. Small intestine dysmotility results from the replacement of smooth muscle tissue by collagen
B. Small intestine involvement is often characterized by luminal dilation
C. The small intestine circular muscle layer is one often involved than the longitudinal muscle layer
D. The small intestine is involved less often that the esophagus and stomach

80. **Barium small intestine radiography may display thickening of the valvulae conniventes in each of the following small intestine disease *except*:**
A. Lymphoma
B. Amyloidosis
C. Whipple disease
D. Celiac sprue

81. **Each of the following statements about abetalipoproteinemia is true *except*:**
A. The plasma cholesterol concentration
B. There is a positive association with acantho-cytosis
C. Enterocytes appear normal under light microscopy
D. It exhibits autosomal recessive inheritance

82. **Each of the following statements concerning microfold (M cells) is true *except*:**
A. They are epithelial cells located in the mucosa overlying lymphoid follicles
B. They selectively “sample” intraluminal antigens
C. They transport microorganisms and large molecules to the underlying lymphoid tissue
D. They express class II antigens on their surface

83. **Intraepithelial lymphocytes are predominantly:**
A. B lymphoblasts
B. B lymphocytes
C. CD4+T cell
D. CD8+cells

84. **Which of the following statement regarding secretory IgA is true?**
A. It facilitates cell-mediated opsonization of infectious organisms
B. It is protective only when the mucosal barrier is intact

C. It is protective as a result of its ability to active complement
D. It prevents the adherence of bacteria of epithelial cells

85. The major mucosal defense system against parasitic infection includes each of the following *except*:
A. Eosinophils
B. IgD
C. IgE
D. Mast cells

86. Histamine secretion by mast cells can be triggered by each of the following *except*:
A. Gastrin
B. Vasoactive intestinal polypeptide
C. Substance P
D. Somatostatin

87. The following statement regarding selective IgA deficiency are true *except*:
A. Most patient with selective IgA deficiency are asymptomatic
B. Selective IgA deficiency is associated with celiac disease and pernicious anemia
C. IgA deficiency is the most common primary immune deficiency
D. Jejunal biopsy specimens are usually histological abnormal

88. A predisposition to the development of diarrhea illness from Giardia lamblia infection exists with each of the following immunodeficiency syndromes *except*:
A. X-lined or Burton hypogammaglobulinemia
B. Severe combined immunodeficiency syndrome
C. Common variable hypogammaglobulinemia

89. Each of the following statement concerning secretary component (SC) is true *except*:
A. SC functions as a receptor for J-chain-Dimeric IgA complexes on the basal surface of the epithelial cells
B. SC serves a protective function of secretory IgA in the intestinal lumen
C. SC is not found by itself in mucosal secretions
D. SC is transported to the apical surface of the epithelial cells in endoplasmic vesicles

90. In the intestinal epithelia, the rate-limiting barrier restricting the passive movement of hydrophobic solutes through the paracellular space is:
A. The plasma membrane
B. The tight junction
C. The intestinal mucus
D. The basement membrane

91. All of the following statements about tight junctions are true *except*:
A. The permeability of tight decreases moving distally from the duodenum to the ileum
B. Water, small molecules with molecular weight less than 300 d, and electrolytes are unable to pass through the tight junctions
C. Tight junctions in the villous regions are less permeable than those in the small intestine crypts
D. The intestinal epithelial cell cytoskeleton is connected directly to the tight junction

92. Gap junction:
A. Behave as conduits to allow the direct passage of ions and small molecules between the cytoplasms of adjancent cells
B. Are located on the apical membrane of cells
C. Consist of homologous proteins that are identical in the epithelia of different organs
D. Are also known as desmosomes

93. All of the following statements concerning chloride channels are true *except*:
A. There are at least three different chloride channels in intestinal epithelial cells
B. The most important channel in the intestine is the calcium-activated chloride channel
C. cAMP-activated chloride channels are defective in cystic fibrosis
D. Calcium-calmoduline is an important intracellular regulator of one type of chloride channel

94. Which of the following statement concerning common variable hypogammaglobulinemia is true?
A. It is the most common primary immunodeficiency in adults
B. Jejunal biopsy specimens are usually normal
C. Nodular lymphoid hyperplasia is a common finding
D. Malabsorption is unusual

95. Each of the following statement about chronic granulomatous disease is true *except*:
A. Catalase-negative organisms (e.g., pneumococci and lactobacilli) are not major pathogens
B. Staphylococci, Serratia species and salmonella species are common pathogens
C. Gastrointestinal symptoms may mimic those of Crohn's disease
D. Liver abscess formation is unusual

96. Hereditary angioedema (CI esterase inhibitor deficiency):

A. Can be effectively treated with anabolic steroid
B. Is characterized by recurrent, pitting edema of the extremities
C. Commonly presents in associated with pruritus
D. Commonly presents with associated leukocytosis

97. Intestinal lymphangiectasia is typically associated with:
A. A rash resembling dermatitis herpetiformis
B. Skin test energy
C. Pruritus
D. Decreased α antitrypsin level in stool

98. A 35-year-old man presents for the evaluation of suspected food allergies. He reports two discrete episodes of periorbital edema and severe wheezing one of which required management in a local emergency department with bronchodilators. Both episodes occurred shortly after the ingestion of peanuts. His past medical history is remarkable only for eczema. Finding from a review of systems and a physical examination at this time are normal which of the following would be the most appropriate method for evaluating this patient for food allergies?
A. Skin tests
B. Radioallergosorbent test (RAST) or enzyme-linked immunosorbent assay (ELISA)
C. Cytotoxicity food allergy test
D. Double-blind placebo-controlled oral challenge with peanuts

99. Eosinophilic gastroenteritis:
A. Typically is associated with normal or low peripheral eosinophil counts
B. May be associated with Charcot-Leyden crystals in the stool
C. Is characterized by eosinophilic infiltration confined to the mucosa
D. Does not affect the colon

100. All of the following statements regarding travelers' diarrhea are true *except*:
A. Most cases of travelers' diarrhea are caused by enterotoxigenic Escherichia coli
B. The treatment of choice for adults in trimethoprimsulfamethoxazole
C. Antibiotics decrease the duration of illness as well as the number of stools per day
D. Bismuth subsalicylate is an effective prophylaxis for travelers' diarrhea

101. All the following statements regarding food-borne illness are true *except*:
A. Shigella species are the most common causes of food-borne illness in the United States
B. The ingestion of fired rice contaminated with Bacillus cereus produces an emetic illness
C. Botulinum toxin produces an illness characterized by nausea, vomiting and mild abdominal pain
D. Food poisoning caused by a staphylococcal toxin typically occurs 6 to 24 hours after ingestion of the affected food

Explanation

1. **Ans. (D)** Celiac sprue typically causes reduction or loss of the valvulae conniventes rather than thickening.

(Sleisenger, 9th edition, P-1799)

2. **Ans. (C)** Enterocytes from patients with abetalipoproteinemia contain numerous small, clear vacuoles that are visible under light microscopy and reflect lipid accumulation within the enterocyte.

(Sleisenger, 9th edition, P-1763)

3. **Ans. (D)** A few intraepithelial lymphocytes (IELs) are CD4* T cells, but most express the CD8 α/β heterodimer, the CD45RO isoform. They have suppressor and cytolytic activities; however, their exact roles are unknown.

(Sleisenger, 8th edition, P-118)

4. **Ans. (D)** Secretory IgA inhibits the adherence of bacteria to epithelial cells, interfering with bacterial colonization and replication.

(Sleisenger, 8th edition, P-118)

5. **Ans. (B)** IgD is not involved in mucosal defense against parasitic infection.

(Sleisenger, 8th edition, P-137)

6. **Ans. (A)** Vasoactive intestinal polypeptide, substance P. and somatostatin can trigger histamine secretion by both connective tissue and intestinal mucosal mast cells.

(Sleisenger, 8th edition, P-137)

7. **Ans. (D)** IgA deficiency is the most common primary immune deficiency. Biopsy specimens from the jejunum in IgA deficient subjects are morphologically normal, whereas immunofluorescence studies show a paucity. of IgA producing cells and an increase in IgM secreting cells.

(Sleisenger, 8th edition, P-2548)

8. **Ans. (B)** Gastrointestinal infection with giardia lamblia occurs in approximately 30% of X-linked hypogammaglobulinemia patients. Severe combined immunodeficiency syndromes show a markedly increased risk of viral infections in early childhood, but giardia infections do not predominate. Giardiasis is a common cause of steatorrhea and malabsorption in common variable hypogammaglobulinemia. Giardiasis has been reported with IgA deficiency, but the incidence is probably the same or only slightly increased in comparison with the general population.

(Sleisenger, 9th edition, Pp-1912-1914)

9. **Ans. (B)** Under most conditions, the apical intercellular tight junctions are the rate-limiting barrier restricting the passive movement of hydrophobic solutes through the paracellular space. The plasma membrane and transmembrane proteins are the rate-limiting barriers to transcellular absorption.

(Sleisenger, 8th edition, P-147)

10. **Ans. (B)** Tight junctions are selective pores that allow the passage of water and small molecules of molecular weight less than 300 D. Tight junctions are the route for the net movement of those substances that are not actively transported to maintain the osmotic and electrical balance of the cell.

(Sleisenger, 8th edition, Pp-146, 152)

11. **Ans. (A)** Gap junctions assist in coordinating the activities of adjacent cells within the epithelial sheet by allowing them to behave as syncytia with respect to the transfer of small molecules.

(Sleisenger, 8th edition, P-146)

12. **Ans. (B)** In the small intestine, the most important chloride channel is the cAMP-activated low conductance channel, which participates in hormone-stimulated chloride secretion. This channel is defective in cystic fibrosis. A separate calcium activated chloride channel has been isolated in airway epithelial cells and in colon cancer cell lines. This appears to be regulated by calcium-calmodulin. The role of the calcium activated chloride channel in intestinal chloride secretion is unclear.

(Sleisenger, 9th edition, Pp-1683-1684)

13. **Ans. (A)** Abdominal pain, vomiting and watery diarrhea are common features of hereditary angioedema. Pitting edema, pruritus and leukocytosis are notably absent. Anabolic steroids can be effective in treating some cases of hereditary angioedema.

(Sleisenger, 8th edition, P-244)

14. **Ans. (B)** Patients with intestinal lymphangiectasia most commonly exhibit lymphopenia, resulting in anergy, and increased excretion of α-antitrypsin in the stool.

(Sleisenger, 9th edition, P-441)

15. **Ans. (B)** Most cases of travelers' diarrhea develop within the first week of travel. Antibiotic prophylaxis reduces the incidence of travelers' diarrhea by about 90%. Bismuth is an effective prophylaxis and has been effective in the treatment of mild to moderate cases of travelers' diarrhea. Because of increasing drug resistance and the high incidence of illness caused by campylobacter jejuni, the quinolones are now the treatment of choice for adults.

(Sleisenger, 8th edition, P-1615)

16. **Ans. (A)** Bacillius cereus is also associated with a diarrheal illness following ingestion is also associated with this toxin is confined to the ingestion of contaminated fried rice; the ingestion of the toxin in other foodstuff is associated with a diarrheal illness. Botulinum toxin blocks acetylcholine at the neuromuscular junction and produces skeletal muscle weakness with a 15% case-fatality rate. There is also a mild associated disturbance of gastrointestinal function. The clinical feature of ingestion of staphylococcus aureus enterotoxin include profuse vomiting and nausea. Typically beginning within 6 to 24 hours of ingestion. S aureus is the most common ingested food-borne pathogen in the United States.

(Sleisenger, 9th edition, Pp-1845-1846)

17. **Ans. (C)** The glucose-amino acid sodium co-transport mechanism is not affected by cholera toxin and in mild to moderate disease, can provide adequate rehydration of patients. Vibrio parahemolyticus is halophilic, or salt-loving, and is usually found in salt water fish or shellfish. Aeromonas infections can be associated with a chronic diarrheal illness that can last as long as a year.

(Harrison, 17th edition, P-975)

18. **Ans. (A)** Although no test is diagnostic for tropical sprue, small intestine biopsy specimens show shortening of the villi and lengthening of the crypts along with infiltration of the lamina propria with chronic inflammatory cells. A completely flat mucosa, similar to that observed with celiac sprue, is seen in less than 10% of cases. Demonstration of lipid droplets adjacent to the surface epithelium with oil red O stain is a more specific finding.

(Sleisenger, 9th edition, P-1648)

19. **Ans. (C)** Tropical sprue results from damage to the small intestine wall from coliform bacteria toxins, leading to malabsorption and megaloblastic anemia resulting from folate and vitamin B12 deficiency.

(Sleisenger, 8th edition, P-1649)

20. **Ans. (D)** Ascariasis may present with any of the clinical manifestations listed with the exception of hepatic granulomas, which are more typical of schistosomiasis

(Sleisenger, 9th edition, Pp-1921-1922)

21. **Ans. (A)** Trichuris trichiura (whipworm) infections are often asymptomatic and result from the ingestion of embryonated ova. The other helminths listed have a component of their lifecycle that includes migration of larvae to the lung, which can be associated with pulmonary hypersensitivity reactions.

(Sleisenger, 9th edition, P-192)

22. **Ans. (C)** Hookworm disease (Necator americanus infection) was once prevalent in the southeastern United States but is now unusual. Persons from an endemic region who present with abdominal pain flatulence, iron deficiency, or pulmonary hypersensitivity reactions should undergo direct fecal examination for ova, which is adequate to detect clinically significant infections.

(Sleisenger, 9th edition, Pp-1925, 1926)

23. **Ans. (B)** Stem cells located near the base of the crypt-villus axis give rise to four major epithelial cell types in the small intestine. The enterocyte is the main functional cell of the crypt-villus axis. Enteroendocrine cells are distributed throughout the intestinal mucosa but are (found predominantly in the crypts. Goblet cells secrete an acidic mucus and are located along the crypts and villi. Paneth cells are serous and zymogenic cells located at the base of the crypt; their exact physiologic function has not been determined. Intraepithelial lymphocytes are also present in a ratio of about lymphocyte for every 5 epithelial cells; however, these lymphocytes are predominantly T-suppressor cells.

(Sleisenger, 9th edition, Pp-1618-1619)

24. **Ans. (D)** Congenital atresias and stenoses can occur anywhere in the small intestine, but 40% of atresias and 70% of stenoses occur in the duodenum. The overall mortality rate for atresias has been reduced to about 20%, but the prognosis worsens with proximal or multiple atresias. A number of cases are associated with other birth defects such as malrotation, annular pancreas, and cardiac anomalies. Thirty percent of duodenal atresias or stenoses are associated with Down syndrome.

(Sleisenger, 9th edition, P-1633)

25. Ans. (D) Malrotation can produce small intestine volvulus with associated obstruction and ischemia. Ladd bands from cecal peritonealization can also obstruct the duodenum. Malrotation has been associated with other anomalies, including small bowel atresia, Hirschsprung disease and abdominal wall defects, but not arteriovenous malformations.

(Sleisenger, 9th edition, Pp-1630-1631)

26. Ans. (B) This is the classic presentation of intussusception, one of the most common causes of abdominal pain in infancy. In addition to confirming the diagnosis, a gentle barium enema will frequently replace the idiopathic intussusception in patients in the pediatric age group.

(Sleisenger, 9th edition, Pp-2114-2115)

27. Ans. (D) A Meckel diverticulum results from a failure of the vitelline duct—the structure that connects the fetal yolk sac to the primitive gut—to be completely resorbed. In adults, gastrointestinal hemorrhage is by far the most frequent presentation and intestinal obstruction is relatively uncommon. Crohn's disease and other inflammatory diseases of the bowel can lead to false-positive readings on it Meckel's scan.

(Sleisenger, 9th edition, P-1628)

28. Ans. (A) Patients with congenital lymphangiectasia (Milroy disease); usually present with asymmetric edema of the extremities as a result of peripheral lymphatic obstruction, or in a manner similar to secondary, lymphangiectasia, with diffuse symmetric edema exacerbated by hypoalbuminemia. Despite lymphocytopenia and delayed hypersensitivity reactions, opportunistic infections resulting in the development of diarrhea are rare.

(Sleisenger, 8th edition, P-1578)

29. Ans. (C) Volvulus of the small intestine occurs in newborns and is rare in adults, unlike the more common colonic volvulus and sigmoid volvulus, which occur in persons of a broad age range, including older persons. Small intestine volvulus is often associated with an underlying defect, such as an inadequate mesenteric attachment in malrotation a fibrous band, or an adhesion. Treatment is surgical, and is often performed emergently evidence of intestinal ischemia is present.

(Sleisenger, 8th edition, P-1576)

30. Ans. (C) The plicae circulares increase the surface area of the small intestine and have no role in small intestine propulsion. The plicae circulares are invaginations of the submucosa and mucosa only, and are most prominent in the duodenum and jejunum.

(Sleisenger, 8th edition, P-1561)

31. Ans. (B) Most evidence, collected using selective antisera and relatively selective receptor antagonists, suggests that vasoactive intestinal polypeptide contributes to the descending relaxation component of peristalsis. Other data support the participation of nitric oxide in smooth muscle relaxation as well.

(Sleisenger, 8th edition, P-97)

32. Ans. (B) Studies using selective antagonists and relatively selective receptor antagonists suggest that tachykinins such as substance P participate in the ascending contraction component of peristalsis. Acetylcholine may also contribute to this contractile event.

(Sleisenger, 8th edition, P-98)

33. Ans. (D) Risk factors for primary small bowel lymphoma include immunodeficiency syndrome celiac sprue, and the human immunodeficiency virus. The gastrointestinal tract is the most common location for primary extranodal lymphoma. Primary small bowel lymphomas are typically of the non-Hodgkin variety: two-third are B-cell and one-third are T-cell derived.

(Sleisenger, 9th edition, Pp-453-454)

34. Ans. (B) Omeprazole is reportedly of benefit in the treatment of congenital chloride diarrhea. Investigators have proposed that the inhibition of gastric chloride secretion reduces exposure of the distal bowel to unabsorbed chloride. In contrast, neither NaCl nor glucose can ameliorate the metabolic abnormalities seen in congenital chloride diarrhea, nor is there any evidence that histamine H_2 receptor blockade is of any benefit.

(Sleisenger, 9th edition, P-1641)

35. Ans. (D) Both the mRNA for apolipoprotein B (apo B) and the apo B protein are expressed in the intestinal mucosa and liver of persons affected with abetalipoproteinemia. The defect resides in the protein complex, microsomal triglyceride transler protein (MTP). Studies of patients with abetalipoproteinemia have shown that the assembly of apo B containing lipoproteins is defective as a result of non-functional MTP.

(Sleisenger, 9th edition, P-1763)

36 Ans. (A) The most likely cause of this man's discomfort is lactose intolerance. The disorder is very common in persons from Asia and Africa. It is characterized by intermittent symptoms that are exacerbated by the ingestion of lactose-containing food. The absence of bloody diarrhea weight loss, fever and metabolic abnormalities render the diagnosis of irritable bowel syndrome, amebiasis or sprue less likely.

(Sleisenger, 9th edition, P-1755)

37. **Ans. (B)** For explanation see Ans. no.36.

(Sleisenger, 9th edition, P-1755)

38. **Ans. (C)** Whipple disease is caused by the bacterium Tropheryma whippelii. It occurs most often in the fifth and sixth decades of life and exhibits a male predominance (male, female, 8: 1). Diarrhea affects 75% of patients. Weight loss is a common presenting symptom. Extraintestinal symptoms may precede the gastrointestinal symptoms by years. Migratory arthritis involving the large and small joints is the most common extraintestinal symptom; fever is second most common. Tropical sprue is associated with chronic diarrhea and malabsorption in patients from an endemic area; extraintestinal manifestations are not common. The diagnosis of Whipple disease is best made by small bowel biopsy, which demonstrates infiltration of the lamina propria with large foamy macrophages that grossly distort the normal villous architecture, giving the villi a blunted clublike appearance. Treatment is with one of several antibiotic regimens, including trimethoprim sulfamethoxazole, penicillin, amoxicillin, or chloramphenicol for 1 year.

(Sleisenger, 9th edition, P-1841)

39. **Ans. (B)** For explanation see Ans. no.38.

(Sleisenger, 9th edition, P-1841)

40. **Ans. (A)** Dermatitis herpetiformis is the most common skin lesion found in celiac disease.

(Sleisenger, 9th edition, Pp-1811-1812)

41. **Ans. (C)** Celiac disease occurs as a consequence of sensitivity of the small bowel mucosa to gluten. There is a strong association with HLA-DQ2 antigen and high circulating levels of antigluten, antireticulum, and antiendomysial antibodies in untreated patients. Persons with celiac disease are at risk for lactose and sucrose intolerance and hyposplenism. Gluten-sensitive enteropathy is closely associated with dermatitis herpetformis; 100% of patients with dermatitis herpetifomis have abnormal jejunal biopsies. Celiac disease is associated with an increased risk of small bowel lymphoma the risk is significantly decreased if the patient adheres to a gluten-free diet. Persons with celiac disease are at increased risk for several other skin disorders including psoriasis, eczema, pustular dermatitis, cutaneous amyloid, cutaneous vasculitis, nodular prurigo, acquired ichthyosis, epidermal necrolysis, pityriasis, rubra pilaris and mycosis fungoides.

(Sleisenger, 9th edition, Pp-1810-1819)

42. **Ans. (C)** For explanation see Ans. no. 41.

(Sleisenger, 9th edition, Pp-1810-1819)

43. **Ans. (B)** The histologic characteristics of celiac sprue include flattening of intestinal villi, loss of normal villous architecture and a reduction in the normal ratio of villous height to crypt depth. The total thickness of the mucosa is increased because of crypt hyperplasia and cellular infiltration of the lamina propria with plasma cells and lymphocytes. The crypt mitotic activity is no longer confined to the base of the crypt to the villous tips shortened to 12 to 24 hours from a normal rate of 3 to 5 days. The ratio of intraepithelial lymphocytes to epithelial cells is also increased.

(Sleisenger, 9th edition, Pp-1799-1800)

44. **Ans. (B)** Hypoalbuminemia in a compliant patient with celiac sprue should heighten suspicion for a complication such as small bowel lymphoma or ulcerative jejunitis. Other possible causes of hypoalbu-minemia in this include disaccharide deficiency, bacterial overgrowth, or the ingestion of foods thought to be gluten-free that in fact contain gluten.

(Sleisenger, 9th edition, Pp-1815-1816)

45. **Ans. (B)** Gluten shock is a rare event and occurs in patients who are rechallenged with gluten-containing foods. These patients develop nausea, vomiting, tachycardia and cardiovascular collapse. Systemic corticosteroids are used in the treatment of this condition. Steroids can be used to treat moderate to severe celiac sprue, but they should not be a part of routine management.

(Sleisenger, 9th edition, Pp-1815-1816)

46. **Ans. (C)** The incidence of gallstones is increased in patients 2 to 3 times with extensive ileal resection. However, the explanation that the bile salt pool is depleted leading to super saturation of bile with cholesterol may be too simplistic. Forty percent of patients with ileostomies have radiopaque calcium-containing stones. In addition, interruption of the enterohepatic circulation may predispose to pigment stones.

(Sleisenger, 9th edition, P-1955)

47. **Ans. (C)** Calcium oxalate stones are formed in the setting of fat malabsorption when terminal ileal disease or resection inhibits bile salt resorption. Fatty acids bind calcium in the lumen, which leaves oxalate,

normally bound to calcium, free to enter the colon where it is absorbed and precipitated in the kidney. The colon is required to absorb the oxalate.

(Sleisenger, 9th edition, P-1955)

48. **Ans. (B)** Neutrophils do not secrete immunoglobulin.

(Sleisenger, 9th edition, P-1955)

49. **Ans. (C)** Olsalazine is composed of two 5-ASA moieties linked by an azo bond. This drug can elicit a secretory response from small bowel epithelium, resulting in watery diarrhea in 5% to 10% of treated patients.

(Sleisenger, 9th edition, P-1961)

50. **Ans. (B)** Diarrhea is a clinical feature in nearly all patients with Crohn's disease. Perianal disease and bleeding occur more commonly in patients with Crohn's colitis and ileocolitis than in patients with isolated ileal disease.

(Sleisenger, 9th edition, P-1953)

51. **Ans. (D)** Whipple disease, predominately involves duodenum and jejunum with sparons of ileum in addition there is also evidence of abdominal lymphadenopathy.

(Sleisenger, 9th edition, P-1836)

52. **Ans. (B)** Irritable bowel syndrome (IBS) is not associated with an increased mortality rate. Symptoms usually persist over a long period. The quality of life for many patients with IBS can be enhanced by appropriate physician intervention. Male patients who exhibit an acute onset but short history of symptoms, a predominant symptom of constipation, and a good initial response to treatment are most likely to achieve long term improvement. Also, patients who are included in detailed discussion about their diagnoses, psychological issues, precipitating factor, and treatments return fewer time to physicians. Education, counseling and a judicious use of medications improve the outcomes for many patients with IBS.

(Sleisenger, 9th edition, P-2103)

53. **Ans. (C)** Tropical sprue is a chronic diarrheal illness associated with malabsorption that often leads to severe nutritional deficiencies. The etiology is presumed to be bacterial over-growth of the small bowel by toxigenic strains of coliform bacteria. The diagnosis is made by small bowel biopsy. Histologic examination reveals partial villous atrophy. Ileal involvement is common. Megaloblastic anemia caused by vitamin B_{12} and folate deficiencies is the hallmark of tropical sprue. Treatment involves a regimen of folic acid and tetracycline for 6 months.

(Sleisenger, 9th edition, Pp-1821-1829)

54. **Ans. (D)** Gastrointestinal tuberculosis is caused by Myco-bacterium tuberculosis and Mycobacterium bovis. Persons at increased risk for tuberculosis infection include those infected with human immunodeficiency virus, older people, persons from endemic areas, persons who abuse intravenous drugs. The most common presenting symptom is abdominal pain. The differential diagnosis includes Crohn's disease, lymphoma and infections including mycobacterium avium complex enteritis, histoplasmosis and cryptosporidiasis.

(Sleisenger, 9th edition, Pp-1877-1878)

55. **Ans. (D)** Gastrointestinal tuberculosis involves areas of high lymphoid density, especially the distal small bowel, the cecum and the appendix. The diagnostic procedure of choice of colonoscopy with biopsies of the terminal ileum and cecum. The organism can frequently be identified on intestinal biopsy specimens using an acid-fast stain.

(Sleisenger, 9th edition, Pp-1877-1878)

56. **Ans. (A)** Mycotic infection of gastrointestinal tract can result from the dissemination of pulmonary infections. Histoplasmosis can disseminate in immunocompetent as well as immuno compromised persons. Intestinal aspergillosis, candidiasis and mucormycosis affect only severely immunocompromised persons.

(Sleisenger, 9th edition, P-527)

57. **Ans. (C)** Viral ulceration is the most common cause of bleeding in patient who have undergone bone marrow transplant. Peptic-appearing gastroduodenal ulcers that are resistant of standard ulcer therapy may be caused by cytomegalovirus. Epstein-Barr virus does not cause direct mucosal ulcerations but often presents with large small intestine mucosal nodules and diffuse mucosal immunoblast infiltration. In acute graft-versus host disease, the most common sources of bleeding are esophagitis and gastric erosions.

(Sleisenger, 9th edition, Pp-531-532)

58. **Ans. (A)** Acid-peptic disease is the most common of occult-gastrointestinal bleeding in western countries. Hookworm infection is the most common cause worldwide, but it is rare in the industrialized countries of the western.

(Sleisenger, 9th edition, Pp-286-290)

59. **Ans. (A)** Although Giardia lamblia is a common cause of enteric infection worldwide, it is not considered a

particularly important pathogen in acquired immuno-deficiency syndrome. In the United States, G lamblia is the most commonly identified intestinal parasite with prevalence rates as high as 16% in some communities. Diagnosis of Giardia infection can be made by examining fresh stool for trophozoites or preserved stool for cysts, which provide diagnostic yields of approximately 50%.

(Sleisenger, 9th edition, Pp-1911-1914)

60. **Ans. (C)** Diarrhea resulting from colonic disease commonly presents with 3 to 30 bowel movements per day, whereas diarrhea from small intestine pathology usually presents with only about 3 to 8 bowel movements per day. Stool volumes are variables but are often large in small intestine disease and small in colonic disorders. Diarrhea from small intestine diseases commonly occurs at irregular intervals, especially at night and in the early morning and does not commonly contain blood. Diarrhea from colonic disease occurs at more regular intervals throughout the day and night and is often associated with an inflammatory colitis which results in occult or gross blood loss.

(Sleisenger, 9th edition, P-216)

61. **Ans. (C)** Pinworm (Enterobious vermicularis) is the most prevalent small intestine helminths, followed by Ascaris lumbricoides.

(Sleisenger, 9th edition, Pp-1921-1939)

62. **Ans. (C)** Visceral larva migrans is a syndrome that produces the clinical triad of eosinophilia, hepatomegaly, and hypergammaglobulinemia that results from infection by Toxocara ova found in dog or cat feces. It most commonly seen in children with a history of pica, but it is occasionally seen in adults.

(Sleisenger, 9th edition, Pp-1921-1939)

63. **Ans. (C)** Evidence of increased intestinal permeability of inflammation is found in upto 70% of patients taking non-steroidal anti-inflammatory dugs (NSAIDs). Non-specific small intestine ulcers have been observed in 8.4% of patients prescribed NSAIDs in the 6 months prior to their death. NSAID- associated intestinal injury primarily occurs in the distal small intestine. Stricture formation occurs in 5% of patients on chronic NSAID therapy and can mimic the presentation of Crohn's disease in the small intestine. NSAIDs have been associated with several other small intestine disorders, including collagenous colitis, celiac sprue and non-celiac flattening of the small intestine mucosa.

(Sleisenger, 9th edition, Pp-2052-2053)

64. **Ans. (C)** The basic mechanism of action of cocaine-induced ischemia is inhibition of the presynaptic reuptake of norepinephrine, dopamine and serotonin as well as an increased synthesis of norepinephrine and dopamine. Therefore, this drug may lead to arterial vasoconstriction and subsequent intestinal ischemia. There have been several reports of intestinal ischemia secondary to the administration ergot alkaloids with subsequent splanchnic vasoconstriction. Oral contraceptives can cause mesenteric thrombosis leading to small bowel cause mesenteric thrombosis leading to small bowel infraction. Angiotensin-converting enzyme inhibitors do not cause intestinal ischemia.

(Sleisenger, 9th edition, P-2030)

65. **Ans. (C)** A high index of suspicion is necessary to make the diagnosis of an aortoenteric fistula as a source of gastrointestinal hemorrhage, because the fistula is difficult to discern by endoscopy or angiography. Aortoenteric fistulas almost always involve the third portion of the duodenum. In patients with Dacron grafts, the fistula usually arises from the proximal portion of the graft.

(Sleisenger, 9th edition, P-306)

66. **Ans. (A)** Necrotizing entercolitis is seen in premature, low birth-weight babies and is believed to be caused by the entry of bacteria into damaged intestinal mucosa. Breast feeding may be protective by providing additional antibody protection not afforded by cow's milk or formula feeding. Pneumatosis intestinalis secondary to bacterial gas formation can be seen on abdominal radiography and is characteristic of necrotizing enterocolitis. The condition is most common in the ileocecal region.

(Sleisenger, 9th edition, Pp-2248-2249)

67. **Ans. (A)** Radiation enteritis is uncommon when the total radiation dose is less than 45 Gy. A dose of 60 Gy increases the risk of intestinal damage to 25% to 50% in the early stages of radiation enteritis, the most common symptom is diarrhea. Later, the patient may present with obstructive symptoms. The radiographic evaluation may be normal or reveal dilated, edematous loops of small bowel.

(Sleisenger, 9th edition, Pp-639-652)

68. **Ans. (A)** The patient has acute jejunitis secondary to infection with clostridium perfringens. Epidemics of this type of infection have been described in New Guinea. Patients are typically observed with a 3- to

10-day history of upper abdominal cramps, vomiting and often bloody diarrhea. Stool cultures are usually positive for C perfringens and leukocytosis is often present. Patients often present. Patients often require surgical intervention, although medical management, including antibiotics is frequently successful in patients who have not developed fulminant toxemia.

69. **Ans. (A)** In the absence of nephritic syndrome or significant liver disease, hypoalbuminemia associated with lower exremity edema suggests protein-losing enteropathy (PLE). Although lower extremity deep vein thrombosis may cause edema this would not explain the hypoalbuminemia noted in this patient. PLE may secondary to lymphatic obstruction (e.g., lymphoma, tuberculosis, right-sided heart failure) or enterocyte barrier breakdown (e.g., Crohn's disease, celiac sprue). The diagnostic evaluation should focus on these consideration. The fecal á$_1$-antitrypsin is highly resistant to proteolytic digestion and therefore is elevated in conditions that lead to intestinal protein loss. Significant steatorrhea is commonly associated with many of the disorders that cause PLE.

(Sleisenger, 9th edition, Pp-437-444)

70. **Ans. (C)** Hereditary hemorrhagic telangiectasia is an autosomal dominant disease characterized by vascular ectasias of the skin and mucosus membranes. Other connective tissue disorders are seen in association with this syndrome. Patients often present with epistaxis of gastrointestinal hemorrhage from either upper of lower sources.

(Sleisenger, 9th edition, Pp-600-601)

71. **Ans. (B)** Giardia lamblia, isospora belli, and diverticulitis would be unlikely causes for melena and guaiac positive stools in a patient with acquired immunodeficiency syndrome. The most likely diagnosis is Kaposi sarcoma, which may present with gastrointestinal tract bleeding.

(Sleisenger, 9th edition, Pp-528-532)

72. **Ans. (C)** Pneumatosis intestinalis is often benign, occurring in association with hematologic cancer or acquired immunodeficiency syndrome and following chemotherapy or organ transplantation. This diagnosis does not necessarily represent a severe form of enteritis. It can also be associated with scleroderma, in which gas accumulation assume a cystic pattern and in some cases the rupture of the cysts pattern and in some cases, the rupture of the cysts may lead to pneumoperitoneum. In the setting of intestinal ischemia, gas may accumulate in the bowel wall in a linear pattern. This may be associated with gas in the portal system and likely represents intestinal infarction.

(Sleisenger, 9th edition, P-2141)

73. **Ans. (B)** Ischemic injury to the gut wall may largely occur at the time of tissue reperfusion. The breakdown of ATP leads to the production of free readicals by xanthine oxidase. Reperfusion supplies the oxygen needed to catalyze this reaction. The already damaged mucosa may be further injured by luminal toxins such as hydrochloric acid in the stomach, proteases and bacterial toxins. Superoxide dismutase dose not exacerbate ischemic injury.

(Sleisenger, 9th edition, Pp-2027-2028)

74. **Ans. (B)** The sympathetic rather than the parasympathetic nervous system contribute to the modulation of gastrointestinal blood flow.

(Sleisenger, 9th edition, Pp-1646-1647)

75. **Ans. (C)** Most small intestine tumors are benign and remain asymptomatic, whereas at least 80% of malignant small intestine tumors produce symptoms. Small intestine tumors account for approximately 1% of all gastrointestinal malignancies and are more common in western industrialized nations than in other parts of the world. Japanese who migrate to Hawaii population.

(Sleisenger, 9th edition, Pp-2145-2153)

76. **Ans. (A)** Symptoms of carcinoid syndrome are improved or abolished in more than 90% of patients during treatment with octreotide. Although plasma serotonin levels are not altered. Octreotide reduces the urinary excretion of 5-hydroxyindoleacetic acid (5-HIAA) in 66% of patients. Claims that long term octreotide therapy retards or reverses tumor growth have not been substantiated.

(Sleisenger, 9th edition, P-489)

77. **Ans. (C)** The prevalence of prior infection with adenovirus serotype 12 is higher in patients with celiac sprue compared with healthy controls. In addition there is significant amino acid homology between A gliadin and 1:16 protein of adenovirus serotype 12. The D region of the HLA gene, i.e., HLA-DR and HLA DQ, has the highest association with celiac sprue. These genes are necessary, but not sufficient for the development of celiac sprue.

(Sleisenger, 9th edition, P-1801)

78. **Ans. (C)** There are multiple underlying causes for adynamic ileus, including inflammatory disorders, metabolic abnormalities and vascular insufficiency. The intraluminal pressures generated with an ileus are not great enough to compromise the mucosal blood flow. Focal pain, borborygmi and multiple air fluid levels are more characteristic ileus.

(Sleisenger, 9th edition, Pp-2121-2126)

79. **Ans. (D)** The small intestine is the second most frequently involved gastrointestinal organ in scleroderma after the esophagus. Small intestine dysmotility is presumably caused by collagen and is characterized by dilation of the small intestine, delayed intestine transit and occasionally an accordion appearance of the small intestine mucosa on radiographic evaluation. The circular muscle layer is more often involved than is the longitudinal muscle layer.

(Sleisenger, 9th edition, Pp-693-695)

80. **Ans. (D)** Celiac sprue typically causes a reduction or loss of the valvulae conniventes rather than thickening.

(Sleisenger, 9th edition, P-1799)

81. **Ans. (C)** Enterocytes from patients with abetalipoproteinemia contain numerous small, clear vacuoles that are visible under light microscopy and reflect lipid accumulation within the enterocyte.

(Sleisenger, 9th edition, P-577)

82. **Ans. (D)** Microfold (M) cell transport but do not process antigens. M cells lack class II antigens on their surface but express MHC class II molecules in lysosomal organelles, suggesting that under certain circumstances they may serve as antigen-presenting cells.

(Sleisenger, 9th edition, Pp-23-29)

83. **Ans. (D)** A few intraepithelial lymphocytes (IELs) are CD4 T cells, but most express the CD8 áâ heterodimer, the CD45RO isoform. They have suppressor and cytolytic activities; however their exact roles are unknown.

(Sleisenger, 9th edition, P-28)

84. **Ans. (D)** Secretory IgA inhibits the adherence of bacteria to epithelial cells, interfering with bacterial colonization and replication.

(Sleisenger, 9th edition, P-23)

85. **Ans. (B)** IgD is not involved in mucosal defense against parasitic infection.

(Sleisenger, 9th edition, Pp-23-24)

86. **Ans. (A)** Vasoactive intestinal polypeptide, substance P, and somatostatin can trigger histamine secretion by both connective tissue and intestinal mucosal mast cells.

(Sleisenger, 9th edition, Pp-817-825)

87. **Ans. (D)** IgA deficiency is the most common primary immune deficiency. Biopsy specimens from the jejunum in IgA-deficiency subjects are morphologically normal of IgA-producing cells and an increase in IgM secreting cells.

(Sleisenger, 9th edition, P-514)

88. **Ans. (B)** Gastrointestinal infection with Giardia lamblia occurs in approximately 30% of X-linked hypogammaglobulinemia patients. Severe combined immunodeficiency syndrome show a markedly increased risk of viral infection in early childhood, but Giardia infection do not predominate. Giardiasis is a common cause of steatorrhea and malabsorption in common variable hypogammaglobulinemia. Giardiasis has been reported with IgA deficiency, but the incidence is probably the same or only slightly increased in comparison with the general population.

(Sleisenger, 9th edition, Pp-1911-1914)

89. **Ans. (C)** Secretory component is released into external secretions bound to IgA, although it may also occur in a free form.

(Sleisenger, 9th edition, Pp-23-24)

90. **Ans. (B)** Under most conditions the apical intercellular tight junctions are the rate-limited barrier restricting the passive movement of hydrophobic solutes through the paracellular space. The plasma membrane and transmembrane proteins are the rate-limiting barriers to transcellular absorption.

(Sleisenger, 9th edition, Pp-1676-1677)

91. **Ans. (B)** Tight junctions are selective pores that allow the passage of water and small molecules of molecular weight less than 300 d. Tight junctions are the route for the net movement of those substances that are not actively transported to maintain the osmotic and electrical balance of the cell.

(Sleisenger, 9th edition, P-1676)

92. **Ans. (A)** Gap junctions assist in coordinating the activities of adjacent cells with the epithelial sheet by allowing them to behave as syncytia with respect to transfer of small molecules.

(Sleisenger, 9th edition, P-1676)

93. Ans. (B) In the small intestine, the most important chloride channel is the cAMP-activated low-conductance channel, which participates in hormone-stimulated chloride secretion. This channel is defective in cystic fibrosis. A separate calcium-activated chloride channel has been isolated in airway epithelial cells and in colon cancer cell lines. This appears to be regulated by calcium-calmodulin. The role of the calcium activated chloride channel in intestinal chloride secretion is unclear.

(Sleisenger, 9th edition, Pp-1682-1684)

94. Ans. (C) In contrast to patients with selective IgA deficiency, upto 60% of patients with common variable hypogammaglobulinemia have chronic recurrent diarrhea and two-thirds of these have malabsorption. Nodular lymphoid hyperplasia is frequently found in common variable hypogammaglobulinemia, and is rare in selective IgA deficiency. Selective IgA deficiency is the most common primary immunodeficiency syndrome in adults.

(Sleisenger, 9th edition, P-1830)

95. Ans. (D) Every organ is vulnerable to infection, but hepatic gastrointestinal disorders are a prominent feature of chronic granulomatous disease. Hepatomegaly is very common and liver abscess formation occurs in more than 30% of patients.

(Sleisenger, 9th edition, P-1830)

96. Ans. (A) Abdominal pain, vomiting and watery diarrhea are common features of hereditary angioedema. Pitting edema, pruritus and leukocytosis are notably absent. Anabolic steroids can be effective in treating some cases of hereditary angioedema.

(Sleisenger, 9th edition, P-1830)

97. Ans. (B) Patients with intestinal lymphagiectasia most commonly exhibit lymphopenia, resulting in anergy and increased excretion of $á_1$-antitrypsin in the stool.

(Sleisenger, 9th edition, P-441)

98. Ans. (B) Skin tests of oral challenges with peanuts should not be performed in those with suspected allergy to peanuts because of the risk of anaphylaxis.

(Sleisenger, 9th edition, Pp-139-148)

99. Ans. (B) Eosinophilic gastroenteritis can involve the mucosa muscularis or serosa in any region of the gastrointestinal tract. The condition commonly results in the release of Charcot-Leyden crystals into the stool.

(Sleisenger, 9th edition, Pp-425-433)

100. Ans. (B) Most cases of travelers' diarrhea develops within the first week of travel. Antibiotic prophylaxis reduces the incidence of travelers' diarrhea by about 90%. Bismuth is an effective prophylaxis and has been effective in the treatment of mild to moderate cases of travelers' diarrhea. Because of increasing drug resistance and the high incidence of illness caused by Campylobacter jejuni, the quinolones are now the treatment of choice for adults.

(Sleisenger, 9th edition, Pp-1841-1868)

101. Ans. (A) Bacillus cereus is also associated with a diarrheal illness following ingestion of a performed toxin. The emetic illness associated with this toxin is confined to the ingestion of contaminated fried rice the ingestion of the toxin in other foodstuffs is associated with a diarrheal illness. Botulinum toxin blocks acetylcholine at the neuromuscular junction and produces skeletal muscle weakness with a 15% cases–fatality rate. There is also a mild associated disturbance of gastrointestinal function. The clinical features of ingestion of Staphylococcus aureus enterotox include profuse vomiting and nausea, typically beginning within 6 to 24 hours of ingestion. S aureus is the most common ingested food-borne pathogen in the United States.

(Sleisenger, 9th edition, Pp-1841-1868)

Chapter 4

Colonic Diseases

1. **Acute appendicitis is best characterized by which of the following statements?**
   A. Older patients generally have significantly better outcomes than younger patients
   B. To make an accurate diagnosis of acute appendicitis, ultrasonographic examination of the right lower quadrant is required
   C. Acute appendicitis has a high rate of spontaneous peforation within the first 3 hours of the onset of abdominal pain
   D. Acute appendicitis can be treated non-operatively if complicated by the development of an appendiceal abscess

2. **Which one of the following statements regarding pregnancy and inflammatory bowel disease is true?**
   A. Women with Crohn's disease have a slightly increased rate of infertility, which may be closely related to disease activity and nutritional status
   B. Infertility is greater in patients with ulcerative colitis than in the normal population
   C. Inflammatory bowel disease management using total parenteral nutrition is detrimental to the fetus
   D. Steroids should be tapered off and discontinued during pregnancy

3. **Microscopic colitis/collagenous colitis (MC/CC) is distinguished from inflammatory bowel disease (IBD) by each of the following *except:***
   A. Typically, the colonic mucosa appears endoscopically normal in MC/CC but not in IBD
   B. Histologic evaluation of biopsy specimens reveals an increased number of intraepithelial lymphocytes in MC/CC relative to IBD
   C. Crypt distortion is seen in IBD but is rarely seen in MC/CC
   D. Ulcerative colitis presents with a more abundant inflammatory cells infiltrate of the lamina propria than does MC/CC

4. **Which one of the following syndromes is associated with hamartomatous gastrointestinal polyposis and hair loss?**
   A. Gardner syndrome
   B. Peutz-Jeghers syndrome
   C. Familial adenomatous polyposis
   D. Cronkhite Canada syndrome

5. **Which one of the following statements concerning Peutz-Jeghers syndrome is true?**
   A. The most common location of polyps is the small intestine
   B. There is no significant increased risk of the development of gastrointestinal malignancies
   C. Mucocutaneous pigmentation typically occurs in the third decade of life
   D. Glands often show epithelial invasion into the submucosa, indicating malignancy

6. **Each of the following statements regarding bacterial infections of the colon is true *except:***
   A. Small-volume diarrhea (IL/day) is typical
   B. The results of a fecal leukocyte test are considered positive if 3 or more leukocytes per high-power microscopic field are present in four or more
   C. The presence of fecal leukocytes makes ulcerative colitis an unlikely diagnosis
   D. Presenting symptoms often include fever and crampy abdominal pain

7. **Which one of the following statements concerning colonic transit is true?**
   A. In general, markers ingested within a 48 hours period of time leave the colon in the same order in which they entered
   B. The transit of markers through the colon is dependent upon whether or not they are ingested with a meal
   C. Normally, 80% of ingested markers are passed by the fifth day after ingestion
   D. Segmental colonic transit can be measured by counting number of markers in the stool

8. **Each of the following statements regarding diverticular bleeding is true *except:***
   A. Hemorrhage arises from an arterial source as a result of a detect in the vasa recta
   B. Histologic studies reveal that most cases of bleeding are not associated with inflammation in the bleeding diverticulum

C. Bleeding occurs in about 5% of all patients with diverticulosis
D. Recurrence of bleeding occurs in 20% of patients after one episode and in 50% of patients after recurrent bleeding
E. Diverticular bleeding is occult in 50% of patients

9. **Each of the following statements regarding diverticulitis is true *except:***
A. Recurrence of diverticulitis occurs in about 5% of patients
B. Surgical treatment is necessary in 15% to 30% of patients
C. Peritonitis, abscess and fistula are indications for surgery
D. Broad-spectrum antibiotic coverage for both aerobic and anaerobic organisms is necessary

10. **All of the following statements regarding colonic angiodysplasia are true *except:***
A. Angiodysplasia occurs in 5% of subjects undergoing colonoscopy for unrelated indications
B. Angiodysplasia is a frequent cause of recurrent lower gastrointestinal bleeding in elderly subjects
C. Histologic features of gastric angiodysplasia are distinguishable from those of right colon angiodysplasia
D. Bleeding from angiodysplastic lesions is usually chronic and low-grade

11. **A 26-year-old man presents to the emergency department with acute bloody diarrhea, crampy abdominal pain and fever. The differential diagnosis includes infection with each of the organisms listed *except:***
A. Shigella species
B. Campylobacter species
C. Giardia lamblia
D. Escherichia coli O157:H7

12. **Each of the following statements concerning shigella infections of the colon is true *except:***
A. They are endemic in nursing homes and day care centers
B. Most strains are not highly contagious
C. The bacteria produce enterotoxins
D. The most severe infections are usually located in the rectosigmoid region, with infections of diminished severity in the proximal colon

13. **Each of the following statements regarding campylobacter jejuni infections of the colon is true *except:***
A. They are primarily a disease of children and young adults
B. Fecal leukocytes and erythrocytes are present
C. Diagnosis is by culture of stool
D. Oral antibiotics are required for most patients

14. **Which one of the following statements regarding Hirschsprung disease is true?**
A. Symptoms usually present during toilet training
B. It is diagnosed by deep sigmoid biopsy
C. It can usually be ruled out if the rectoanal inhibitory reflex is present during anorectal manometry
D. It requires a subtotal colectomy in the majority of cases

15. **Causes of painful anorectal lesions in AIDS patients include each of the following *except:***
A. Tuberculosis
B. Kaposi sarcoma
C. Squamous cell carcinoma
D. Yersinia enterocolitica

16. **Important functions of the gut microflora include all of the following *except:***
A. Drug metabolism
B. Vitamin synthesis
C. Suppression of pathogens
D. Metabolism of dietary triglycerides

17. **All of the following statements regarding Shigella infections of the colon are true *except:***
A. The virulence of Shigella infection is related to invasiveness, whereas diarrhea is related to toxin production
B. The typical clinical course of shigellosis in adults is onset of fever and diarrhea 4 to 6 days after ingestion of the bacterium, followed by a 5 to 7-day illness
C. Hemolytic-uremic syndrome is associated with Shigella infection
D. Most patients with symptomatic Shigella infection should be treated with tetracycline or ciprofloxacin

18. **All of the following statements regarding sexually transmitted rectal, anal and perianal infection are true *except:***
A. Rectal Neisseria gonorrhoeae infections are usually asymptomatic
B. Diarrhea is the most frequent symptom of gonorrheal proctitis
C. Chlamydia trachomatis proctitis may mimic Crohn's proctitis
D. The differential diagnosis of perianal warts includes secondary syphilis

19. Which of the following is the best initial management of a case of diarrhea?

A. Obtain a complete blood count: examine a stool specimen for fecal leukocyte count ova and parasites and culture for bacteria; have the patient return in 1 week or sooner if his symptoms worsen

B. Counsel the patient about maintaining proper hydration and advise him to return promptly if he develops bloody diarrhea, fever or other systemic symptoms or if he is not able to maintain proper hydration; schedule a return visit in 2 weeks if the diarrhea persists

C. Obtain a stool specimen for culture and for fecal leukocyte count; start an empiric regimen of doxycycline 100 mg twice daily; schedule a return visit in 1 week

D. Measure levels of serum electrolytes, blood urea nitrogen and creatinine; examine stool specimens for sodium, potassium, osmolality, ova, parasites, and fecal leukocytes and culture for bacterial; have the patient return in 1 week or sooner if his symptoms worsen; base treatment on the test results

20. A 67-year-old man presents with diarrhea after a 2-week course of antibiotics. A stool examination is negative for fecal leukocytes and flexible sigmoidoscopy shows no pseudomembranes but does show friability, erythema and exudates. Which one of the following statements is true?

A. The lack of fecal leukocytes makes the diagnosis of pseudomembranous colitis unlikely

B. A stool culture positive for Clostridium difficile and C difficile cytotoxin would confirm the diagnosis of antibiotic-associated colitis unlikely

C. Lack of pseudomembranes on flexible sigmoidoscopy makes the diagnosis of antibiotic associated colitis unlikely

D. If C difficile colitis is successfully treated the likelihood of relapse is 15% to 20%

21. Acute amebic proctocolitis is characterized by each of the following *except:*

A. Progressively more severe and frequent diarrhea

B. Abdominal pain and tenderness

C. Watery diarrhea with little or no blood

D. Weight loss

22. Complications of amebic liver abscess include each of the following *except:*

A. Serous pleural effusions

B. Peritonitis

C. Pulmonary embolism

D. Pericarditis

23. Recommended surveillance colonoscopy with random biopsy for adenocarcinoma in patients with ulcerative colitis involving most of the colon should begin after:

A. 5 to 7 years of disease

B. 8 to 10 years of disease

C. 11 to 15 years of disease

D. More than 15 years of disease

24. The best estimate of normal daily blood loss from the gastrointestinal tract is approximately:

A. 0.01 mL/day
B. 0.7 mL/day
C. 5.5 mL/day
D. 10.0 mL/day

25. The lifelong likelihood of an American developing a colon cancer is approximately:

A. 1%
B. 5%
C. 10%
D. 25%

26. A 24-year-old man with chronic ulcerative colitis is referred for the consideration of surveillance screening for colon cancer. His disease was diagnosed 15 years ago with inflammation to the level of the midtransverse colon. His symptoms have been mild and three sigmoidoscopic examinations over the past 5 years have revealed only quiescent colitis. You should advise the patient that:

A. Mild, well-controlled disease that involved less than the entire colon is not associated with a substantially increased incidence of neoplasia

B. He should undergo a screening barium enema radiographic examination at this time

C. The fact that his disease has been mild does not reduce his risk of dysplasia and cancer

D. If low-grade dysplasia is found, a colectomy will be recommended

27. The following groups of bacteria each account for more than 1% of the fecal flora *except:*

A. Facultative gram-negative organism (e.g. Escherichia coli)

B. Bacteroides species

C. Clostridium species

D. Peptostreptococcus species

28. Therapy for diminutive colonic polyps:

A. Cold snaring is acceptable, however, it is associated with a high rate of hemorrhage

B. Hot biopsy forceps are more likely to produce a complication in the left as compared to the right colon

C. Cold biopsy is a safe, acceptable technique for polyp removal
D. Snare cautery should not be used unless the polyp is larger than 5 mm

29. **Therapy for large sessile polyps:**
A. Saline injection has been associated with tumor seeding
B. When assisting polypectomy, an injection with saline should be made directly into the mucosa
C. Polyps smaller than or equal to 1.5 cm should be removed by a snare in 2 or 3 pieces, if possible
D. The risk of metastasis after snare resection of malignant large sessile polyps is greater than that for pedunculated malignant polyps

30. **The best and most practical way to determine passage of the colonoscope to the cecum is by:**
A. The length of endoscope inserted
B. Finger plapation and transillumination in the right lower quadrant
C. Fluoroscopic confirmation
D. Apparent landmarks in the cecal region (i.e. ileocecal valve, appendiceal orifice)

31. **Appropriate preparation for colonoscopy includes:**
A. Discontinue iron preparations for several days prior to the procedure
B. Administer antibiotics if biopsy or polypectomy is possible
C. Discontinue aspirin for 2 weeks prior to the procedure
D. Administer a balanced electrolyte solution such as oral sodium phosphate

32. **Which portion of the colon is not a retropritoneal structure?**
A. Ascending colon
B. Transverse colon
C. Descending colon
D. Rectum

33. **All of the following have a positive association with adenomatous colorectal polyps *except*:**
A. Ureterosigmoidoscopy
B. Acromegaly
C. Streptococcus bovis infection
D. Cholecystectomy

34. **If one were to characterize adenomas based on their predominant histology, the most common would be:**
A. Villous
B. Hyperplastic
C. Tubulovillous
D. Tubular

35. **In the hereditary non-polyposis colorectal cancer syndrome, the responsible defect lies in the:**
A. APC gene
B. K-ras gene
C. P53 gene
D. Micro satellite instability due to DNA mismatch repair

36. **Colonoscopy is an appropriate screening tool for all of the following groups of patients *except:***
A. Patients with multiple first-degree relatives with colon cancer
B. Patients with a first-degree relative with a tubular adenoma
C. Patients with long-standing left sided ulcerative colitis
D. A patient with a large (>1 cm) tubular adenoma on prior colonoscopy

37. **Poor prognostic features for a malignant polyp include all of the following *except:***
A. Incomplete resection
B. Poorly differentiated carcinoma
C. Sessile malignant polyps
D. Pedunculated malignant polyps

38. **To be considered a malignant polyp, penetration must be into the:**
A. Mucosa
B. Muscularis mucosae
C. Submucosa
D. Muscularis propria

39. **The most prevalent mutations in colorectal adenomas is the:**
A. P53 gene mutation
B. K-ras mutation
C. APC gene defect
D. DNA mismatch repair defects

40. **All of the following are inherited polyposis syndromes *except:***
A. Hyperplastic polyposis
B. Familial adenomatosis polyposis
C. Peutz-Jeghers syndrome
D. Turcot syndrome

41. **A 25-year-old man is referred to you for evaluation. He is adopted and knows little of his family history, other than a recollection of "multiple polyposis" and "early colon cancer". He does not know his biological parents and is concerned he may be at risk for familial adenomatous polyposis and colon cancer. What type of genetic testing would help identify his risk for familial adenomatous polyposis?**

A. Flow cytometry of colonic epithelium from biopsy specimens
B. Linkage testing
C. In vitro protein synthesis (IVPS)
D. Mutation identification

42. **In Gardner syndrome the extracolonic lesion include all of the following *except*:**
A. Ovarian carcinoma
B. Osteomas
C. Desmoid tumors
D. Dental abnormalities such as unerupted and supernumerary teeth

43. **The mutation in familial adenomatous polyposis involves a mutation in:**
A. DNA repair enzymes
B. APC protein
C. C282y
D. ATP7B

44. **The polyps in juvenile polyposis are:**
A. Tubular adenomas
B. Hyperplastic polyps
C. Desmoid polyps
D. Non-neoplastic hamartomatous polyps

45. **All of the following have been associated with an increased risk for colorectal cancer *except:***
A. Smoking
B. Consumption of alcohol, specifically beer
C. High dietary intake of animal fat
D. Radiation for gynecologic cancer

46. **Which of the following drug has been approved by FDA for regression of adenomas in patients with familial adenomatous polyposis?**
A. Acetaminophen
B. Interferon
C. COX-2 inhibitors
D. Mesalamine

47. **Which one of the following hamartomatous gastrointestinal polyposis have characteristic histological finding of excessive proliferation of lamina propria with cystically dilated submucosal glands?**
A. Gardner syndrome
B. Peutz-Jeghers syndrome
C. Juvenile polyposis
D. Familial adenomatous polyposis

48. **Which one of the following statements concerning Peutz-Jeghers syndrome is false?**
A. This is a hamartomatous polyps
B. There is significant increased risk of the development of gastrointestinal malignancies and breast cancer
C. Mucocutaneous pigmentation typically occurs in the third decade of life
D. Glands often show arborizing pattern of smooth muscle proliferation

49. **Ileal brake by all *except*:**
A. GLP-1
B. PYY
C. GLP-2
D. CCK

50. **Transport of glucose in intestine from enterocyte to interstitium:**
A. GLUT 4
B. GLUT 2
C. SGLT 1
D. GLUT 5

51. **All are true regarding anorectal manometry *except*:**
A. Normal anal pressure is 60-90 mm Hg
B. Pressure may increase to 2-3 times during squeezing
C. Resting anal pressure is mostly contributed by IAS
D. During voluntarily squeezing EAS has least role

52. **Investigation of choice for diverticulosis:**
A. Colonoscopy
B. Barium enema
C. CT colonography
D. None

53. **Investigation of choice for ultrashort segment Hirschsprung disease:**
A. Rectal biopsy
B. Rectal manometry
C. Barium enema
D. None

54. **Anti-VEGF used in colon cancer:**
A. Planitunab
B. Bevacizumab
C. Cetuximab
D. Rituximab

55. **In a normal person on BMFT, diameter of ileum:**
A. 1 cm
B. 2 cm
C. 3 cm
D. 5 cm

56. **A 63-year-old man present with a 2-month history of severe constipation. Which one of the following statements is most accurate?**

A. This patient would be best evaluated with a combination of anorectal manometry, defecography and colonic transit testing
B. Barium enema radiography or an endoscopic procedure of the colon should be performed to rule out a structural lesion
C. A flexible sigmoidoscopy should be performed and if no lesions are noted, a rectal biopsy specimen should be taken
D. A short trial of stimulant laxatives is indicated. An evaluation can be performed at a later date if there is no significant benefit

57. **Which one of the following statements regarding colonic motor function is most accurate?**
A. The predominant pattern of contraction in the right colon is rhythmic peristalsis
B. Tonic circular contractions in the colon can be seen radiographially as haustral markings
C. The predominant contraction pattern in the left colon is anti-peristaltic
D. The internal anal sphincter tonically contracts during defecation

58. **Which one of the following statements concerning the mechanisms of fecal incontinence is most accurate?**
A. The external sphincter muscle contributes to the majority of testing an anal canal tone
B. During acute increases in intra abdominal pressure (i.e., coughing). The internal sphincter has the primary responsibility for maintaining continence
C. Abnormal straightening of the anorectal angle predisposes to fecal incontinence
D. Chronic constipation can cause fecal incontinence except when fecal occurs

59. **A 28-year-old man reports episodes of rectal pain that are unrelated to defecation. The pain occurs once or twice per month and is described as severe and "stabbing" but it lasts for only several seconds. The patient is otherwise healthy, and a review of systems reveals nothing abnormal. Findings on physical examination, including anorectal examination, are normal. The most likely diagnosis is:**
A. Proctalgia fugax
B. Intermittent coccygodynia
C. Anal fissure
D. Levator ani syndorme

60. **A-63-year-old woman complains of a dull, aching rectal pain that lasts for minutes to hours and occurs several times per week. She reports that sometimes she feels like she is "sitting on a ball". Findings from anoscopy and sigmoidoscopy are normal. Which one of the following statements is most accurate?**
A. The most likely diagnosis is proctalgia fugax
B. Digital examination will often yield useful findings despite normal findings from anoscopy and sigmoidoscopy
C. A trial of anti-inflammatory therapy is indicated
D. Surgery is necessary in the minority of cases that do not respond to medical therapy

61. **Acute appendicitis is best characterized by which of the following statements?**
A. Older patients generally have significantly better outcomes than younger patients
B. To make an accurate diagnosis of acute appendicitis, ultrasonographic examination of the right lower quardrant is required
C. Acute appendicitis has a high rate of spontaneous perforation within the first 3 hours of the onset of abdominal pain
D. Acute appendicitis can be treated nonoperatively if complicated by the development of an appendiceal abscess

62. **You have been treating a 24-year-old woman with ulcerative colitis limited to the distal 30 cm of colon for 2 months. Her symptoms were successfully managed with sulfasalazine, but the development of a rash prompted a change to 5-aminosalicylic acid enemas each night at bedtime. After 1 month on this regimen, the symptoms had completely resolved and she discontinued the enemas completely. Two weeks later, she presents with recurrent symptoms of cramping abdominal pain, tenesmus, and increased stool frequency (6 loose stools per day) with occasional bloody stools. She is afebrile and able to eat without nauses. You should perform the following:**
A. Perform colonoscopy to document the extent of disease
B. Start metronidazole or azathioprine because of the progression of her disease and intolerance to sulfasalazine
C. Reinstitute 5 aminosalicylic acid enemas and consider a slow tapering if the patient stabilizes
D. Begin oral prednisone

63. **Chronic radiation-induced proctitis is produced by:**
A. Superinfection of the rectal mucosa with common bacterial pathogens

B. Tissue ischemia as a result of obliterative endarteritis
C. Radiation-induced vascular hyperproliferation leading to extensive telangiectasia formation
D. A direct effect of tissue necrosis as a result of cumulative radiation exposure

64. **Which one of the following statement regarding pregnancy and inflammatory bowel disease is true?**
A. Women with uncomplicated Crohn's disease have a normal infertility
B. Infertility is greater in patients with ulcerative colitis than in the normal population
C. Inflammatory bowel disease management using total parenteral nutrition is detrimental to the fetus
D. Azathioprine and 6-MP are category B drug

65. **True love score in activity of ulcerative colitis includes all *except*:**
A. Hematocrit
B. Albumin
C. Rectal Bleed
D. CRP

66. **Regarding the natural history of ulcerative colitis, all of the following statements are true *except:***
A. Younger patients are more likely than older ones to enter sustained periods of remission
B. Ulcerative colitis most commonly follows a chronic intermittent course, marked by long periods of quiescence interspersed with acute attacks lasting weeks to months
C. The rate of colectomy at 2 years from diagnosis for those patients who initially present with severe disease is 50%
D. The rate of colectomy at 5 years from diagnosis for those patients who initially present with pancolitis is 50%

67. **Which one of the following statements regarding immunosuppressive therapy for inflammatory bowel disease is not true?**
A. Azathioprine use may allow a tapering or gradual withdrawal of corticosteroids
B. Azathioprine and 6-mereaptoparine will generally not provide clinical benefit until after 2 months of drug administration
C. Immunosuppressive therapy is never indicated in ulcerative colitis, because colectomy provides a cure
D. Pancreatitis and leucopenia are major adverse effects

68. **Which one of the following syndromes is associated with hamartomatous gastrointestinal polyposis and macrocephaly?**
A. Gardner syndrome
B. Peutz-Jeghers syndrome
C. Bannayan-Ruvalaca-Riley syndrome
D. Familial adenomatous polyposis

69. **Recto-anal inhibitory reflex includes all *except*:**
A. Relaxation of EAS
B. Contraction of EAS
C. Relaxation of IAS
D. Contraction of rectal muscles

70. **Each of the following statements regarding diverticular bleed is true *except:***
A. Occurs in 3%-5% of diverticular cases
B. Right sided colon is the most common source of bleed in Asian patient
C. Diverticulitis increases the risk of diverticular bleed
D. Surgery is not required in all cases

71. **Rectosigmoid junction from anal verge:**
A. 12 cm
B. 18 cm
C. 24 cm
D. 30 cm

72. **All of the following causes malabsorption *except*:**
A. E. histolytica
B. Cryptosporidium
C. Giardia lamblia
D. Microsporidium

73. **Normal bacterial content in terminal ileum:**
A. 10^8
B. 10^3
C. 10^5
D. 10^{11}

74. **RDA of Vitamin D for adult male:**
A. 1000 IU
B. 4000 IU
C. 8000 IU
D. 10000 IU

75. **Ideal site of biopsy in hirschprung disease:**
A. 4 cm from anal verge
B. 6-7 cm from anal verge
C. 8 cm from anal verge
D. 12 cm from anal verge

76. **Most common type of biliary stones in PSC:**
A. Mixed
B. Black
C. Brown
D. Cholesterol

77. **Statements that are true concerning pathogenic mechanisms for diarrhea in patients treated with broad spectrum antibiotics include all of the following:**
A. An accumulation of gastrointestinal mucin, normally hydrolyzed by colonic flora, presents an osmotic load to the colon
B. The antibiotics and antibiotic metabolites present an osmotic load to the colon
C. The normal balance between anaerobic and aerobic bacteria is disturbed
D. Infection with clostridium difficile develops

78. **Colonoscopy contraindicated in all *except*:**
A. Aortic aneurysm
B. Coagulopathy
C. Diverticulitis
D. Peritonitis

79. **True about physiology of gut *except*:**
A. Ph of ileum is more acidic than jejunum
B. Redox potential of stomach is more negative than small intestine
C. Jejunum has zero anaerobes bacterial count
D. In normal colon anaerobes exceeds aerobes

80. **Clostridium difficile all are true *except*:**
A. Causes bloody diarrhea
B. Metronidazole is the drug of choice
C. Diagnosis by clostridium difficile toxins
D. Exacerbates ulcerative colitis

81. **Most common appendiceal tumor:**
A. Carcinoid
B. Lymphoma
C. Adenocarcinoma
D. GIST tumor

82. **A 4-year-old girl is admitted for bloody diarrhea and dehydration. She recently ate at a fast-food restaurant. On admission, her creatinine level is 2.0 mg/DL and her leukocyte count is 22,000/mm^3. The next day after hydration, her creatinine level is 3.4 mg/DL, and her leukocyte count is 18,000/mm^3. Which one of the following statements is true?**
A. If antibiotics have not been started, they should be started now
B. The mechanism of disease for this organism is invasiveness rather than toxin production
C. Cattle appear to be a common reservoir for the agent that causes this infection
D. Renal insufficiency occurs as a complication in 15% to 20% of cases of this infection

83. **Patients subsets that have a high risk for the acquisition of amebiasis in developed countries include each of the following *except:***
A. Immigrants or travelers from South America, Africa and India
B. Homosexual males and AIDS patients with diarrhea
C. Institutionalized individuals
D. Individuals with selective IgA deficiency

84. **Most characteristic ulcer of intestine in Crohn's disease:**
A. Transverse
B. Apthous ulcer
C. Longitudinal
D. None

85. **Calcium absorption increased by all *except*:**
A. MCT
B. Tetracycline
C. Lactulose
D. Berilium

86. **A 36-year-old woman complains of embarrassment from excessive flatulence. Weight loss and recent dietary changes are denied. In discussing this problem with the patient, which of the following statements would be most accurate?**
A. The expelled gas is largely the result of dietary intake and bacterial fermentation
B. Passage of flatus more than 15 times per day is abnormal
C. The patient should be evaluated for malabsorption
D. Oral simethicone will usually reduce the flatulence

87. **Ideal age of screening for colorectal cancer in asian patient:**
A. 40
B. 45
C. 50
D. 55

88. **The minimum amount of GI bleed detected by angiography:**
A. 0.01 mL/min
B. 1 mL/min
C. 0.5 mL/min
D. 10.0 mL/min

89. **A 62-year-old man with aortic stenosis is admitted to the hospital with a fever of 39.4°C. Physical examination reveals an aortic insufficiency murmur. Echocardiography reveals vegetations on the aortic valve. Blood cultures grow**

streptococcus bovis. Which one the following statement is true?

A. A search for colonic neoplasia should be undertaken
B. A search for gastric neoplasia should be undertaken
C. Stool should be collected and examined for streptococcus species
D. Telangiectasias in the colon are associated with this infection

90. **With respect to the endoscopic treatment of gastrointestinal lesions. All of the following statements are true *except*:**

A. Endoscopic strip biopsy allows the removal of a large area of mucosa and limits significant associated complications
B. Photodynamic therapy uses photosensitizing agent that are activated by the standard visible light source of the endoscope
C. Endoscopic ultrasonography has been shown to add useful diagnostic information to that obtained by computed tomography in the assessment of tumor respectability
D. Laser therapy can be used to ablate tumors and recanalize obstructing lesions

91. **Pregnancy all of the following *except*:**

A. Gastric emptying delayed
B. Colon transit time increased
C. No effect on gastric acid secretion
D. Small bowel transit increased

92. **A 44-year-old man with chronic ulcerative colitis is referred for the consideration of surveillance screening for colon cancer. His disease was diagnosed 15 years ago with inflammation to the level of the mid transverse colon. His symptoms have been moderate and colonoscopic biopsy have revealed high grade dysplasia. Most appropriate management strategy:**

A. Periodic colonoscopy surveillance
B. Colectomy should be offered to patient
C. Follow up is not required
D. None

93. **A 59-year-old college professor presents with painless hematochezia. Colonoscopy is normal except for a 2.5 cm pedunculated polyp in the sigmoid colon that is completely removed with snare polypectomy. The pathologist reports that the head of the polyp is largely replaced by an invasive cancer that penetrates into the stalk. The stalk is 3 cm long and is examined carefully by the pathologist, who notes that the cancer extends only 5 mm into the stalk and that the margin is free of neoplasm. The cancer is well-differentiated, and no vascular invasion is noted. The patient is otherwise in good health and plans to continue teaching for antoher 5 to 10 years. You should advise his patient that:**

A. The colonoscopic resection of the malignant polyp was adequate, and not additional treatment is needed at this time
B. A low anterior resection is a low-risk procedure in this patient, and to be safe, the operation should be offered
C. Recurrence is likely at the polypectomy site, and surveillance is indicated every 6 months
D. Little information is available on the management of these polyps and a surgical consultation is the best option

94. **The following groups of bacteria each account for more than 1% of the fecal flora *except*:**

A. Facultative gram-negative organisms (e.g. Escherichia coli)
B. Bacteroides species
C. Clostridium species
D. Peptostreptococcus species

95. **A healthy 33-year-old man presents at the emergency department with rectal pain. He finally sheepishly admits to the inability to extricate a lightbulb from his rectum. Which one of the following statements is true?**

A. The lightbulb was probably placed in the rectum in a misguided attempt to relieve a particular symptom
B. If the object is palpable on digital examination, abdominal radiography is probably unnecessary
C. Because the object is glass transanal removal is unsafe
D. Proctosigmoidoscopy should be performed after the object is successfully removed

96. **Regarding diminutive colonic polyps, all are true *except*:**

A. Size usually <5 mm
B. Usually contains villous component
C. More malignant in the setting of HNPCC
D. Snare cautery should not be used unless the polyp is of villous histology

97. Adenoma may lead to carcinoma in all *except*:
A. Site
B. Size
C. Dysplasia
D. Villous component

98. The best and most practical way to treat a patient of isolated ileal Crohn's disease:
A. Infliximab
B. Steroid
C. Budesonide enema
D. AZA/6-MP

99. Prokinetics drug used for preparation of colon for colonoscopy in massive lower gastrointestinal bleeding:
A. Erythromycin
B. Domperidone
C. Metoclopramide
D. None

100. Not responding to colectomy in ulcerative colitis patient:
A. PSC
B. PG
C. Uveitis
D. Urinary calculus

101. CD (Crohn's disease) activity index suggestive of remission:
A. <100
B. <150
C. 200
D. >250

102. In the hereditary non-polyposis colorectal cancer syndrome, the most common defect is:
A. hMsh2
B. hMsh1
C. P53 gene
D. hMlh1

103. Poor prognostic features for colorectal carcinoma includes all of the following *except:*
A. Incomplete resection
B. Poorly differentiated carcinoma
C. Microsatellite instability
D. Mucinous histology

104. What is the sensitivity of flexible sigmoidoscopy for detecting colorectal polyps/cancer?
A. 10%-20%
B. 30%-50%
C. <10%
D. >90%

105. In prospective human studies, which of the following have failed to show any benefit for prevention of colorectal neoplasia?
A. Celecoxib
B. Lowfat high fiber diet
C. Estrogen replacement therapy
D. Calcium

106. The genetic abnormality in majority of patients with colorectal carcinoma, adenomas even smaller adenomas and dysplastic lesion is:
A. K-ras mutations
B. Loss of tumor suppressor gene activity on chromosome 18q
C. APC gene mutations
D. Loss of P53 gene

107. Good prognostic clinical indicator in colon cancer is:
A. Age <30 years
B. Bowel obstruction
C. Short duration of symptoms
D. Rectal bleeding as presenting symptom

108. DNA mis-match repair genes associated with hereditary non-polyposis colorectal carcinoma are located on chromosome:
A. 2 and 3 B. 5 and 12
C. 6 and 11 D. 17 and 18

109. Good prognostic indicator for colorectal carcinoma is:
A. Mircosatellite instability
B. Increased tumor DNA content
C. Mutation in BAX gene
D. Mucinous or colloid carcinoma on histology

110. Which of the following statement is false for a 35 years old adult with familial adenomatous polyposis who underwent subtotal colectomy with ileorectal anastomosis?
A. 5% of those with rectal polyps will develop carcinoma in 5 to 23 years
B. 60% will develop carcinoma of rectal stump on 20 years follow up despite semiannual sigmoidoscopic surveillance and fulguration of all polyps
C. Carcinoma of rectal stump have good prognosis
D. Risk of carcinoma of recta stump is higher in patients with APC mutation between codons 1250 and 1464

111. Least useful drug for adjuvant chemotherapy of colorectal carcinoma after surgery is:
A. 5 Flurouracil B. Cisplatin
C. Levamisole D. Levcovorin

112. Which of the following statement is NOT correct for adjuvant chemotherapy for colorectal carcinoma after surgical resection, on 5 years follow up:
A. Reduces recurrence by 40%
B. Reduces recurrences at liver and lungs
C. Improve survival
D. Mostly useful for Dukes B2 (Stage II) tumors after surgical resection

113. In person with family history of hereditary non-polyposis colon cancer the guidelines for early detection of cancer is to perform colonoscopy and consider genetic testing beginning at:
A. Puberty
B. 21 years age
C. 40 years age
D. 10 years before the youngest case in the immediate family

114. Carcinoembryonic antigen in carcinoma colon has following utility, *except*:
A. Pre-operative staging
B. Post-operative follow up
C. Screening large asymptomatic population
D. Prognostic marker

ANORECTAL DISEASE

115. Which of the following statement regarding solitary rectal ulcer syndrome is false?
A. Multiple ulcers may be seen
B. Commonly located on anterior rectal wall 5-10 cms from anal verge
C. Ulcers are always confined to rectum
D. Biofeedback may be helpful in patients with associated non-relaxing puborectalis muscle

116. Guaiac test for fecal occult blood test is false-positive in following conditions, *except*:
A. Red meat ingestion
B. Cauliflower ingestion
C. Aspirin ingestion
D. Radish ingestion

117. Which of the following statement is false regarding hemorrhoids?
A. Haemorrhoids are normal part of human anatomy
B. Internal hemorrhoids originate above the dentate line and are covered by transitional mucosa
C. First line treatment of external hemorrhoids is rubber band ligation
D. Infrared photocoagulation is useful in treatment of internal hemorrhoids

118. Which of the following statement is false for fissure in ano?
A. About 90% of anal fissures are located in mid posterior portion of anus
B. Botulinum toxin A has a role in treatment of chronic anal fissure
C. The standard treatment of chronic anal fissure is surgery
D. 80% of anal fissures start at dentate line and extends proximally to a variable length

119. Rectal prolapse may be associated with all of the following, *except*:
A. Cauda equina syndrome
B. Schistosomiasis
C. Down syndrome
D. Solitary rectal ulcer syndrome

120. In pruritis ani:
A. Anal itching is invariably idiopathic
B. Anal itching is due to autoimmune disorder
C. Methylene blue ingestion helps in some patients
D. Relapse is common

121. Which of the following is true for perianal warts?
A. Perianal warts due to human papilloma virus (HPV) type 6 and 8 have oncogenic potential
B. Topical application of 2% podophyllin is the most effective medical therapy
C. Surgical excision is the preferred therapy and is useful in preventing recurrences
D. Intralesional interferon alpha may be an important adjunct to surgical method

122. Which of the following is true for fistula in ano due to Crohn's disease?
A. These are cryptoglandular in origin
B. These follow Goodsall's rule
C. These are curved with multiple tracts
D. Anorectal suppuration if any is associated with marked tenderness like an anorectal abscess

123. First line treatment for anal canal cancer is:
A. Abdominal-perineal resection with permanent colostomy
B. Abdominal-perineal resection with radiation therapy
C. Abdominal-perineal resection with chemotherapy
D. Radiation therapy with chemotherapy

MEGACOLON IN ADULTS

124. Hirschsprung's disease presenting in adult life has following feature/features:
A. Acute intestinal obstruction
B. Severe constipation recurrent fecal impaction

C. Diarrhoea in 20% causes due to pseudomembranous enterocolitis
D. All of the above

125. Which of the following does not discriminate between acquired megacolon in adults from congenital type?
A. Evidence of voluntary withholding
B. Presence of overflow soiling
C. Evidence of fecal impaction on X-ray or physical examination
D. Palpable stool at internal sphincter

126. Most convincing evidence for acquired megacolon is:
A. Demonstration of ganglion cells on rectal biopsy
B. Dilated colon and rectum on barium enema
C. Presence of reactional inhibitory response on anorectal manometry
D. Absence of delayed colonic transit

127. Medical management acquired megacolon in adults are following *except*:
A. Stool disimpaction, all even manually under anesthesia
B. Bulking agents are useful
C. Bisacodyl as laxative is preferred
D. Large volumes of water intake is encouraged

128. Which of following is incorrect for Ogilvie's syndrome?
A. Trauma or orthopedic surgery is often a predisposing event
B. Sudden onset abdominal distension in post operative patient uneventfully recovering
C. Massive gaseous distension of colon on X-ray
D. The caecal diameter is usually 12 cm or more

ACUTE APPENDICITIS

129. Patients with uncomplicated acute appendicitis usually present with following *except*:
A. Emesis, 4 to 6 hours later followed by epigastric or periumbilical pain
B. Mild fever
C. Pain in right lower quadrant after 12 to 24 hours of onset
D. High fever and rigors are uncommon

130. Physical sign in uncomplicated acute appendicitis may include following *except*:
A. Tachycardia
B. Rebound tenderness
C. Rectal tenderness
D. Point tenderness with a cough

131. Which of the following statement regarding pathogenesis of acute appendicitis is not correct?
A. Classic hypothesis holds that obstruction of the appendiceal human in most cases, but obstructive lesion is found in minority of cases
B. Most convincing evidence in favour of obstruction raised intraluminal pressure at appendectomy
C. Ulceration of appendiceal mucosa has been noted in 75%, which could get infected and result in appendicitis
D. Decrease intake of fiber has been postulated but recent reports does not confirm this view

132. Most common Burne's described the surface anatomy of appendix. According to his description the appendix is located at the junction of:
A. Lateral one third and medial two third of line joining right anterior superior iliac spine and symphysis pubis
B. Lateral two third and medial on third of line joining right anterior superior iliac spine and symphysis pubis
C. Lateral one third and medial two third of line joining right anterior superior iliac spine and umbilicus
D. Lateral two third and medial one third of line joining right anerior superior iliac spins and umbilicus

133. Which of the following statements regarding diagnostic tests for acute appendicitis is not correct?
A. Polymorphonuclear leucocytosis with shift to left is a sensitive and useful test
B. CRP estimation though improves diagnostic accuracy but is less sensitive and accurate than blood counts
C. Urine analysis and microscopy is most useful test to exclude the differential diagnosis of urinary tract infection
D. Ultrasound and CT scan has about 80% sensitivity and about 90% specificity in diagnosing acute appendicitis

134. Major complication of appendicitis is perforation. Which of the following statement is not correct about appendiceal perforation?
A. It is common is infants and may be as high as 90%
B. High fever, leucocytosis and signs of peritonitis can predict perforation preoperatively but lack specificity
C. Free intraperitoneal air on abdominal radiography excludes appendix as the site of bowel perforation
D. It can cause portal pyelophlebitis

Explanation

1. **Ans. (D)** Acute appendicitis is a clinical diagnosis supported by carefully selected laboratory and radiographic studies. Abdominal ultrasonography may be helpful in ambiguous cases. Perforation should be suspected if symptoms have been present for more than 24 hours. If the temperature exceeds 38°C, or if the leukocyte count exceeds 15,000/mm^3. The prognosis is related to age; mortality rate higher in patients older than 50 years. Appendiceal abscesses can be treated either operatively or non-operatively, depending on the clinical setting. Some surgeons favor a non-surgical approach initially, draining the fluid percutaneous and treating the patient with potential antibiotics.

(Sleisenger, 9th edition, Pp-2059-2070)

2. **Ans. (A)** There is little evidence of fertility problems with ulcerative colitis; however, studies suggest that women with Crohn's disease have a slightly increased rate of infertility that may be closely related to disease activity and nutritional status. Total parenteral nutrition by itself has not been shown to be detrimental to the fetus. Steroids have been widely used for many diseases during pregnancy and have not been shown to increase the risk of fetal abnormalities.

(Sleisenger, 9th edition, Pp-629-630)

3. **Ans. (D)** Both diseases commonly exhibit inflammatory cell infiltration of the lamina propria. The prominence of intraepithelial lymphocytes has led to use of the term lymphocytic rather than microscopic colitis. A prominent subepithelial collagen band larger than 10 to 15 im in diameter is abnormal and is responsible for the sterno collagenous colitis.

(Sleisenger, 9th edition, Pp-2239-2242)

4. **Ans. (D)** Cronkhite-Canada syndrome is a non-inherited condition of unknown etiology characterized by generalized hamartomatous gastrointestinal polyposis, mucocutaneous hyperpigmentation, nail atrophy and hair loss.

(Sleisenger, 9th edition, P-2188)

5. **Ans. (A)** Peutz-Jeghers syndrome has been associated with gastrointestinal malignancies as a result of adenomatous change in some polyps. Mucocutaneous pigmentation often begins during the first or second year of life. Polyps in Peutz-Jeghers syndrome are hamartomas and lack cellular atypia. The arborization of the epithelium lead to the unique microscopic picture of benign glands surrounded by smooth muscle extending well into the submucosa. This characteristic is called pseudoinvasion and is not indicative of malignancy. The most common location of polyps is the small intestine, followed in frequency by the colon and stomach.

(Sleisenger, 9th edition, Pp-2185-2186)

6. **Ans. (C)** Although fecal leukocytes are often seen with bacterial infections of the colon, they are also a common finding in ulcerative colitis and in other chronic inflammatory disease of the colon.

(Sleisenger, 9th edition, Pp-1844-1850)

7. **Ans. (C)** In general, markers ingested over a 2 to 3-day period are mixed together in the stool and passed in a random manner. No significant differences in marker transit have been found when given either before or with meal. Segmental colonic transit can be measured only if abdominal radiographs are taken to count markers in normal volunteers, 80% of markers are passed by the fifth day after ingestion.

(Sleisenger, 9th edition, P-1755)

8. **Ans. (C)** Colonic diverticula should not be considered a source of occult bleeding.

(Sleisenger, 9th edition, Pp-2073-2089)

9. **Ans. (A)** Recurrence of diverticulitis is relatively common, occurring in 27% of 45% of patients.

(Sleisenger, 9th edition, Pp-2073-2089)

10. **Ans. (C)** Angiodysplasia from the stomach and right colon are histologically indistinguishable.

(Sleisenger, 9th edition, Pp-593-599)

11. **Ans. (C)** Giardia lamblia typically infects the small bowel and does not result in dysentery.

(Sleisenger, 9th edition, P-1849)

12. **Ans. (B)** Shigella species invade the colonic epithelium and produce enterotoxins, although the toxin is not essential for the development of colitis. Endoscopically, the severity of disease diminishes in more proximal regions of the colon. The entire colon is involved in 15% of patients. Shigella infection is highly contagious; the ingestion of even small number of organisms causes disease.

(Sleisenger, 9th edition, Pp-1858-1860)

13. **Ans. (D)** Campylobacter jejuni infections are usually self-limited and frequently resolve by the time culture results are positive. Therapy is usually conservative and includes replacement of fluid and electrolytes. Weak evidence suggests that antibiotics (e.g., erythromycin ciprofloxacin) may decrease the duration of symptoms if instituted within 3 days of the onset of diarrhea: however, most patients do not benefit from antibiotic administration.

(Sleisenger, 9th edition, Pp-1867-1869)

14. **Ans. (C)** Hirschsprung disease is diagnosed by a deep mucosal biopsy performed in the distal rectal region. If the aganglionic segment is relatively short, a biopsy in the proximal rectum or sigmoid colon will miss the area of abnormality. If the rectoanal inhibitory reflex is present during anorectal manometry, the disease can be ruled out without a rectal biopsy. Symptoms usually present in infants and not during toilet training. Surgery is required to treat this condition, but the majority of the colon is left in place.

(Sleisenger, 9th edition, Pp-1636-1639)

15. **Ans. (D)** Patients with acquired immunodeficiency syndrome may present with painful anorectal lesions caused by typical veneral organisms. Other etiologies include tuberculosis, Kaposi sarcoma, Cloacogen's carcinoma, squamous cell carcinoma and lymphoma but not yersinia enterocolitica.

(Sleisenger, 9th edition, P-531)

16. **Ans. (D)** The gut microflora synthesizes vitamin K and plays an essential role in the metabolism of drugs such as sulfasalazine and metronidazole. Probably the most important function of the colonic microflora is to suppress populations of other bacteria that are more pathogenic.

(Sleisenger, 9th edition, Pp-1769-1770)

17. **Ans. (B)** The toxin produced by Shigella species inhibits colonocyte protein synthesis and leads to diarrhea through the secondary failure of fluid absorption.The clinical course of adult infection begins with the onset of fever within 1 to 3 days of ingestion, followed by diarrhea within an additional day. The typical duration of the illness is 5 to 7 days. Shigella infections are associated with the hemolytic-uremic syndrome and with Reiter syndrome. Most patients with symptomatic Shigella infections should be treated, except for selected patients with mild disease. Tetracycline therapy is effective for most infections acquired in North America, whereas ciprofloxacin will also treat cases acquired outside the United States, which may be caused by tetracycline-resistant organisms.

(Sleisenger, 9th edition, Pp-1858-1860)

18. **Ans. (B)** The most frequent symptoms of gonorrheal proctitis are constipation and obstipation, although asymptomatic rectal carriage occurs in upto 53% of patients. Chlamydia trachomatis is responsible for up to 20% of proctitis in gay men. The conditions may become chronic with fistula formation and clinically mimic Crohn's proctitis. The perianal warts of secondary syphilis are known as condyloma lata, while those caused by human papillomavirus are known as condyloma acuminate.

(Sleisenger, 9th edition, P-1848)

19. **Ans. (B)** The most common causes of acute diarrhea are infectious agents. In the United States, most cases of infectious diarrhea are self-limited and are not caused of significant morbidity. Attempting to determine the etiologic agent in all cases is not warranted for numerous reasons, including cost, the inability to make a definitive diagnosis in a large number of cases and result that will not influence patients care. A thorough evolution is warranted for patients who are likely to benefit from a specific diagnosis, such as for those with fever higher than 39° C, systemic illness, bloody diarrhea, dehydration or a prolonged course.

(Sleisenger, 9th edition, Pp-1846-1849)

20. **Ans. (D)** About 50% of patients with pseudomembranous colitis (PMC) or antibiotic associated colitis (AAC) do not have fecal leukocytes on stool examination, in cases of antibiotic associated diarrhea, 15% to 25% have clostridium difficile cytotoxin in their stool and upto 40% are culture-positive. In about 30% of PMC cases, pseudomembranes are not seen in the rectum but are found more proximal in the colon. Pseudomembranes are not necessary for the diagnosis of AAC, which is confirmed by evidence of systemic illness of by evidence of colitis on flexible sigmoidoscopy.

(Sleisenger, 9th edition, Pp-1896-1897)

21. **Ans. (C)** Acute amebic proctocolitis is commonly characterized by 1 to 3 weeks of increasingly frequent bloody diarrhea associated with abdominal pain and tenderness. Fever is present in about 33% of patients. Weight loss is common.

(Sleisenger, 9th edition, Pp-1906-1907)

22. **Ans. (C)** Atelectasis, elevation of the right hemi-diaphragm serous pelural effusion, and peritonitis are all common manifestations of amoebic liver abscess. Pericarditis is an unusual complication that results from the direct spread of the liver abscess. Pulmonary embolism is not known to be specifically associated with amebic liver abscess formation.

(Sleisenger, 9th edition, Pp-1368-1369)

23. **Ans. (B)** Surveillance for dysplastic changes in chronic ulcerative pancolitis should begin 8 to 10 years after symptom onset.

(Sleisenger, 9th edition, Pp-2005-2008)

24. **Ans. (B)** Physiologic losses of blood from the gastrointestinal tract in normal subjects range from 0.5 to 1.0 mL/day.

(Sleisenger, 9th edition, P-2173)

25. **Ans. (B)** The lifetime risk of the development of colon cancer is approximately 5% for the average American.

(Sleisenger, 9th edition, Pp-2191-2193)

26. **Ans. (C)** Extensive disease extending proximal to the splenic flexure is usually treated the same as pancolitis involving the entire colon. This patient has had disease for 15 years and even if just isolated to the left side, a colonoscopy is indicated. Despite the mild, well controlled nature of the disease, he is at substantial risk for the development of cancer because of the duration and extent of the disease. A barium enema radiographic study is not sufficiently sensitive for the detection of dysplasia, or cancer and sigmoidoscopy is an incomplete examination. The finding of high grade dysphasia, when reviewed by an expert pathologist, is an indication of colectomy, whereas low-grade dysplasia requires careful follow-up but not necessarily resection.

(Sleisenger, 9th edition, Pp-2005-2008)

27. **Ans. (A)** The overwhelming majority of colonic bacteria are anaerobic. Facultative gram-negative organisms account for only 0.1% to 0.5% of the fecal flora.

(Sleisenger, 9th edition, P-2101)

28. **Ans. (C)** For diminutive polyps, cold snaring and cold biopsy are safe and hemorrhage is rare, in comparison with hot cautery techniques. Hot biopsy forceps are five times more likely to produce a complication in the right than in the left colon. Snare cautery effectively removes the entire polyp is smaller than 5 mm. Cold biopsy may be used to completely remove small polyps.

(Sleisenger, 9th edition, P-2158)

29. **Ans. (D)** Only saline injection into the submucosa would raise an effective mound. This technique has not been associated with a risk of tumor seeding or peritonitis. Lesions smaller than 1.5 cm should be removed in a single piece if possible. The incidence of residual cancer and even of metastasis from sessile malignant polyps is clearly greater than that associated with pedunculated malignant polyps.

(Sleisenger, 9th edition, Pp-2168-2170)

30. **Ans. (D)** Finger palpation and transillumination in the right lower quadrant are sometimes effective in confirming passage of the endoscope tip to the cecum: however they can on occasion be misleading. Using the length of endoscope inserted as a gauge is unreliable. Fluoroscopic confirmation may be helpful, but it is not practical and exposes the patients to unnecessary radiation. The ideal way to identify passage of the scope to the cecum is by using cecal landmarks.

(Sleisenger, 9th edition, Pp-2224-2225)

31. **Ans. (A)** Antibiotics are completely unnecessary even if a biopsy or polypectomy is performed, unless the patient has certain unusual risk factors for endocarditis. Routine avoidance of aspirin is discontinued because of a planned polypectomy, discontinuation 1 week prior is sufficient. Oral sodium phosphate is not a balanced electrolyte solution. It is reasonable to avoid iron preparations for several days prior to colonoscopy, because they can produce a black, stickly residue in the colon, which makes the procedure difficult.

(Sleisenger, 9th edition, Pp-658-660)

32. **Ans. (B)** The cecum, transverse colon and sigmoid colon are all intraperitoneal structures and are prone to volvulus because of their location and relative lack of fixation.

(Sleisenger, 9th edition, Pp-1615-1616)

33. **Ans. (D)** All have a strong association with adenomas, with the exception of cholecystectomy.

(Sleisenger, 9th edition, Pp-2164-2165)

34. **Ans. (D)** Tubular adenomas are most common comprising 80% to 85% of all adenomas, followed by

tubulovillous adenomas (10%) and villous adenomas (5%).

(Sleisenger, 9th edition, P-2155)

35. **Ans. (D)** Microsatellite instability due to DNA mismatch repair is the hallmark defect in hereditary non-polyposis colorectal cancer syndrome.

(Sleisenger, 9th edition, P-2206)

36. **Ans. (B)** Tubular adenomas are relatively common; therefore, a first degree relative with only an adenoma is not an indication for colonoscopy (except in certain hereditary syndromes with multiple polyps).

(Sleisenger, 9th edition, Pp-2208-2210)

37. **Ans. (D)** All are poor prognostic factors except pedunculated malignant polyps. Some studies suggest that the outcome for patients with pedunculated malignant polyps is improved.

(Sleisenger, 9th edition, P-2208)

38. **Ans. (C)** Once the polyp penetrates the submucosa, metastatic spread is possible because the lymphatics are located in the submucosa.

(Sleisenger, 9th edition, P-2208)

39. **Ans. (B)** This mutation occurs in approximately half of colorectal adenomas larger than 1 cm.

(Sleisenger, 9th edition, P-2200)

40. **Ans. (A)** All are inherited in an autosomal dominant fashion except hyperplastic polyposis, which is not an inherited syndrome. However upto one-third of newly diagnosed cases of familial adenomatous polyposis appear to represent de novo mutations.

(Sleisenger, 9th edition, P-2177)

41. **Ans. (C)** In vitro protein synthesis (IVPS) would be the most reasonable initial genetic test. Linkage testing requires blood from two or more known affected persons in a family to identify DNA markers that associate with the mutant gene. Mutation identification on uses direct DNA sequencing at gene sites to determine the precise gene mutation; however, it is primarily limited to research laboratories, and it is not commercially available at present. IVPS testing requires that only a single individual be tested. It has been shown to identify a protein truncation successfully in 80% of families with familial adenomatous polyposis tested.

(Sleisenger, 9th edition, Pp-2226-2227)

42. **Ans. (A)** All of the extra colonic lesions listed are seen in Gardner syndrome except ovarian carcinoma.

(Sleisenger, 9th edition, P-2177)

43. **Ans. (B)** The APC gene (located on the long arm of chromosome 5) is mutated in familial adenomatous polyposis. The resultant mutation almost always causes a truncation of APC protein, which is thought to function as a tumor suppressor gene.

(Sleisenger, 9th edition, P-2177)

44. **Ans. (D)** Juvenile polyposis is characterized by ten or more juvenile polyps. Juvenile polyps are considered non-neoplastic hamartomatosis polyps, usually occurring in the colons of children between ages of 4 and 14 years.

(Sleisenger, 9th edition, P-2177)

45. **Ans. (A)** Tobacco use has been associated with a 2 to 3 fold increase in adenoma prevalence, but not in colorectal cancer. Regular consumption of beer has been associated with a 2 to 3 fold increased risk. The ingestion of animal fat has been associated with a modest but statistically significant increased risk. Women who have received radiation therapy for gynecologic cancer have a 2 to 3 fold increased risk of colorectal cancer.

(Sleisenger, 9th edition, Pp-2193-2196)

46. **Ans. (C)** COX2 inhibitors such as celecoxib and rofecoxib are recommended by FDA for regression of polyps in familial adenomatous polyposis.

(Sleisenger, 9th edition, P-2198)

47. **Ans. (C)** Juvenile polyps are mucosal tumors that primarily consists of excess of lamina propria and dilated cystic submucosal gland.

(Sleisenger, 9th edition, P-2174)

48. **Ans. (C)** Peutz-Jeghers syndrome has been associated with gastrointestinal and breast malignancies as a result of adenomatous change in some polyps. Mucocutaenous pigmentation often begins during the first or second year of life. Polyps in Peutz-Jeghers syndrome are hematomas and lack cellular atypia. The arborization of the epithelium leads to the unique microscopic picture of benign glands surrounded by smooth muscle extending well into the submucosa. This characteristic is called pseudoinvasion and is not indicative of malignancy. The most common location of polyps is the small intestine, followed in frequency by the colon and stomach.

(Sleisenger, 9th edition, P-2175)

49. **Ans. (D)** Ileal brake probably mediated by a neurohumoral mechanism for which various neurotransmitters and hormones have been implicated including PYY, GLP1 and GLP2.

(Sleisenger, 9th edition, P-1697)

50. Ans. (B) GLUT-2 expressed in basolateral membrane and transport glucose from enterocytes to interstitium through facilitated diffusion.

(Sleisenger, 9th edition, Pp-1710-1711)

51. Ans. (D) Normal resting anal pressure is 60-90 mm of Hg mostly contributed by IAS (Internal Anal Sphincter) upto 70% pressure contributed by it. During voluntary squeezing IAS contribute only 40% of total pressure but majorities are contributed by EAS and levator ani muscles.

(Sleisenger, 9th edition, Pp-241-243)

52. Ans. (A) Colonoscopy has more sensitivity and specificity in detecting uncomplicated diverticulosis.

(Sleisenger, 9th edition, P-2076)

53. Ans. (B) Hirschsprung disease is diagnosed by a deep mucosal biopsy performed in the distal rectal region. If the aganglionic segment is relatively short, a biopsy in the proximal rectum or sigmoid colon will miss the area of abnormality. If the rectoanal inhibitory reflex is present during anorectal manometry, the disease can be ruled out without a rectal biopsy. Anal manometry is the most reliable method by which diagnosis of ultrashort segment HD is made.

(Sleisenger, 9th edition, Pp-1636-1639)

54. Ans. (B) Bevacizumab is a recombinant humanized monoclonal antibody that acts by binding all isoforms of circulating VEGF-A thus decreasing angiogenesis phase III trial for colon cancer.

(Sleisenger, 9th edition, P-2235)

55. Ans. (C) Normal ileum diameter is 3 cm.

(Sleisenger, 9th edition, P-2142)

56. Ans. (B) All adults older than 50 years who present with constipation should undergo a colonoscopy, flexible sigmoidoscopy and barium enema or CT colonography to screen for colorectal cancer as widely recommended flexible sigmoidoscopy is probably sufficient for evaluation of constipation younger than 50 years without alarm features.

(Sleisenger, 9th edition, P-272)

57. Ans. (B) Tonic ring contraction of circular muscles of colon responsible for Haustral marking. They have no tendency to migrate.

(Sleisenger, 9th edition, Pp-1668-1670)

58. Ans. (C) The internet anal sphincter (IAS) contributes approximately 70% to 85% of resting anal sphincter pressure but only 40% of pressure after sudden distention of the rectum so, IAS is responsible chiefly for maintaining continence of rest.

(Sleisenger, 9th edition, Pp-242-243)

59. Ans. (B) Most likely diagnosis in this patient is levator ani syndrome. Even if all investigations are normal. Levator ani might feel like a tight, tender bad on rectal examination.

(Sleisenger, 9th edition, Pp-2272-2273)

60. Ans. (D) Acute appendicitis with appendicular abscess can be treated conservatively of not associated with rupture or perforation.

(Sleisenger, 9th edition, Pp-2068-2069)

61. Ans. (C) Clinical condition listed above is a case of ulcerative colitis with mild exacerbation of symptoms due to non-compliance to medication so, best management at this stage is reinstitute 5-ASA enema and consider slow tapering if patient stabilizes.

(Sleisenger, 9th edition, Pp-1992-1994)

62. Ans. (B) Chronic radiation proctitis occur when total dose of radiation exceeds 80 Gx. Tissue ischemia leading to obliterative endarteritis.

(Sleisenger, 9th edition, P-650)

63. Ans. (A) Pregnancy does not appear to increase the severity of morbidity due to preexisting IBD, disease activity prior to conception seems to most important.

(Sleisenger, 9th edition, P-629)

64. Ans. (A) There is little evidence of fertility problems with ulcerative colitis; however, studies suggest that women with Crohn's disease have a slightly increased rate of infertility that may be closely related to disease activity and complication. Total parenteral nutrition by itself has not been shown to be detrimental to the fetus. Steroids have been widely used for many diseases during pregnancy and have not been shown to increase the risk of fetal abnormalities. AZA/6-MP are category D drugs.

(Sleisenger, 9th edition, Pp-2241-2242)

65. Ans. (B) Stool frequencies, temperature, heart rate, hematocrit, acute phase reactant (ESR,CRP) are used for classification of severity of ulcerative colitis.

(Sleisenger, 9th edition, P-1991)

66. Ans. (C) Azathioprine used for maintenance of remissions in ulcerative colitis. Maintenance therapy with azathioprine decreases the rate colectomy.

(Sleisenger, 9th edition, Pp-1996-1999)

67. Ans. (C) Cronkhite-Canada syndrome characterized by diffuse gastrointestinal polyposis, dystrophic changes in the fingernails, alopecia, cutaenous hyperpigmentation.

(Sleisenger, 9th edition, P-2188)

68. Ans. (C) Bannayan-Ruvalacab Riley syndrome is a familial hamartomatous polyposis syndrome with Macrocephaly and developmental delay.

(Sleisenger, 9th edition, P-2185)

69. Ans. (A) Recto-anal inhibitory reflex occurs in response to rectal distension. Relaxation of EAS not occur as a part of recto-anal inhibitory reflex.

(Sleisenger, 9th edition, P-235)

70. Ans. (C) Diverticular bleed occur in only 3-5% of diverticulosis patient. Diverticulitis never increases risk of diverticular bleed. Surgery is not indicated in all cases. Right sided colon is the most common source of diverticular bleed in asian patient.

(Sleisenger, 9th edition, Pp-2085-2087)

71. Ans. (A) Rectosigmoid junction lies 12-16 cm above anal verge.

(Sleisenger, 9th edition, P-2113)

72. Ans. (A) E. histolytica infection usually never causes malabsorption syndrome.

(Sleisenger, 9th edition, Pp-1907-1910)

73. Ans. (A) Normal bacterial count of terminal ileum is 10^8/ml of stool.

(Sleisenger, 9th edition, P-1770)

74. Ans. (C) Normal daily Vitamin D requirement 8000 IU.

(Sleisenger, 9th edition, P-1868)

75. Ans. (B) Rectal biopsy should be taken 2-3 cm above ano-rectal junction in Hirshsprung's disease.

(Sleisenger, 9th edition P-1639)

76. Ans. (C) Calcium bilirubinate stone (Brown stone) is the most common type of stone in PSC.

(Sleisenger, 9th edition P-1343)

77. Ans. (B) Multiple mechanism involved in pathogenesis of antibiotic associated diarrhea. Antibiotics and antibiotics metabolites never increases osmotic load of the colon.

(Sleisenger, 9th edition, Pp-1889-1890)

78. Ans. (B) Diagnostic colonoscopy is not contraindicated in coagulopathy. However it is contraindicated in perforation peritonitis, diverticulitis and aortic aneurysm.

(Sleisenger, 9th edition, Pp-658-660)

79. Ans. (C) Ileum is more acidic than jejunum because of anaerobic fermentation leads to more acid production. Jejunum also contains large numbers of anaerobic bacteria.

(Sleisenger, 9th edition, Pp-1769-1770)

80. Ans. (A) Clostridium difficile causes watery diarrhea. It also exacerbates acute exacerbation of ulcerative colitis. Metronidazole and vancomycin are useful in treatment.

(Sleisenger, 9th edition, P-1895)

81. Ans. (A) Carcinoid tumor is the most common appendiceal tumor.

(Sleisenger, 9th edition, P-2152)

82. Ans. (C) This is due to poisoning with EHEC 0157:H7 leading to Hus, Verotoxin mediated with disease transmitted due to uncooked cattle meat.

(Sleisenger, 9th edition, P-1856)

83. Ans. (C) Severe combined immunodeficiency (SCID) is a risk factor for amoebiasis. Selective IGA deficiency is not a risk factor.

(Sleisenger, 9th edition, P-1908)

84. Ans. (B) Intestinal apthous ulcer is the most characteristic feature of Crohn's disease.

(Sleisenger, 9th edition, P-1948)

85. Ans. (B) Tetracycline decreases the absorption of calcium.

(Sleisenger, 9th edition, P-1548)

86. Ans. (A) The excessive flatus is due to dietary intake and bacterial fermentable.

(Sleisenger, 9th edition, Pp-233-237)

87. Ans. C. Asian Pacific Gastroenterology Society recommend colorectal cancer screening should be started at the age of 50 years.

(Sleisenger, 9th editon P-2007)

88. Ans. (C) Minimal amount of blood loss detected on angiography is 0.5 ml/min.

(Sleisenger, 9th edition, P-2088)

89. Ans. (A) It is suggested that patient with streptococcus bovis bacteremia should undergo thorough colonoscopic examination to rule out colonic malignancy.

(Sleisenger, 9th edition, P-2165)

90. Ans. (B) Photodynamic therapy uses three principles:

1. Photosensitizer agent.
2. A separate light source.
3. Re-active oxygen species.

The light source is different from the light source of endoscope.

(Sleisenger, 9th edition, P-656)

91. **Ans. (A)** Gastric emptying is usually not altered during pregnancy. However small intestinal and large intestine transit time increased during pregnancy.

(Sleisenger, 9th edition, P-625-630)

92. **Ans. (B)** In view of high grade dysplasia colectomy should be offered to this patient.

(Sleisenger, 9th edition, P-2007)

93. **Ans. (A)** Singly pedunculated malignant polyp with cancer free margin, without any invasion to surrounding tissue does not require any further treatment at present. Only periodic follow-up required.

(Sleisenger, 9th edition, P-2064)

94. **Ans. (A)** Fecal flora (Anaerobes) accounts for more than 99% of total no. of bacterial load.

(Sleisenger, 9th edition, P-1769)

95. **Ans. (D)** Proctosigmoidoscopy should be recommended after the foreign body is removed to rule out the severity and extent of local anorectal injury.

(Sleisenger, 9th edition, Pp-658-659)

96. **Ans. (B)** 30%-50% of diminutive polyp is adenoma. Diminutive polyp in the setting of hereditary non-polyposis colorectal cancer should be respected. Cold biopsy is safe and acceptable technique for polyp removal. However only 4% of cases contain villous components.

(Sleisenger, 9th edition, P-2158)

97. **Ans. (A)** Site is not a risk for malignant transformation of colonic adenoma. However, polyp size, Villous histology and dysplasia components are definite risk factor for malignant transformation of colonic polyps.

(Sleisenger, 9th edition, P-2170)

98. **Ans. (A)** Anti-TNF-alpha agents are most effective drugs for induction and maintenance of ileal Crohn's disease.

(Sleisenger, 9th edition, P-1967)

99. **Ans. (C)** Metoclopramide is used along with PEG for urgent colonoscopic preparation in case of massive hematochezia to facilitate urgent colonoscopy.

(Sleisenger, 9th edition, P-293)

100. **Ans. (A)** Colectomy is not effective for PSC resolution in ulcerative colitis. Rest all symptoms resolve on colectomy in ulcerative colitis.

(Sleisenger, 9th edition, P-2012)

101. **Ans. (B)** Remission criteria for CD includes:
   a. Decreasing of CDAI (Crohn's disease activity index) by 70 after 4 weeks of starting treatment.
   b. CDAI (Crohn's disease activity index) <150.

(Sleisenger, 9th edition, P-1960)

102. **Ans. (A)** The most common mutation in HNPCC is hMsh2 (40-45%) of cases on chromosome 2.

(Sleisenger, 9th edition, P-2206)

103. **Ans. (C)** Presence of MSI (Microsatellite instability) is associated with good prognosis in colorectal cancer.

(Sleisenger, 9th edition, P-2216)

104. **Ans. (B)** Flexible sigmoidoscopy is able to detect upto 50% of colorectal cancer.

(Sleisenger, 9th edition, P-2224)

105. **Ans. (B)** Benefit of dietary fiber in prevention of colorectal neoplasms appears in epidemiological and observational studies, but prospective human trials have given equivocal or negative results. Other (A,C,D) have been found to reduce the incidence of adenomatous polyp recurrence of carcinogenesis.

(Harrison, P-443;
Sleisenger, 8th edition, Pp-2221-2222)

106. **Ans. (C)** APC gene mutation is an early and gate keeping event for development of colorectal neoplasia, hence C is present in very early lesions like smallest of adenomas and dysplasia. A, B and D are associated with later event and present only with larger adenomas or when adenomas transform into carcinoma.

(Sleisenger, 8th edition, P-2224)

107. **Ans. (D)** Rectal bleeding is associated with better prognosis. A and B are associated with poor prognosis. C (duration of symptoms) have no impact on outcome.

(Sleisenger, 9th edition, Pp-2216-2217)

108. **Ans. (A)** MSH2 gene on chromosome 2 (in 40-50%) and MLH1 gene on chromosome 3 (in 20-30%) in HNPCC.

(Sleisenger, 9th edition, Pp-2206-2207)

109. **Ans. (A)** Microsatellite instability are associated with poor prognosis.

(Sleisenger, Pp-2216-2217)

110. **Ans. (C)** Prognosis is dismal; A, B and D are correct.

(Sleisenger, 8th edition, P-2220)

111. **Ans. (B)** Cisplation is not used for colorectal cancer ACD-5FU+Levamisole or 5FU+ Leucovorin is used.

(Sleisenger, 9th edition, Pp-2234-2237)

112. **Ans. (D)** Equivocal benefit in stage II most useful in stage III 8th.

(Sleisenger, 9th edition, Pp-2234-2237)

113. **Ans. (B)** A for FAP, C and D for colorectal cancer or Adenomatous polyp in first degree relative of <60 years age.

(Sleisenger, 8th edition, P-2248)

114. **Ans. (C)** Not useful in detecting asymptomatic cases.

(Sleisenger, 8th edition, Pp-2238, 2246)

115. **Ans. (C)** Sometimes ulcers may not be confined to rectum.

(Sleisenger, 9th edition, Pp-2050-2051)

116. **Ans. (C)** Aspirin ingestion causes upper GI bleeding hence FOBT is true positive (It may be false positive in context of colorectal carcinoma screening). B and D are peroxidase containing vegetables and A contains non-human globin, so give false positive results.

(Sleisenger, 8th edition, P-2244)

117. **Ans. (C)** External hemorrhoids are covered with skin hence does not bleed so do not require banding.

(Sleisenger, 8th edition, P-2280)

118. **Ans. (D)** Anal fissures start at anal verge and extend upto dentate line.

(Sleisenger, 8th edition, P-2282)

119. **Ans. (C)** A, B and D are associated with rectal prolapse.

(Sleisenger, 8th edition, Pp-2294, 2297)

120. **Ans. (D)** Anal itching is primary in 50% and secondary in 50% injection of methylene blue is useful in some cases and relapse is common.

(Sleisenger, 8th edition, Pp-2288-2289)

121. **Ans. (D)** An HPV type 16 and 18 are associated with neoplasia, 25% podophyllin application gives only 20-50% success rate. C recurrences are common even after surgery which is used only for extensive lesions. D surgery along with cautery or intralesional interferon checks recurrences.

(Sleisenger, 9th edition, Pp-2270-2271)

122. **Ans. (C)** These may be related to increased lymphoid tissue, B: do not follow goodsall's rule and D: anorectal suppuration is less tender.

(Sleisenger, 8th edition, P-2286)

123. **Ans. (D)** Resulted in 94% cure rate surgical options are for residual and recurrent cancers. Chemoradiotherapy is the treatment of choice.

(Sleisenger, 8th edition, P-2286)

124. **Ans. (B)** Acute obstruction and its complication pseudomembranous enterocolitis is uncommon in adults.

(Sleisenger, 8th edition, P-2133)

125. **Ans. (C)** A, B and D are present in acquired megacolon, C present both in congenital and acquired megacolon.

(Sleisenger, 8th edition, P-2130)

126. **Ans. (C)** Ganglion cells can be positive even in Hirschsprung's if biopsy has not been taken from agnonflionic segment, B can be a feature of Hirschsprung's and acquired megacolon and D colonic transit is usually delayed.

(Sleisenger, 8th edition, P-2130)

127. **Ans. (C)** Bisacodyl is a stimulant laxative which should be avoided.

(Sleisenger, 8th edition, P-2136)

128. **Ans. (D)** Caecal diameter is 8-10 cm and ABC are correct.

(Sleisenger, 8th edition, P-2137)

129. **Ans. (A)** Pain is first and followed by Emesis.

(Sleisenger, 9th edition, Pp-2059-2071)

130. **Ans. (A)** Tachycardia is unusual in uncomplicated appendicitis.

(Sleisenger, 9th edition, Pp-2059-2071)

131. **Ans. (B)** Intraluminal pressure is raised in minority only.

(Sleisenger, 8th edition, P-2090)

132. **Ans. (C)** Mc Burney's point lies at the junction of medial two third and lateral one third of the line joining right anterior superior iliac spine and umbilicus.

(Sleisenger, 8th edition, P-2090)

133. **Ans. (C)** Abnormalities or urine microscopy (hematuria and pyuria) has been noted in upto 50% cases.

(Sleisenger, 9th edition, Pp-2059-2071)

134. **Ans. (C)** Free gas in peritoneum on plain X-ray may be seen in appendiceal perforation as well.

(Sleisenger, 8th edition, P-2096)

Chapter 5

LIVER PHYSIOLOGY AND METABOLISM

1. **All of the following are true regarding bilirubin *except:***
   A. Production in adults averages 250 to 350 mg/d
   B. Derived primarily from senescent erythrocytes
   C. Liver and spleen are the site of bilirubin production
   D. "Early-labeled bilirubin" constitutes 40% of bilirubin

2. **All of the following are true regarding heme oxygenase enzyme *except:***
   A. Converts heme to biliverdin
   B. The rate of heme oxygenase activity is relatively low in the spleen
   C. Cytochrome C cannot be cleared by heme oxygenase
   D. Sn-protoporphyrin (i.e. tin) is a powerful competitive inhibitor of heme oxygenase

3. **All of the following are true regarding in the formation of bilirubin from heme *except:***
   A. Biliverdin is reduced to bilirubin by biliverdin reductase
   B. Biliverdin reductase exhibits two pH optima (pH 6.7 and 8.5) using NADH at the lower pH and NADPH at the higher pH
   C. The three catalyzing the conversion of heme to bilirubin (microsomal located at the cytosol-endoplasmic reticulum interface
   D. Complete biotransformation of heme to biliary excretion of bilirubin is of the order of half an hour

4. **All of the following are true regarding plasma transport of bilirubin *except:***
   A. At molar ratios below 1:1 bilirubin binds to a primary high affinity site on albumin
   B. Affinity between bilirubin and albumin increases as the chloride concentration increases
   C. In healthy individuals bilirubin conjugates are detectable in low levels (0.1 mg/dl)
   D. "Delta fraction" or "biliprotein" explains the disappearance of bilirubin conjugates from the urine while remaining detectable in the plasma

5. **All of the following are true regarding hepatic uptake of bilirubin *except:***
   A. Hepatic uptake of bilirubin is a rate limiting step
   B. Human OATP2 and OATP3 are expressed exclusively in the live and are capable of mediating the hepatocellular uptake of bilirubin conjugates BSP
   C. In normal persons, about 40% of the bilirubin taken up by hepatocytes in a single pass returns unchanged back into plasma
   D. Conjugated bilirubin appears to be taken up from the plasma even more rapidly than unconjugated bilirubin

6. **All of the following are true regarding intracellular transport and storage of bilirubin *except:***
   A. Fatty acid binding protein, has a lower binding affinity but a greater binding capacity than ligandin for bilirubin
   B. Ligandin is a basic protein that constitute upto 5% of the cytosolic protein in human liver
   C. In humans the "Maturation" of hepatic ligandin to adult levels during the first 1 year of life coincides with maturation of hepatic uptake mechanisms
   D. Ligandin may function as a regulatory mechanism to slow the cytosolic diffusion of bilirubin and perhaps decrease efflux back into plasma

7. **All of the following are true regarding bilirubin metabolism *except:***
   A. Bilirubin diglucuronide is the principle bilirubin conjugate in bile (80%)
   B. Bilirubin uridine diphosphate glucuronosyl-transferase (UGT1A1) in present only in the liver
   C. UGT1AZ gene lows is on chromosome 2q37
   D. UGT1A1 adult levels are attained by 14 weeks of age

8. **All of the following are true regarding bilirubin metabolism:**
   A. UGTs deamidation greatly diminishes enzyme activity
   B. Fasting increases the UDP-glucuronic acid concentration

C. UIGT1A1 is relatively more efficient in converting bilirubin to DMG than in converting BMG to BDG
D. N-acetylglucosamine enhances UGT activity toward virtually all substrates

9. **All of the following are true regarding the transport of bile pigments across the canalicular membrane *except:***
A. Biliary concentrations of bile pigments exceed those in plasma upto 40 fold
B. Canalicular excretion is rate limiting step
C. In the canalicular membrane primary transporter is multidrug resistance protein 3 (MRP 3)
D. Microtubules are inhibited in drug induced cholestasis

10. **All of the following are true regarding intestinal metabolism of bilirubin *except:***
A. The absorption of conjugated bilirubin in both the gallbladder and intestine is negligible
B. Only about 5% of the daily turnover of bilirubin is recovered as fecal urobilinogen
C. 50% of the urobilinogen undergoes on entero-hepatic circulation
D. Upto 4 mg/d of bile pigments are excreted in the urine as urobilinogen

11. **All of the following are true regarding renal excretion of bilirubin metabolite *except:***
A. Bilirubin is undetectable in patients with an unconjugated hyperbilirubinemia
B. Salicylate and sulfisoxazole decrease the renal excretion of bile pigments
C. In addition to glomerular filtration, tubular secretion and tubular absorption are involved
D. Urobilinogen absorbed more efficiently from the small intestine and then from the colon

12. **All of the following are true regarding central nervous system (CNS) interactions with bilirubin *except:***
A. CNS is the only system in which bilirubin is directly toxic
B. A fundamental mechanism of bilirubin neurotoxicity appears to be inhibition of protein phosphorylation
C. Kernicterus occurs in 1% to 3% of untreated premature newborns
D. Albumin bound bilirubin is the ultimate determinant of CNS toxicity

13. **All of the following are true regarding bilirubin metabolism in hemolytic disorder *except:***
A. Hemolysis generally given rise to a modest elevation in the plasma levels of unconjugated bilirubin (1-41 mg/dl)
B. Bilirubin is elevated in all patients with a 50% reduction in red cell survival
C. Formation of pigment gallstones is the major complication of long standing excess production of bilirubin
D. Unconjugated bilirubin may also play a role in the initation of cholesterol stones

14. **All of the following are true regarding ineffective erythropoiesis *except:***
A. A marked increase in early labeled bilirubin (EBL) is seen in disease associated with ineffective erythropoiesis
B. Red cell destruction is increased
C. Hepatic component of ELB is unchanged in most dyserythropoietic anemias
D. Markedly ineffective erythropoiesis is the basis of the rare disorder known as primary shunt hyperbilirubinemia or idiopathic dyserythropoietic jaundice

15. **All of the following are true regarding neonatal hyperbilirubinemia *except:***
A. 97% of healthy full term infants manifest biochemical hyperbilirubinemia (>1.0 mg/dl)
B. Plasma bilirubin return to normal within the first 10 days
C. A definite cause can be defined in 80% with bilirubin in a "pathologic" range (>12 mg/dl)
D. In the absence of an identifiable cause a course of phototherapy may be all that is warranted

16. **All of the following are true regarding drug induced hyperbilirubinemia *except:***
A. Rifampicin causes hyperbilirubinemia by impairing the bile secretory apparatus
B. Flavaspidic acid induce unconjugated hyper-bilirubinemia per se by diminishing the hepatic uptake of bilirubin
C. Probenecid competes with bilirubin for binding to ligandin or Z protein
D. Plasma bilirubin concentration reverts rapidly to normal following discontinuation of the offending drug

17. **All of the following are true regarding Crigler-Najjar syndrome Type I *except:***
A. Extremely rare
B. Causes severe jaundice and severe neurologic impairment

C. Primarily metabolic defect involves the secretion of bilirubin
D. In vitro assay of UGT1A1 activity reveals a virtually complete absence of bilirubin glucuronide formation

18. **All of the following are true regarding Crigler-Najjar syndrome Type I *except:***
A. Glucoronide formation in vivo is typically reduced, but not absent
B. Bilirubin production is consistently increased in these patients
C. The plasma bilirubin levels generally exceed 20 mg/dl
D. Higher bilirubin values are seen in the winter and during intercurrent illness

19. **All of the following are true regarding Crigler-Najjar syndrome Type I *except:***
A. Hepatic clearance of bilirubin is greatly diminished (1%-2% of normal)
B. Half life of circulating bilirubin exceeds 156 hours
C. Excretion of pigment into bile is markedly increased
D. Trace amounts of conjugated bilirubin may present in bile, predominantly as BMG

20. **All of the following are true regarding Crigler-Najjar syndrome Type I *except:***
A. Concentration of fecal urobilinogen is usually markedly reduced
B. Liver histology is essentially normal
C. Death usually occur in teen years
D. Phototherapy to maintain the serum bilirubin level below 21 mg/dl prevents brain damage

21. **All of the following are true regarding Crigler-Najjar syndrome Type I *except:***
A. Inherited as an autosomal-recessive trait
B. The first mutation identified involved the creation of a premature stop codon in the common exon 3 of the UGT1 locus
C. Phototherapy is not effective
D. Liver transplantation has become the treatment of choice

22. **All of the following are true regarding Crigler-Najjar syndrome Type I *except:***
A. Plasma bilirubin concentration usually ranges from 6 to 25 mg/dl
B. Plasma bilirubin levels may also increase progressively with age
C. Circulating bilirubin is virtually unconjugated
D. Red cell survival is decreased

23. **All of the following are true regarding Crigler-Najjar syndrome Type II *except:***
A. These patients do not respond to phenobarbital
B. BMGs predominate in the bile of patients with Type II disease
C. Clinical impact is usually to the social discomfort of chronic jaundice
D. Mode of inheritance is autosomal recessive

24. **All of the following are true regarding Gilbert's syndrome *except:***
A. Most often recognized in the second or third decade
B. Incidence is 3% to 7% of the population
C. Females are commonly affected
D. Hyperbilirubinemia is mild, by definition below 6 mg/dl

25. **All of the following are true regarding Gilbert's syndrome *except:***
A. Plasma bilirubin level may be normal on occasion in up-to one third of patient
B. Bilirubinuria present
C. Fecal excretion of urobilinogen is usually normal but may be slightly decreased
D. Accumulation of lipofusion like pigment, predominantly around the terminal hepatic venules is noted

26. **All of the following are true regarding Gilbert's syndrome *except:***
A. Mode of inheritance is both autosomal-recessive and autosomal-dominant
B. Two fold to three fold increase of unconjugated bilirubin seen after calorie deprivation test
C. Daily intake of 400 kcal is given for 48 hours in calorie deprivation test
D. Increase of unconjugated bilirubin in calorie deprivation is specific for Gilbert's syndrome

27. **All of the following are true regarding Glibert's syndrome *except:***
A. Fasting induced hyperbilirubinemia is multi-factorial
B. UV nicotinic acid causes 2 to 3 fold increase of plasma unconjugated bilirubin
C. Phenobarbital normalizes bilirubin
D. Corticosteroids increase plasma bilirubin

28. **All of the following are true regarding Gilbert's syndrome *except:***
A. In upto 60% of patients mild and fully compensated state of hemolysis is present
B. Increase in hepatic heme production is seen

C. Calorie deprivation test is positive in all patients
D. Most important aspect of management is reassurance

29. All of the following are true regarding conjugated hyperbilirubinemia *except:*
A. Bilirubin conjugated may be present in plasma at low levels in healthy adults (0.1 mg/dl)
B. In obstructive jaundice bilirubin in plasma usually exceed 30 mg/dl
C. In obstructive jaundice diconjugate is often the major pigment in plasma
D. Because of "delta fraction" jaundice may resolve slowly despite improvement in all liver functions

30. All of the following are true regarding Dubin-Johnson syndrome *except:*
A. Subclinical hyperbilirubinemia is often unmasked by pregnancy or the use of total contraceptives
B. Pigment disappears from the liver during the course of acute viral hepatitis
C. Hepatic pigment is lipofuscin
D. Plasma bilirubin concentration is usually between 2 and 5 mg/dl

31. All of the following are true regarding Dubin-Johnson syndrome *except:*
A. Biliary excretion of both conjugated bilirubin and BSP is markedly impaired
B. Coproporphyrin III excretion is more in the urine
C. MRP2/cMOAT gene is located on chromosome 10q24
D. Inheritance is autosomal recessive

32. All of the following are true regarding Rotor syndrome *except:*
A. Usually apparent before the age of 20 years
B. The liver is normal on histology and pigmentation is lacking
C. BSP storage capacity is normal
D. Urinary excretion of coproporphyrin I is proportionally greater than that of coproporphyrin III

Explanation

1. **Ans. (D)** Although most of the labeled bile pigment is excreted in the feces between 90 and 150 days after administration, corresponding to the end of the erythrocytes life span, between 10% and 20% of the labeled pigment appear within the first few days after administration. The production of "early labeled bilirubin" (ELB) which begins within minutes after the administration of heme precursors is attributable to the rapid turnover of free heme pools in the liver and bone marrow erythroid cells.

(Sleisenger, 9th edition, Pp-323-324)

2. **Ans. (B)** The rate of heme oxygenase activity is relatively high in the spleen; heme oxygenase is also present in both parenchymal and Kupffer cells in the liver and to a lesser extent in bone marrow, the proximal renal tubular cells, macrophages and the choroids plexus.

(Sleisenger, 9th edition, Pp-323-324)

3. **Ans. (D)** Studies in vivo indicate that the total time required for the complete biotransformation of heme to biliverdin, the reduction of biliverdin to bilirubin and conjugation and biliary excretion of bilirubin is of the order of 1 to 2 minutes.

(Sleisenger, 9th edition, Pp-323-324)

4. **Ans. (D)** Electrolyte concentration also affects bilirubin and albumin binding; affinities decrease as the chloride concentration increase. The fact that lysine residues play an important role in establishing salt linkages between the albumin polypeptide and bilirubin may be relevant to the effect of electrolytes on albumin affinity.

(Sleisenger, 9th edition, Pp-323-324)

5. **Ans. (A)** The hepatic uptake system normal operates well below saturation, and its maximum capacity greatly exceeds that of bilirubin excretion, so that uptake is not rate-limiting in hepatic bilirubin transport.

(Sleisenger, 9th edition, Pp-323-324)

6. **Ans. (C)** In humans the "maturation" of hepatic ligandin to adult levels during the first 5 to 10 days of life coincides with the maturation of the hepatic uptake mechanisms for organic anions.

(Sleisenger, 9th edition, Pp-323-324)

7. **Ans. (B)** The liver is the major biologic source of bilirubin glucornoides and has the highest content of UGT1a1. Functional data, immunohistochemical techniques and molecular biologic studies have demonstrated the presence of UGT1A1 in jejunum, rat kidney and skin.

(Sleisenger, 9th edition, Pp-323-325)

8. **Ans. (B)** Fasting decreases the UDP glucuronoic acid concentration and may be a contributing mechanism to the fasting hyperbilirubinemia of Gilbert's syndrome.

(Sleisenger, 9th edition, P-325)

9. **Ans. (C)** The primary transporter in canalicular membrane is multi-drug resistance protein 2 (MRP2) also known as canalicular multispecific organic anion transporter (cMOAT). A transporter system is also present on the basolateal plasma membrane, multidrug resistance protein 3 (MRP3) that is capable of secreting bilirubin conjugates into the sinusoidal blood.

(Sleisenger, 9th edition, P-324)

10. **Ans. (C)** Urobilinogen undergoes an enterohepatic circulation, although less than 20% of the amount produced daily is reabsorbed because it is formed mostly in the colon, where the absorption rate is low, about 90% of this promptly excreted by the liver into bile; the remaining 10% reaching the systemic circulation is excreted in the urine approximately 2% of the urobilinogen produced daily.

(Sleisenger, 9th edition, P-324)

11. **Ans. (B)** Compounds that compete with conjugated bilirubin for protein binding, such as salicylate, sufisoxazole and bile salts, increase the amount of diffusible conjugated bilirubin and augment the renal excretion of bile pigments.

(Sleisenger, 9th edition, Pp-324-325)

12. **Ans. (D)** It appears that "free" bilirubin is the ultimate determinants of central nervous system toxicity because this is the form of bilirubin that is exchanged with cell membranes and intracellular organelles.

(Sleisenger, 9th edition, P-324)

13. **Ans. (B)** Although the level of plasma bilirubin increases linearly in relation to the production of bilirubin the plasma concentration of bilirubin may still be nearly normal in patients with a 50% reduction in red cell survival provided that the hepatic clearance of bilirubin is normal.

(Sleisenger, 9th edition, P-324)

14. **Ans. (B)** In patients with ineffective erythropoiesis characterized by abnormalities in heme biosynthesis within the developing normoblast, red cell destruction is not increased but total bile pigment turnover is significantly increased.

(Sleisenger, 9th edition, P-325)

15. **Ans. (C)** Of these infants with plasma bilirubin in a "pathologic" range (>12mg/dl), a definite cause can be defined in fewer than 50%.

(Sleisenger, 9th edition, Pp-323-325)

16. **Ans. (A)** Although numerous drugs may cause hyperbilirubinemia by impairing the bile secretory apparatus drugs such as rifampicin and other rifamycin antibiotics, bunamiodyl, flavaspidic acid and probenecid occasionally may induce unconjugated hyperbilirubinemia per se by diminishing the hepatic uptake of bilirubin and possibly by competing with bilirubin for binding to ligandin or Z protein.

(Sleisenger, 9th edition, P-325)

17. **Ans. (C)** The primary defect in Crigler-Najjar syndrome Type I involves the conjugation of bilirubin.

(Sleisenger, 9th edition, P-326)

18. **Ans. (B)** Bilirubin production is consistently normal in these patients, as assessed by the plasma hemoglobin concentration, reticulocyte count, and erythrocyte survival, the magnitude and kinetics of the ELB fraction and the plasma bilirubin turnover.

(Sleisenger, 9th edition, P-326)

19. **Ans. (C)** The excretion of pigment into bile is markedly reduced, with unconjugated bilirubin-IX comprising 30% to 57% of the total bile pigment excreted (<1% in normal subjects) although the absolute amount of unconjugated bilirubin in bile is only one to seven times that observed in normal adults and constitutes only a minor fraction of the total bilirubin produced.

(Sleisenger, 9th edition, Pp-325-326)

20. **Ans. (C)** When the condition is untreated, death usually occurs within 18 months after birth, although rarely patients' survival beyond puberty before bilirubin encephalopathy develops.

(Sleisenger, 9th edition, P-326)

21. **Ans. (C)** The efficacy of phototherapy in the management of neonatal jaundice is well established, with documented excretion of essentially all photoisomers of bilirubin in urine. This therapeutic modality has also been successful in reducing plasma bilirubin levels to less than 10 mg/dl in some infants with Crigler-Najjar syndrome Type I.

(Sleisenger, 9th edition, Pp-325-326)

22. **Ans. (D)** Red cell survival and bilirubin production are normal, but hepatic clearance is markedly diminished.

(Sleisenger, 9th edition, P-326)

23. **Ans. (A)** Unlike patients with Crigler-Najjar syndrome Type I, those with Type II respond to phenobarbital which presumably acts tropically on the endoplasmic reticulum and increases UGT1A1 activity, although the precise mechanism of the response to phenobarbital has not yet been defined.

(Sleisenger, 9th edition, P-326)

24. **Ans. (C)** Male to female ratio is 2:1 to 7:1 population studies have shown that in generally the plasma bilirubin level is higher in men than women, possibly as a consequence of hormonal effects of UGT1A1 activity or other factors, including sex differences inorganic anion uptake by the liver.

(Sleisenger, 9th edition, P-326)

25. **Ans. (B)** Because the plasma bilirubin is virtually all unconjugated, bilirubinuria is absent.

(Sleisenger, 9th edition, P-326)

26. **Ans. (D)** Fasting also has been shown to increase plasma levels of unconjugated bilirubin in patients with liver disease or hemolysis, the magnitude of this rise is considerably less that observed in persons with Gilbert's syndrome.

(Sleisenger, 9th edition, Pp-325-326)

27. **Ans. (D)** Corticosteroids administration significantly reduces the plasma concentration of bilirubin in patients with Gilbert's syndrome via an increase in the hepatic uptake or storage of bilirubin.

(Sleisenger, 9th edition, Pp-325-326)

28. **Ans. (C)** Not all patients with Gilbert's syndrome respond to calorie deprivation test which appear less

sensitive and specific for female than for male subjects.

(Sleisenger, 9th edition, Pp-325-326)

29. **Ans. (C)** In obstructive jaundice, the concentration of bilirubin in plasma gradually increases and if the obstruction is complete, plateaus between 10 and 30 mg/dl. Concentrations above 30 mg/dl are more likely to be found in hepatocellular disease than in biliary obstruction.

(Sleisenger, 9th edition, P-326)

30. **Ans. (C)** The chemical nature of the pigment remains unclear. Earlier investigators assumed that the pigment belonged to the ill-defined group of lipofuscin and later histochemical, spectroscopic and physiochemical analysis suggested that it was closely related to melanin. More recent studies with electron spin resonance spectroscopy indicate that the pigment is not melanin and probably not a porphyrin but it possibly made up of polymers of adrenaline (epinephrine) metabolites.

(Sleisenger, 9th edition, P-326)

31. **Ans. (B)** The urine of healthy persons contains copro-porphyrin isomers I and III with about 75% in the form of isomer III, reflecting the fact that the isomers in series III are precursors in heme biosynthesis. In Dubin-Johnson syndrome, urinary excretion of coproporphyrin is normal or only slightly increased but more than 80% is coproporphyrin I.

(Sleisenger, 9th edition, P-326)

32. **Ans. (C)** The BSP transport maximum is modestly reduced, whereas the relative hepatic storage capacity for BSP may be decreased by as much as 90%. In contrast, the transport maximum is almost zero and storage capacity is normal in Dubin-Johnson syndrome.

(Sleisenger, 9th edition, P-326)

Chapter 6

LIVER DISEASES

1. **Mean fall of portal vein pressure following TIPS:**
   A. 30% B. 50%
   C. 70% D. 100%

2. **TIPS is a type of:**
   A. End to end shunt B. Side to side shunt
   C. End to side shunt D. Mesocaval shunt

3. **Diagnosis of ischemic cholangitis following liver transplant is by:**
   A. Liver biopsy B. MRI
   C. CT scan D. Spiral CT

4. **Hepatic veins within fatty liver are best visualized by:**
   A. CT scan without contrast
   B. Doppler US
   C. Contrast enhanced CT
   D. MRI

5. **The lipid solubility of bilirubin is explained by:**
   A. Hydrogen bonds
   B. Tetra pyrrole ring
   C. A bridge carbon atom
   D. IX a biliverdin

6. **Benign liver tumor associated with CCF:**
   A. Juvenile hemangioendothelioma
   B. Cavernous hemangioma
   C. Nodular regenerative hyperplasia
   D. Multiple hepatic adenoma

7. **Multiple hepatic adenomas are associated with glycogen storage disease:**
   A. Type I B. Type II
   C. Type III D. Type IV

8. **The following are para-neoplastic manifestations of HCC *except:***
   A. Hypothyroidism
   B. Erythrocytosis
   C. Peripheral neuropathy
   D. Acquired porphyria

9. **Immune histochemical stain revealing factor VIII antigen on hepatocytes is diagnostic of:**
   A. Fibro lamellar carcinoma
   B. Hepatoblastoma
   C. Hemangiosarcoma
   D. Hemangioendothelioma

10. **Hepatic toxin causing zone I necrosis:**
    A. Phosphorus + iron
    B. CCl_4
    C. Halothane
    D. Acetaminophen

11. **Maximum quantity of alcohol that can be metabolized by liver per day:**
    A. 100 g B. 180 g
    C. 220 g D. 120 g

12. **One gram of alcohol gives:**
    A. 4 cal B. 7 cal
    C. 10 cal D. No cal

13. **All are bad prognostic indicators in alcoholic liver disease on liver biopsy *except:***
    A. Zone II fibrosis
    B. Megamitochondria
    C. Perivenular sclerosis
    D. Cholestasis

14. **Copper rich foods include all *except:***
    A. Shell fish B. Chocolates
    C. Mushroom D. Egg

15. **Normal daily dietary intake of copper is:**
    A. 4 mg B. 2 mg
    C. 1 mg D. 5 mg

16. **Wilson's disease can present clinically as all *except*:**
    A. Sensory neuropathy
    B. Primary amenorrhoea
    C. Recurrent abortions
    D. Schizophrenia

17. **All are copper containing enzymes *except:***
    A. Cytochrome oxidase
    B. Tyrosinase
    C. Superoxide dismutase
    D. Glutathione-S-transferase

18. **Earliest histological feature of Wilson's hepatic involvement is:**
    A. Bile duct proliferation

B. Increased glycogen/fat deposition
C. Portal inflammation
D. Perivenular fibrosis

19. **Locus of Wilson's disease:**
A. 13q14-q21 B. 13q7-q22
C. 13q11-q18 D. 13q6-q18

20. **The first joints to be involved in hemochromatosis are:**
A. First and second metacarpophalangeal joints
B. Second and third metacarpophalangeal joints
C. Knee joints
D. Temporomandibular joints

21. **In hemochromatosis phlebotomy improve all the following *except:***
A. Liver function B. Survival
C. Diabetes D. Arthropathy

22. **For each increase in 1 mg/l of ferritin, the increase in body iron stores is approximately:**
A. 45 mg B. 65 mg
C. 85 mg D. 500 mg

23. **The most common psychiatric manifestation of Wilson's disease is:**
A. Schizophrenia
B. Maniac depressive psychosis
C. Neurosis
D. Bizarre behaviour

24. **Fatty liver is defined as triglycerides more than of total liver weight:**
A. 2% B. 5%
C. 10% D. 15%

25. **Zone I fatty infiltration of liver is seen with all *except:***
A. PEM B. TPN
C. Methotrexate D. Obesity

26. **Colourless bile is seen in:**
A. Crigler-Najjar-I
B. Crigler-Najjar-II
C. Dubin-Johnson syndrome
D. Lucy-Driscoll syndrome

27. **In normal pregnancy all the following parameters can be deranged *except:***
A. Alkaline phosphates
B. Amino transferases
C. BSP retention
D. Serum bilirubin

28. **Which one of the following is a non-enveloped virus?**
A. HAV
B. HDV
C. HCV
D. HBV

29. **The hepatitis virus with the largest genome is:**
A. HAV B. HBV
C. HCV D. HDV

30. **The following hepatitis viral antigen is present in the nucleus:**
A. HBSAg B. HCV
C. HDV D. HEV

31. **In acute HCV infection the antibody to which viral protein is not detected is:**
A. C33c B. C100-3
C. C22-3 D. NS 5

32. **Sexual transmission is not seen with:**
A. HAV B. HCV
C. HDV D. HEV

33. **The indication for liver transplant which has maximum recurrence rate of HBV is:**
A. HBV DNA +ve cirrhosis
B. FHF with HBV
C. Cirrhosis due to HDV
D. Cirrhosis due to HDV
E. FHF with HDV

34. **Least recurrence rate of HBV after liver transplant is for:**
A. HBV DNA +ve cirrhosis
B. FHF with HBV
C. Cirrhosis due to HDV
D. FHF with HDV

35. **Most common indication for liver transplantation in adults is:**
A. PBC
B. HCV related cirrhosis
C. Alcoholic cirrhosis
D. Fulminant hepatitis

36. **Elevated alkaline phosphates with normal GGT is seen in all the following *except:***
A. Elderly males B. Pregnancy
C. Byler's disease D. BRIC

37. **All the following increase cyclosporine levels *except:***
A. Erythromycin B. Omeprazole
C. Ketoconazole D. Metoclopramide

38. **The mean time for sonographic disappearance of amoebic liver abscess is:**
A. 2-4 months B. 4-6 months
C. 6-9 months D. 10-12 months

39. **Rarest congenital hyperbilirubinemia is:**
A. Crigler-Najjar I
B. Crigler-Najjar II
C. Rotor syndrome
D. Dubin-Johnson syndrome

40. **Drug causing unconjugated hypebilirubinemia:**
A. Cholorpromazine
B. Methimazole
C. Rifampicin
D. PAS

41. **AST/ALT ratio is typically less than 1 in:**
A. Alcoholic hepatitis
B. NASH
C. Cirrhosis
D. Fatty liver of pregnancy

42. **Highest levels of transaminases are seen in:**
A. Prolonged hypotension
B. CAH
C. Cirrhosis
D. Hepatic metastases

43. **All the following cause increased aminotransferase *except:***
A. Acute MI B. Myopathy
C. Toxins D. Uremia

44. **All are infectious cause of Budd-Chiari syndrome *except:***
A. Actinomyces
B. Syphilis
C. TB
D. Amoebic liver abscess

45. **Prevalence of portal vein thrombosis in cirrhosis is:**
A. 6% B. 10%
C. 16% D. 25%

46. **P450 II D6 is the antigen for:**
A. Anti-SLA B. Anti-LKM
C. Anti-LKM1 D. AMA

47. **One of the following is not a risk factor for SBP:**
A. Low ascitic protein B. UTI
C. Paracentesis D. GI bleed

48. **Non-nitrogenous precipitating factor for hepatic encephalopathy include all *except:***
A. Hypothyroidism B. Anaemia
C. Sedatives D. Infection

49. **Frontline tumor marker for HCC in low incidence areas is:**
A. AFP
B. Fucosylated AFP
C. α-1 Fucosidase
D. Des-γ-carboxy prothrombin

50. **Tumor marker for fibrolamellar variant of HCC is:**
A. Fucosylated AFP
B. α_1-Fucosidase
C. Neurotensin
D. Isoenzymes of GGT

51. **The minimum level of AFP which is strongly suggestive of HCC is:**
A. 500 ng/ml B. 500 ng/l
C. 1000 ng/ml D. 1000 mg/ml

52. **All are major risk factors for HCC *except:***
A. Hemochromatosis
B. Cirrhosis
C. Aflatoxin B
D. Chronic hepatitis C

53. **All are major risk factors for HCC *except:***
A. Hemochromatosis
B. Cirrhosis
C. Aflatoxin B
D. Chronic-C

54. **All are risk factors for HCC *except:***
A. Ataxia telangiectasia
B. Membranous obstruction of IVC
C. Cigarette smoking
D. Type IV glycogen disorder

55. **Risk factor for HCC in a non-cirrhotic liver occurs in:**
A. Hemochromatosis
B. Type I glycogen storage disease
C. Type I tyrosinemia
D. α_1 - AT deficiency

56. **Risk of liver cancer in a cirrhotic liver per year is:**
A. 0.5% B. 1%
C. 6% D. 3%

57. **Pathognomonic histologic lesion in liver of cystic fibrosis is:**
A. Inspissated granular material in portal bile ductules
B. Focal biliary cirrhosis
C. Ductular proliferation with inflammatory infiltrate
D. Paucity of bile ducts

58. **All cause increased serum ceruloplasmin levels *except:***
A. Pregnancy
B. Decompensated cirrhosis
C. Oestrogen therapy
D. Large bile duct obstruction

59. For significant decrease in variceal bleeding HPVG should be reduced to a minimum of baseline:
A. 10%
B. 20%
C. 30%
D. 50%

60. The false statement regarding C3 complement levels is:
A. It is normal in chronic hepatitis
B. Increased in PBC
C. Decreased in cirrhosis
D. Increased in FHF

61. Hepatic enlargement in Type I diabetes is predominantly due to:
A. Increased triglycerides
B. Increased glycogen
C. A + B
D. None

62. The type of 'Glycogenoses' that does not affect liver:
A. Type V only
B. Type VII only
C. Type V and VI
D. Type V and VII

63. All the following liver abnormalities occur in Type I glucogenoses (von-Gierke's disease) *except:*
A. Cirrhosis
B. Hepatic adenoma
C. HCC
D. Fatty liver

64. Sex linked glycogen storage disorder is:
A. Type I
B. Type V
C. Type VI
D. Type IX

65. Liver transplantation is definitive treatment for the following type of amyloidosis:
A. Secondary amyloidosis
B. Primary type with myeloma association
C. Primary type without myeloma association
D. Familial amyloidotic polyneuropathy

66. One of the following is not associated with hepatic granulomas:
A. Q fever
B. PBC
C. Infectious mononucleosis
D. Primary syphilis

67. Treatment of pyogenic liver abscess includes:
A. IV broad spectrum antibiotics alone
B. Antibiotics with percutaneous drainage
C. Percutaneous drainage alone
D. Antibiotics with open drainage

68. A 50-year-old man with liver cirrhosis of unknown cause has reported to the clinic. Which one of the following factors is most likely to indicate poor prognosis?
A. ALT>200 IU/L
B. Caput medusa
C. Ascites
D. Gynecomastia
E. Splenomegaly

69. You wish to screen for hepatitis B infection. Which of the following is the most suitable test to perform ?
A. HBsAg
B. HBcAg
C. Hepatitis B viral load
D. Anti-HBsAb
E. HBeAg

70. A 52-year-old man is diagnosed as NAFLD following a liver biopsy. What is the single most important step to help prevent progression of the disease?
A. Life style changes
B. Diet
C. Metformin
D. Pioglitazone

71. In patients of hemochromatosis which is the first useful investigation?
A. Transferring saturation + ferritin
B. Hematocrit + ferritin
C. Liver biopsy with pearl's stain
D. Serum iron + ferritin
E. Serum iron + hematocrit

72. A 54-year-old woman presents with jaundice shortly after being discharged from hospital. The liver function tests show serum bilirubin 20 mg/dl, ALT 66 IU/L, ALP 280 IU/L, GGT 529 U/L, 49 gm/L. Which is the most likely antibiotic which may cause derangement of liver functions?
A. Flucloxacillin
B. Gentamycin
C. Ciprofloxacillin
D. Trimethoprim
E. Ceftazidime

73. A 22-year-old blood donor reported with the following liver function report–bilirubin 2.1 mg% with predominant unconjugated pattern, ALP 84 U/L, ALT 23U//L, Albumin 41 gm/L; dipstick urinalysis-no hemoglobinuria. Which is the most likely diagnosis?

A. Gilbert's disease
B. Dubin-Johnson's syndrome
C. Rotor syndrome
D. Hepatitis C
E. Infectious mononucleosis

74. A 23-year-old nurse is referred to occupational health following a needle stick injury from a man known to be carrier of hepatitis B. Which one of the following marker will appear on the first few days of acute hepatitis B infection?
A. HBsAg
B. Anti-HBc
C. HBeAg
D. HBV DNA

75. A 42-year-old man is referred with abnormal LFT and hepatitis screening is done which shows:

Anti-HAV IgG negative

HBSAg negative

Anti-HBS positive

Anti-HBc negative

Anti-HCV positive

Which does the result demonstrate?
A. Hepatitis B infection
B. Hepatitis C infection
C. Previous vaccination to hepatitis B
D. Hepatitis C infection with previous hepatitis B vaccination
E. Hepatitis B and C infection

76. Which of the following is the most useful prognostic marker in paracetamol induced acute liver failure?
A. ALT
B. Prothrombin time
C. Paracetamol level at presentation
D. Paracetamol level at 24 hours

77. Primary sclerosing cholangitis is mostly associated with:
A. PBC
B. Crohn's disease
C. Hepatitis C infection
D. Ulcerative colitis
E. Celiac disease

78. All the following suitable factors for interferon treatment for chronic hepatitis B *except:*
A. Elevated ALT
B. Immune competence
C. Compensated liver disease
D. Pro-core mutants

79. Which of the following side effect of interferon treatment is irreversible?
A. Bone marrow suppression
B. Alopecia
C. Auto immune thyroiditis
D. Emotional lability

80. Most potent nucleoside analogue against HBV is:
A. 3' Thiacytidine
B. Stavudine
C. Ganciclovir
D. Famciclovir

81. HBV is a:
A. Single stranded DNA virus
B. Partially double stranded DNA virus
C. Complete double stranded DNA virus
D. Double stranded RNA virus

82. Prevalence of HBsAg is increased in all the conditions *except:*
A. Down's syndrome
B. Lepromatous leprosy
C. PAN
D. Diabetes

83. All are features of replicative phase chronic hepatitis B *except:*
A. Presence of HbeAg
B. Intrahepatocytic HbcAg
C. Integrated HBV DNA
D. Severe chronic hepatitis on biopsy

84. Blumberg discovered:
A. HBsAg
B. IgM anti HBC
C. Antibodies to Hep B
D. Anti-HCV antibody
E. None of the above

85. The false statement regarding virion of hepatitis B is:
A. The core is formed in hepatocyte nucleus
B. Surface particle is formed in cytoplasm
C. Core contains DNA polymerase
D. Core contains core antigen and E antigen
E. DNA structure is single stranded and circular

86. Serological marker that is not detected in serum of patients with HBC infection is:
A. Anti Hbs antibodies
B. E antigen
C. Anti HBe antibodies
D. HBcAg
E. DBV DNA

87. HBV precore mutants exhibit all these markers *except:*

A. HBsAg B. HBeAg
C. HBV DNA D. All are absent

88. Incidence of acute and chronic hepatitis B is high in all these *except:*
A. Neonates of HBsAg mothers
B. Patients with immunosuppression
C. Post-transfusion
D. Amyloidosis

89. The arthropathy in HBV is:
A. Asymmetrical non-migratory affecting small joints
B. Symmetrical migratory affecting hand joints
C. Symmetrical non-migratory affecting foot joints
D. Asymmetrical non-migratory affecting large joints

90. Extrahepatic associations of HBV are:
A. Polyarteritis, golmerular nephritis
B. Guillain-Barré syndrome
C. Polymyalgia rhematica, myocarditis
D. Essential mixed cryoglobulinaemia
E. All the above

91. The correct statement about hepatitis B infection is:
A. 10% of the patients in adults will not clear HBsAg
B. 90% of those infected as neonates will become chronic
C. Males are more likely to become carriers than females
D. Healthy carriers may show minimal to chronic hepatitis or cirrhosis
E. All the statements are correct

92. Surface mutants show all these *except:*
A. Seen in infants born to HBsAg positive mothers even after vaccination
B. There is substitution of arginine for glycine at amino acid 145
C. Genetic mutation in 5 gene
D. HBeAg is absent

93. Hepatitis B vaccination is indicated in:
A. Patients and staff of oncology, haematology. kidney, liver disease
B. Close family and sexual contacts of patients with HBsAg positive
C. Babies born to HBsAg positive mother
D. Drug abusers, homosexually active men, travellers to high risk areas
E. All the above groups

94. In a healthy individual, HB vaccine of 10 μg IM at 0, 1 and 6 months induces antibodies in:
A. 40% B. 60%
C. 75% D. 90%
E. 100%

95. Failure of antibody response to Hep B vaccine is seen in:
A. Age more than 50 years
B. Patients with underlying immunosuppression
C. Buttock injection, frozen vaccine
D. HIV positives, genetics (HLA B 8)
E. All the above

96. All are correct combination *except:*
A. HAV-Flavivirus like
B. HBV-Hepadna virus
C. HCV-Flavivirus
D. HDV-Resembles viroids
E. HEV-Alpha virus

97. All are correct regarding replicative stage of HBV infection *except:*
A. E antigen is qualitative marker
B. HBV DNA is quantitative marker
C. In early chronic HBV infection, HBV DNA is in serum and hepatocyte nucleus
D. Replicative stage does not give way to non-replicative stage
E. All are correct

98. Hepatitis A vaccine is necessary for all the following *except:*
A. Nurses working in intensive care centers
B. Food handlers and sewage workers
C. School children and staff in day care centers
D. Military working in areas hygiene is poor
E. None of the above

99. Replication of HAV occurs in:
A. Blood B. Stool
C. Bile D. Liver

100. All are correct about hepatitis A virus *except*:
A. Envelope virus
B. 27 nm
C. Heat, acid and either resistant RNA
D. Contains four capsid poly peptides, VP1-VP4

101. Fulminant hepatitis is most common with:
A. Hepatitis A virus
B. Hepatitis B virus
C. Hepatitis C virus
D. Hepatitis D virus
E. Hepatitis E virus

102. All are correct regarding prophylactic immunoglobulin in hepatitis A *except:*
A. Administered before exposure of during early incubation IG is effective in preventing A
B. Dose administered is 0.02 ml/kg

C. It has no role in limiting the frequency of secondary cases
D. High dose and repeated approach is recommended for personnel who work with HAV
E. Vaccine is used above age of 2 years and provide protection after four weeks of inoculation

103. All of the following are true regarding primary biliary cirrhosis (PBC) *except:*
A. Female: Male ratio is 9:1
B. Median age of onset is 50 years
C. Second common cholestatic disorder in children
D. HLA DR8 is most frequently observed

104. All of the following regarding autoantibodies in primary biliary cirrhosis are true *except:*
A. Pyruvate dehydrogenase complex (PDC-E_2) is located on the inner mitochondrial membrane
B. PDC-E_2 reacting antibodies are present in more than 90% of PBC patients
C. AMAs are predominantly IgM class
D. PBC-specific autoantibodies against protein gp210 carrier specificity of above 99% for PBC

105. All of the following are true regarding symptomotology of PBC *except:*
A. Fatigue is the most common symptom
B. Pruritus worsens as the disease progresses
C. Jaundice occurs later and associated with a poor prognosis
D. Symptoms may also be related fat soluble vitamin deficiency

106. All of the following are true regarding disease associated with primary biliary cirrhosis *except:*
A. Keratoconjunctivitis sicca is seen in 72-100% of patients
B. Cause of renal tubular acidosis may relate to excess copper deposition within the kidney
C. Gall stones can be found in 1/3rd of the patients
D. Risk for HCC is not increased

107. All of the following are true regarding the diagnosis of PBC *except:*
A. Aminotransferases level are usually more than five times than normal
B. AMA of M2 type has a sensitivity rate of 98% and specificity rate of 96%
C. Most important diagnostic clue is ductopenia defined as the absence of interlobular bile ducts in more than 50% of portal tracts
D. Lymphadenopathy in hilar area is noted in about 24% of PBC patients

108. All the following are true regarding ursodeoxycholic acid (UDCA) usage in PBC *except:*
A. UDCA constitutes less than 4% of total bile acids in human bile
B. It reduces the expression of major histocompatibility (MHC) class I and class II antigens on the biliary epithelium
C. It does not decrease the risk of gastroesophageal varices or delays progression to cirrhosis
D. The most cost effective dose of UDCA in PBC is 13 to 15 mg/kg/day

109. All of the following are true regarding complication of chronic cholestasis in PBC *except:*
A. Most PBC patients who have osteopenia as a result of cholestasis have underlying osteoporosis rather than osteoalacia
B. Vitamin E deficiency in PBC primarily affects the posterior columns and is characterized by areflexia or loss of proprioception and ataxia
C. Surgery is the treatment of choice for xanthelasmas that are followed because of hypercholesterolemia
D. Steatorrhea in PBC is mainly caused by decreased delivery of bile acid to intestines other cause are pancreatic insufficiency and celiac sprue in some cases

110. All of the following are true regarding physical examination in a patient with ascites *except:*
A. Approximately 500 ml of fluid must be present before dullness is detected
B. If flank dullness is not present, the chance that the patient has ascites is less than 10%
C. Ultrasonography can detect as little as 100 ml of fluid
D. The presence of large veins on the patients back suggests inferior vena cava blockage

111. All of the following are true regarding abdominal paracentesis in cirrhotics *except:*
A. Coagulopathy should preclude paracentesis only when there is clinically evident fibrinolysis or disseminated intravascular coagulation
B. Fresh frozen plasma and platelets are routinely transfused before paracentesis in cirrhotic patients with coagulopathy
C. Preferred site is the left lower quadrant two fingerbreadths cephalad and two fingerbreadths medial to the anterior superior iliac spine
D. To prevent leakage of ascites, the needle is inserted using iliac spine

112. High serum ascites albumin gradient ascites (SAAG) is seen in all of the following conditions *except:*

A. Massive liver metastasis
B. Nephrotic syndrome
C. "Mixed" ascites
D. Myxedema

113. All of the following are true regarding serum ascites albumin gradient (SAAG) *except:*
A. If the SAAG is greater than or equal to 1.1 g/dl (11 g/l) the patient can be diagnosed with portal hypertension with an accuracy of approximately 97%
B. Arterial hypotension may result in falsely low SAAG
C. Chylous ascites may result in falsely low SAAG
D. Serum hyperglobulinemia can narrow the albumin gradient

114. All of the following are true regarding ascitic fluid analysis *except:*
A. Bedside inoculation of blood culture bottles with ascitic fluid detects growth in approximately 80%
B. In the setting of gut perforation into ascitic fluid, the ascitic glucose concentration usually drops to 0 mg/dl
C. In secondary peritonitis ascitic fluid LDH level is lower than the serum LDH level
D. In acute pancreatitis or gut perforation ascetic fluid amylase concentration is elevated markedly, usually greater than 200 U/L

115. All of the following are true in the differential diagnosis of ascites *except:*
A. In patients with ascites a cause other than liver disease is found in approximately 40% patients
B. Chlamydia peritonitis occurs in young women with fever and it is neutrocytic, high protein and low gradient ascites
C. Cirrhosis is the cause of chylous ascites in more than 90% of the patients
D. Ovarian hyperstimulation syndrome can cause ascites

116. All of the following are true regarding ascitic fluid infection *except:*
A. The diagnosis of spontaneous bacterial peritonitis (SBP) is made when there is a positive ascitic fluid culture and an elevated ascitic fluid PMN count (i.e. at least 250 cells/mm^3) without evidence of an intra-abdominal surgical treatable source of infection
B. In secondary bacterial peritonitis ascitic fluid culture is positive (Usually for multiple organisms)
C. In polymicrobial bacterascites the PMN count is higher than 250 cells/mm^3
D. SBP can occur in fulminant hepatic failure also

117. All of the following are true regarding ascitic fluid infection *except:*
A. Low protein ascetic fluid (e.g.<1 g/dl) is particularly susceptible to SBP
B. Monomicrobial non-neutorcytic bacterascites (MNB) probably represent an early stage of ascitic fluid infection, which can resolve to culture negative neutrocytic ascites (NNA) or progress to spontaneous bacterial peritonitis (SBP)
C. Inoculation into blood culture bottles can detect a single organism in the cultured aliquot of fluid
D. More than 50% of patients with SBP are asymptomatic

118. All of the following are true regarding ascitic fluid infection *except:*
A. E. coli, streptococci (mostly pneumococci) and klebsiella cause most episodes of SBP and MNB
B. In selective intestinal decontamination patients gram-positive organisms are usually cultured
C. Needle induced ascitic fluid infection occurs in one in 1000 taps
D. Gastrointestinal hemorrhage is not a risk for SBP

119. All of the following are true regarding ascitic fluid infection *except:*
A. Convincing symptoms or signs of infection are an indication for empirical antibiotic therapy
B. Culture of ascitic fluid in gallbladder rupture disclose multiple organisms
C. Total protein greater than 1 g/dl glucose less than 50 mg/dl and LDH greater than upper limit of normal for serum indicates secondary bacterial peritonitis
D. Bilirubin greater than 6 mg% and greater than serum level is indicative of biliary or upper gut perforation into ascites

120. All of the following are true regarding treatment of SBP *except:*
A. In monomicrobial non-neutrocytic bacterascites (NNB) treatment is required if the patient is symptomatic or culture is persistently positive
B. Approximately 50% of gram stains demonstrate organisms in SBP
C. Fully 98% of causative organisms were susceptible of cefotaxime
D. Intravenous albumin plus antibiotic reduce the risk of renal failure and improve survival

121. All of the following are true regarding ascites *except:*
A. For the primary prevention of ascetic fluid infection in patients with low protein ascites, it is appropriate to restrict the use of prophylactic antibiotics to in patients only
B. Hepatic hydrothorax sometimes can occur as unilateral left side effusion
C. TIPS is a reasonable second line treatment in hepatic hydrothorax
D. Control of ascites is required before umbilical hernia repair

122. All of the following are true regarding treatment of ascites *except:*
A. Low SAAG ascites responds to salt restriction and diuretics
B. Dietary sodium restriction of 2 gram (88 mmol per day is recommended)
C. Severe hyponatremia (e.g. serum sodium concentration <120 mmol/L) does warrant fluid restriction
D. Symptoms of hyponatremia develop if serum sodium concentration is below 110 mmol/L

123. All of the following are true regarding treatment of ascites *except:*
A. Random urine sodium/potassium ratio greater than 1 predicts good natriuresis
B. Half life of spironalactone is markedly prolonged in patients with cirrhosis: almost 1 month is required to reach a steady state
C. Without edema a reasonable maximum weight loss is probably 1 kg/day
D. Encephalopathy, hyponatremia less than 120 mmol/L despite fluid restriction, or a serum creatinine level greater than 2 mg/dl should result in cessation of diuretics

124. All of the following are true regarding primary sclerosing cholangitis (PSC) *except:*
A. 80% of patients with PSC have concomitant inflammatory bowel disease
B. Occurs more commonly in patients with ulcerative colitis (UC) than in those with Crohn's disease
C. PSC occurs with a frequency of 3% of 5.6 of patients with UC and 12% of those with Crohn's disease
D. UC may run a severe course in patients with PSC than in those without PSC

125. All of the following are true regading PSC *except:*
A. Female preponderance is seen
B. Inverse relationship between smoking and the incidence of PSC is noted
C. Predominately extrahepatic disease is seen in 6%
D. Upto 44% of patients will be asymptomatic at the time of diagnosis

126. All of the following are true regarding PSC *except:*
A. Concentric fibrosis with obliteration of the small ducts (obliterative fibrous cholangitis)–a virtually diagnostic histopathologic lesion is found in fewer than 10% of specimens
B. Small duct PSC is seen in 20% of the PSC patients
C. Caudate pseudotumor (a low attenuation ring like appearance of the right lobe of the liver in the presence of hypertrophy of the caudate lobe) is found only in patients with PSC
D. Position emission tomography (PET) is able to detect small cholangiocarcinomas

127. All of the following are true regarding cholangiographic features of PSC *except:*
A. Intrahepatic ducts alone are involved in 15% to 30% of patients
B. Extrahepatic ducts alone are involved in less than 10% of patients
C. In the presence of IBD extrahepatic duct involvement is more common
D. Dominant strictures occur with greatest frequency (75%) in the area of hepatic duct bifurcation

128. All of the following are true regarding PSC *except:*
A. Jaundice, pruritus, abdominal pain and fever may remit spontaneously and for prolonged periods
B. Asymptomatic PSC constitute 10% of patients
C. Normal alkaline phosphates level is seen in 6% of the patients
D. ANCA is positive in 65% to 84% of cases

129. All of the following are true regarding occurrence of malignancy in PSC *except:*
A. Cholangiocarcinoma most commonly occurs around the common hepatic duct and its bifurcation
B. Longer duration of PSC increases the risk of cholangiocarcinoma
C. Fibrolamellar variant of HCC can occur
D. Proximal colonic neoplasm are common

130. All of the following are true regarding recurrent pyogenic cholangitis *except:*

A. Characterized by intrahepatic pigment stone formation and recurrent bouts of suppurative cholangitis

B. Other names are oriental cholangiohepatitis and hepatolithiasis

C. Common in males

D. Has a peak prevalence in the third and fourth decades

131. All of the following are true regarding recurrent pyogenic cholangitis *except:*

A. Left hepatic duct particularly the left lateral segmental duct is most severely affected

B. Majority of the intrahepatic duct stones composed of cholesterol

C. Biliary stones are absent in 20% to 25%

D. Gallbladder stones are seen in 50% to 70% of patients

132. All of the following are true regarding refractory ascites *except:*

A. Seen in 30% of cirrhotic patients

B. 12 months survival is only 25%

C. Incidence of encephalopathy increase after TIPS

D. Paracentesis induced circulatory dysfunction can occur after large volume paracentesis

Explanation

1. **Ans. (B)** TIPS reduces portal venous pressure by approximate 50%.

(Sheila Sherlock, 11th edition, P-180)

2. **Ans. (B)** A percutaneous transjugular approach is used to insert the shunt. A TIPS functions as a side-to-side portacaval shunt and has been used to treat complications of portal hypertension, mainly variceal bleeding and refractory ascites, as well as Budd-Chiari syndrome, hepatic hydrothorax and hepatorenal syndrome.

(Sleisenger, 9th edition, P-1504)

3. **Ans. (A)** For the occasional patient with presumed acute cellular rejection who fails to have a biochemical response to glucocorticoids, enhancement of immunosuppression may be necessary with the monoclonal antibody OKT3. Liver biopsy should be repeated to confirm a lack of histologic response before more intensive therapy is initiated and to exclude other important causes of graft dysfunction such as ischemia.

(Sleisenger, 9th edition, P-2051)

4. **Ans. (A)** Main hepatic veins may be visualized by USG, colour Doppler, enhanced CT and MR. A CT scan without contrast enhancement in a patient with fatty liver shows excellent hepatic venous anatomy.

(Sheila Sherlock, 11th edition P-191)

5. **Ans. (B)** Bilirubin formed in the reticuloendothelial cells is virtually insoluble in water. This is due to tight internal hydrogen bonding between the water-soluble moieties of bilirubin, proprionic acid carboxyl groups of one dipyrrolic half of the molecule with the imino and lactam groups of the opposite half. This configuration blocks solvent access to the polar residues of bilirubin and places the hydrophobic residues on the outside. To be transported in blood, bilirubin must be solubilized. This is accomplished by its reversible, noncovalent binding to albumin.

(Harrison, 17th edition, P-261)

6. **Ans. (A)** The course of infantile hemangioendothelioma is characterized by tumor growth during the early months of life, followed by gradual involution. If the child survives, the tumor involutes completely. Life-threatening aspects of the disorder are intractable congestive heart failure and, to a lesser extent, consumptive coagulopathy or rupture of the tumor. Cardiac failure should be treated by conventional means initially, but if these measures fail, more aggressive forms of treatment, such as embolization, ligation of the hepatic artery, surgical resection, or liver transplantation should be considered.

(Sleisenger, 9th edition, P-1587)

7. **Ans. (A)** Hepatic adenomas develop in 22% to 75% of patients, as early as 3 years of age but most commonly in the second decade of life, and tend to increase in both size and number as the patient ages. Rarely, adenomas can transform to hepatocellular carcinoma; unfortunately, serum α-fetoprotein levels and features of the lesions on hepatic imaging are not predictive of malignant transformation.

(Sleisenger, 9th edition, Pp-1584-1585)

8. **Ans. (A) Paraneoplastic Syndromes Associated with Hepatocellular Carcinoma**
   - Hypoglycaemia
   - Polycythemia (erythrocytosis)
   - Hypercalcemia
   - Sexual changes: Isosexual precocity, gynecomastia, feminization
   - Systemic arterial hypertension
   - Watery diarrhea syndrome
   - Porphyria
   - Carcinoid syndrome
   - Osteoporosis
   - Hypertrophic osteoarthropathy
   - Thyrotoxicosis
   - Thrombophlebitis migrans
   - Polymyositis
   - Neuropathy

(Sleisenger, 9th edition, P-1571)

9. **Ans. (D)** Epitheloid hemangioendothelioma (EHE).

This rare vascular tumor of adults is also usually multifocal and can also be associated with prolonged survival, even in the presence of metastases, which are commonly in the lung. There is usually no underlying cirrhosis. Histologically, these tumors are usually of borderline malignancy and express factor VIII antigen, confirming their endothelial origin. OLTX may be associated with prolonged survival.

(Sleisenger, 9th edition, P-1583)

10. **Ans. (A)** Hepatocellular Zone 1 necrosis (periportal) is caused by toxicity of ferrous sulfate and phophorus. Zone 3 necrosis is caused by paracetamol, halothane, mushrooms, carbon tetrachloride etc.

(Sheila Sherlock, 11th edition, P-345)

11. **Ans. (B)** Healthy individual cannot metabolize more than 160/180 gm of alcohol per day.

(Sheila Sherlock, 11th edition, P-383)

12. **Ans. (B)** One gram of alcohol gives 7 calories. The empty calories provide only energy with no contribution to nutrition.

(Sheila Sherlock, 11th edition, P-383)

13. **Ans. (B)** In alcoholic hepatitis, there is all gradation of severity. Cholestasis in bile canalicula is a feature of all types of alcoholic liver disease, strongly associated with decreased survival. Giant mitochondria form globular intracytoplasmic inclusion. Perivenular sclerosis is a precursor of cirrhosis collagen deposition.

(Sheila Sherlock, 11th edition, P-387)

14. **Ans. (D)** Copper plays a role in iron metabolism, melanin synthesis, energy production, neurotransmitter synthesis and CNS function; the synthesis and cross-linking of elastin and collagen; and the scavenging of superoxide radicals. Dietary sources of copper include shellfish, liver, nuts, legumes, bran and organ meats.

(Harrison, 17th edition, P-449)

15. **Ans. (A)** Normal daily dietary intake of copper is 4 mg of with 2 mg is absorbed and excreted in bile.

(Sheila Sherlock, 11th edition, P-413; Sleisenger, 9th edition, P-1250)

16. **Ans. (A)** Sensory loss and pyramidal tract signs are absent in Wilson's disease.

(Sheila Sherlock, 11th edition, P-471; Sleisenger, 9th edition, P-1252)

Memory loss, migraine-type headaches and seizures may occur. Patients have difficulties focusing on tasks, but cognition is not usually grossly impaired. Sensory abnormalities and muscular weakness are not features of the disease.

(Harrison, 17th edition, P-2450)

17. **Ans. (D)** Trace amounts of copper are required for essential enzymes that affect connective tissue and elastin cross-linking (lysyl oxidase), free radical scavenging (superoxide dismutase), electron transfer (cytochrome oxidase), pigment production (tyrosinase), and neurotransmission (dopamine β-monooxygenase). Copper in hepatocytes and other cells is bound to metallochaperones, low-molecular-weight proteins that each deliver copper to a specific target molecule.

(Sleisenger, 8th edition, P-1601)

18. **Ans. (B)** In the earliest stages before cirrhosis develops, histologic findings in the liver consist of steatosis, focal necrosis, glycogenated nuclei in hepatocytes, and sometimes apoptotic bodies. As parenchymal damage progresses, possibly through repeated episodes of lobular necrosis, periportal fibrosis develops. Cirrhosis is usually macronodular but may be micronodular.

(Sleisenger, 9th edition, P-1252)

19. **Ans. (B)** Cloning of the Wilson disease gene (ATP7B) was accomplished by a combination of conventional linkage analysis, physical mapping of the relevant region of chromosome 13q14, and recognition of its high homology with the Menkes disease gene. The coding region of the Wilson disease gene is 4.1 kilobases in length, with messenger RNA (mRNA) of about 8 kilobases.

(Sleisenger, 9th edition, P-1250)

20. **Ans. (B)** Characteristic of the arthropathy of HFE-related HH are changes in the second and third metacarpophalangeal joints. Joint space narrowing, chondrocalcinosis, subchondral cyst formation, osteopenia, and swelling of the joints may be seen. Unfortunately, the arthritic symptoms of HFE-related HH typically do not improve with phlebotomy.

(Sleisenger, 9th edition, P-1243)

21. **Ans. (D)** With repeated phlebotomy, the liver decreases in size, liver function improves, pigmentation of skin decreases, and cardiac failure may be reversed. Diabetes improves in about 40%, but removal of excess iron has little effect on hypogonadism or arthropathy. Hepatic fibrosis may decrease, but established cirrhosis is irreversible.

(Sleisenger, 9th edition, P-1246)

22. **Ans. (D)** The serum ferritin concentration is usually a good index of body iron stores, whether decreased or increased. In fact, an increase of 1 mcg/L in serum ferritin level reflects an increase of about 5 mg in body stores. In most untreated patients with hemochromatosis, the serum ferritin level is significantly increased (Fig. 351.2 and Table 351.1). However, in patients with inflammation and hepatocellular necrosis, serum ferritin levels may be elevated out of proportion to body iron stores due to increased release from tissues.

(Harrison, 17th edition, P-2432)

23. **Ans. (B)** As many as 20% of patients may present with purely psychiatric symptoms. These symptoms are highly variable, although depression is common. Phobias and compulsive behaviors have been reported; aggressive and antisocial behaviors may also be seen.

(Sleisenger, 9th edition, P-1252)

24. **Ans. (B)** Fatty liver is defined as triglycerides more than 5% of total liver weight.

(Sheila Sherlock, 11th edition, P-423)

25. **Ans. (B)** Zone 1 Fatty distribution of liver is seen in protein calorie malnutrition, Kwashiorker, TPN, Phosphate poisoning and methoxate poisoning.

(Sheila Sherlock, 11th edition, P-424)

26. **Ans. (C)** Table 297.1.

(Harrison, 17th edition, P-1929)

27. **Ans. (A)** In normal pregnancy, S. ALP is increased in last trimester. S. bilirubin, albumin urea, uric acid is lower, may be due to hemodilution. Serum transminase, Y GGT, fasting bile acid remains within normal limit.

(Sheila Sherlock, 11th edition, P-471)

28. **Ans. (D)** HAV belongs to Enterovirus 72 and non-enveloped and Iscosahedral.

Table 298.1

Icosahedral non-enveloped.

(Harrison, 17th edition, P-1932; Sleisenger, 9th edition, P-1279)

29. **Ans. (C)** Table 298.1.

9.4-kb RNA.

(Harrison, 17th edition, P-1932)

30. **Ans. (C)** Table 298.1.

Defective RNA virus, requires helper function of HBV (hepadnaviruses); HDV antigen present in hepatocyte nucleus.

(Harrison, 17th edition, P-1932)

31. **Ans. (D)** Table 298.1.

Acute diagnosis: Anti-HCV (C33c, C22-3, NS5), HCV RNA.

Chronic diagnosis: Anti-HCV (C100-3, C33c, C22-3, NS5) and HCV RNA; cytoplasmic location in hepatocytes.

(Harrison, 17th edition, P-1932)

32. **Ans. (D)** No sexual transmission with HEV infection although rare reports of percutaneous and sexual transmission for HAV. Table 298.2.

(Harrison, 17th edition, P-1939; Sleisenger, 9th edition, P-1338)

33. **Ans. (A)** Key factors in improving outcomes have included recognition of the key role of active viral replication occurring before liver transplantation, as demonstrated by detection in serum of hepatitis B e-Antigen or HBV DNA by molecular hybridization, as a predictor of recurrent hepatitis B in the graft, and the protective effect of long-term, high-dose hepatitis B immunoglobulin (HBIG). The transplantation candidate with chronic HBV infection is now readily accepted for liver transplantation, with the requirement for long-term immunoprophylaxis following transplantation, with its attendant inconvenience and expense. In a seminal study, Samuel and colleagues observed that patients with a fulminant presentation of acute HBV infection or hepatitis D (delta) virus co-infection had a lower risk of recurrent hepatitis B after liver transplantation than that observed in patients undergoing liver transplantation for HBV-related cirrhosis in the absence of immunoprophylaxis, because of a lower level of HBV replication.

(Sleisenger, 9th edition, P-1599)

34. **Ans. (B)** Key factors in improving outcomes have included recognition of the key role of active viral replication occurring before liver transplantation, as demonstrated by detection in serum of hepatitis B e-Antigen or HBV DNA by molecular hybridization, as a predictor of recurrent hepatitis B in the graft, and the protective effect of long-term, high-dose hepatitis B immunoglobulin (HBIG). The transplantation candidate with chronic HBV infection is now readily accepted for liver transplantation, with the requirement for long-term immunoprophylaxis following transplantation, with its attendant inconvenience and expense. In a seminal study, Samuel and colleagues observed that patients with a fulminant presentation of acute HBV infection or hepatitis D (delta) virus co-infection had a lower risk of recurrent hepatitis B after liver

trans-plantation than that observed in patients undergoing liver transplantation for HBV-related cirrhosis in the absence of immunoprophylaxis, because of a lower level of HBV replication.

(Sleisenger, 9th edition, P-1599)

35. **Ans. (B)** Accounting for upto 40% of all liver transplantation procedures, the most common indication for liver transplantation is end-stage liver disease resulting from chronic hepatitis C. Recurrence of HCV infection after liver transplantation can be documented in almost every patient if sufficiently sensitive virus markers are used.

(Harrison, 17th edition, P-1990)

36. **Ans. (A)** Isolated elevation of serum alkaline phosphatase in the setting of a normal serum GGTP (or 5' NT) level can be associated with rapid bone growth in children, Paget's disease and pregnancy. Additional rare hepatic disorders associated with an isolated AP elevation are PFIC, BRIC, and hereditary defects of bile acid synthesis. Byler's disease, a form of PFIC, is a lethal autosomal recessive cholestatic disease of unclear pathogenesis for which liver transplantation is the only therapeutic option.

(Sleisenger, 8th edition, P-2042)

37. **Ans. (B)** Both cyclosporine and tacrolimus are metabolized by the cytochrome P450 IIIA system, and therefore drugs that induce cytochrome P450 (e.g., phenytoin, phenobarbital, carbamazepine, rifampin) reduce available levels of cyclosporine and tacrolimus; drugs that inhibit cytochrome P450 (e.g., erythromycin, fluconazole, ketoconazole, clotrimazole, itraconazole, verapamil, diltiazem, nicardipine, cimetidine, danazol, metoclopramide, bromocriptine, and the HIV protease inhibitor ritonavir) increase cyclosporine and tacrolimus blood levels.

(Harrison, 17th edition, P-1987)

38. **Ans. (B)** The meantime for disappearance of amoebic liver abscess depends on size. It can vary from 10-300 days.

(Sheila Sherlock, 11th edition, P-500)

39. **Ans. (A)** Crigler-Najjar type I is an exceptionally rare condition found in neonates and characterized by severe jaundice [bilirubin > 342 mol/L (>20 mg/dL)] and neurologic impairment due to kernicterus, frequently leading to death in infancy or childhood.

(Harrison, 17th edition, P-263)

40. **Ans. (C)** Drugs: Rifampicin, probenecid, ribavirin and indinavir.

(Harrison, 17th edition, P-263)

41. **Ans. (B)** Patients with non-alcoholic steatohepatitis (NASH) typically present with an AST/ALT ratio less than or equal to 1 in the absence of cirrhosis.

(Sleisenger, 9th edition, P-1405)

42. **Ans. (A) Table 70.1 — Clinical Significance of Liver Biochemical Tests**

Marked elevations: Hepatitis (viral, toxic, autoimmune and ischemic).

(Sleisenger, 9th edition, P-1576)

43. **Ans. (D)** Patients with azotemia may have a falsely lowered serum AST level. Rarely, AST may form a macroenzyme complex with albumin that results in persistent elevation of the serum AST level.

(Sleisenger, 9th edition, P-1576)

44. **Ans. (A) Table 80.1.**

Infections

- Amebic or pyogenic liver abscess
- Aspergillosis
- Filariasis
- Hydatid cysts
- Pelvic cellulitis
- Schistosomiasis
- Syphilis
- Tuberculosis

(Sleisenger, 8th edition, P-1756)

45. **Ans. (B)** The disorder occurs in at least 10% of patients with cirrhosis, presumably as a result of sluggish portal vein blood flow, but acquired and inherited hypercoagulable states can be identified in many patients with cirrhosis and portal vein thrombosis.

(Sleisenger, 8th edition, P-1762)

46. **Ans. (C)** Type II autoimmune hepatitis, often seen in children, more common in Mediterranean populations, and linked to HLA-DRB1 and HLA-DQB1 haplotypes, is associated not with ANA but with anti-LKM. Actually, anti-LKM represent a heterogeneous group of antibodies. In type II autoimmune hepatitis, the antibody is anti-LKM1, directed against cytochrome P450 2D6. This is the same anti-LKM seen in some patients with chronic hepatitis C.

(Harrison, 17th edition, P-1968)

47. Ans. (C) Low ascitic fluid total protein concentrations, as well as the phagocytic (both motile and stationary) dysfunction associated with cirrhosis, are risk factors for bacterial infection.

Paracentesis itself has been proposed as a risk factor for ascitic fluid infection. This theoretical risk has not been substantiated in prospective studies of paracentesis-related complications. Spontaneous bacterial peritonitis is statistically more likely to be diagnosed on the first paracentesis than on subsequent taps. Needle-induced ascitic fluid infections do not occur unless the bowel is penetrated by the paracentesis needle.

(Sleisenger, 8th edition, P-1950)

48. Ans. (D) Table 89.3—Common Clinical Factors That May Precipitate Hepatic Encephalopathy in Patients with Cirrhosis

Nitrogenous encephalopathy	Non-nitrogenous encephalopathy
Uremia/azotemia	Sedatives, benzodiazepines
Gastrointestinal bleeding	Barbiturates
Dehydration	Hypoxia
Metabolic alkalosis	Hypoglycemia
Hypokalemia	Hypothyroidism
Constipation	Anemia
Excessive dietary protein	Infection

(Sleisenger, 8th edition, P-1970)

49. Ans. (D) Serum concentrations of des-γ-carboxy prothrombin (also known as prothrombin produced by vitamin K absence or antagonism II [PIVKA II]) are raised in a majority of patients with hepatocellular carcinoma. In populations in which the incidence of hepatocellular carcinoma is low, the abnormal prothrombin might arguably be a better marker than alpha-fetoprotein, and it could be used as a first-line tumor marker.

(Sleisenger, 9th edition, P-1572)

50. Ans. (C) Two tumor markers—abnormal Vitamin B_{12}–binding protein and neurotensin—have been linked specifically to the fibrolamellar variant of hepatocellular carcinoma (see later). When present, they provide useful confirmatory evidence of this variant, although the sensitivities of both markers are low.

(Sleisenger, 8th edition, P-2011)

51. Ans. (A) A value of 500 ng/mL (500 mg/L) is used as a diagnostic level because levels below this value may be found in patients with a variety of acute and chronic benign liver diseases, such as acute and chronic hepatitis and cirrhosis. False-positive results also may occur in patients with tumors of endodermal origin and nonseminomatous germ cell tumors.

(Sleisenger, 9th edition, P-1571)

52. Ans. (A) Table 91.4.

Major Risk Factors

- Chronic hepatitis B virus infection.
- Chronic hepatitis C virus infection.
- Cirrhosis.
- Dietary exposure to aflatoxin B_1.

Minor Risk Factors

- Oral contraceptive steroids.
- Cigarette smoking.
- Dietary iron overload in persons of black African ancestry.
- Hereditary hemochromatosis.
- Wilson's disease.
- α_1-Antitrypsin deficiency.
- Type 1 hereditary tyrosinemia.
- Type 1 and Type 2 glycogen storage disease.
- Hypercitrulinemia.
- Ataxia-telangiectasia.
- Membranous obstruction of the inferior vena cava.

(Sleisenger, 9th edition, P-1575)

53. Ans. (A) Table 91.4.

(Sleisenger, 9th edition, P-1575)

54. Ans. (D) Table 91.4.

(Sleisenger, 9th edition, P-1575)

55. Ans. (B) Hepatocellular carcinoma also may develop in patients with other inherited metabolic disorders that are complicated by cirrhosis, such as α_1-antitrypsin deficiency and type 1 hereditary tyrosinemia, and in patients with certain inherited diseases in the absence of cirrhosis, for example, type 1 glycogen storage disease.

(Sleisenger, 9th edition, P-1575)

56. Ans. (B) Risk of HCC progression cirrhosis: 1.3/100 patient year (etiology – unknown).

Cirrhosis (HBV related) = 3.7/100 patient-year.

Cirrhosis (HCV related) = 2.0/100 patient year.

(Sleisenger, 9th edition, P-1577)

57. **Ans. (B)** The pathognomonic lesion of CF, focal biliary cirrhosis (FCC), presumably results from defective function of the cystic fibrosis gene product, which is expressed in bile duct cells. Obstruction of small bile ducts leads to chronic inflammatory changes, bile duct proliferation and portal fibrosis.

(Sleisenger, 9th edition, P-1277)

58. **Ans. (B)** Low values of ceruloplasmin are found in very severe decompensated cirrhosis and Wilson's disease. High values are seen in pregnancy, estrogen therapy, large bile duct obstruction.

(Sheila Sherlock, 11th edition, P-32)

59. **Ans. (B)** Therapy with non-selective beta blockers is the preferred treatment, and either long-acting propranolol or nadolol may be used. Ideally, the hemodynamic response to beta blockers should be monitored with the goal of reducing the HVPG by greater than 20% or to less than 12 mm Hg. If these goals are not achieved, isosorbide mononitrate may be added. The extended-release form of isosorbide mononitrate is preferred, with an initial starting dose of 30 mg per day.

(Sleisenger, 8th edition, P-1922)

60. **Ans. (D)** Low values of C3 complement levels in FHF and alcoholic cirrhosis with or without hepatitis reflect reduced hepatic synthesis. It is normal in chronic hepatitis and increased in PBC.

(Sheila Sherlock, 11th edition, P-428)

61. **Ans. (B)** The hepatic enlargement in type 1 diabetes is due to increased glycogen. In type 2 DM, it is due to increased deposition of hepatic fat.

(Sheila Sherlock, 11th edition, P-432)

62. **Ans. (D)** Type V (muscle phosphoxylase) and VII (Phosphofructokinase) involve only muscle or muscle and kidney respectively.

(Sheila Sherlock, 11th edition, P-434; Sleisenger, 9th edition, P-1262)

63. **Ans. (A)** Hepatomegaly in GSD type I results from increased glycogen storage in the liver as well as a large degree of fatty infiltration; the latter likely develops because of a wide array of perturbations in lipid metabolism, including increased free fatty acid flux into the liver. Patients demonstrate mild elevations in serum aminotransferase levels but generally do not develop cirrhosis or liver failure.

(Sleisenger, 9th edition, P-1263)

64. **Ans. (C)** Type VI (Her's disease) is predominantly X-linked.

(Sheila Sherlock, 11th edition, P-437)

65. **Ans. (D)** Liver transplantation is definitive treatment for familial amyloidotoic poly neuropathy with 75% 5- year survival rate.

(Sheila Sherlock, 11th edition, P-442)

66. **Ans. (D)** Hepatic granulomas are associated with drugs, infection, chemical, sarcoidosis, PBC, granulomatous hepatitis. Infection include mycobacteria (tuberculosis, leprosy), brucella, Treponema palladium, Rickettsial (Q fever), helminth, fungal, Hepatitis A, C and CMV. Liver is involved in the secondary septicemia stage of syphilis with production of miliary granuloma.

(Sheila Sherlock, 11th edition, Pp-482, 487)

67. **Ans. (B)** Treatment of a hepatic abscess requires antibiotic therapy directed at the causative organism(s) and, in most cases, drainage of the abscess, usually percutaneously with radiologic guidance.

(Sleisenger, 9th edition, P-1367)

68. **Ans. (C)** Presence of ascites, coagulopathy, feature of portal hypertension, advancing age are the known poor prognostic factor in patient of cirrhosis.

(Sleisenger, 9th edition, Pp-1498-1503)

69. **Ans. (A)** HBsAg is used for screening of asymptomatic hepatitis B carrier.

(Sleisenger, 9th edition, P-1289)

70. **Ans. (A)** Exercise, diet, life style modification are the most important measures which will prevent progression of NAFLD.

(Sleisenger, 9th edition, P-1499)

71. **Ans. (A)** In case of hemochromatosis the first parameter to be affected is transferrin saturation. If transferrin saturation is more than 45%, then genetic screening for hereditary hemochromatosis may be recommended.

(Sleisenger, 9th edition, P-1245)

72. **Ans. (A)** This is a classic presentation of drug induced cholestasis. Chlopromazine, flucloxacilin, OCP, amoxicillin + clavunate are the most commonly implicated drugs in causation of drug induced cholestasis.

(Sleisenger, 9th edition, P-1423)

73. **Ans. (A)** Asymptomatic young male with predominant unconjugated hyperbilirubinemia with increased jaundice during stress and fasting is the classic presentation of Gilbert syndrome.

(Sleisenger, 9th edition, P-274)

74. **Ans. (A)** HbsAg is the earliest hepatitis B marker elevated in acute hepatitis B infection.

(Sleisenger, 9th edition, Pp-1289-1292)

75. **Ans. (D)** Presence of anti-HbsAg and anti-HCV suggestive of hepatitis C infection on the background of previous hepatitis B vaccination.

(Sleisenger, 9th edition, P-1299)

76. **Ans. (B)** Prothrombin Time (PT>100) is one of the most important parameter used for selecting the patient for liver transplantation in paracetamol poisoning.

(Sleisenger, 9th edition, Pp-1427-1429)

77. **Ans. (D)** Upto 5% of patient of ulcerative colitis patients are having associated primary sclerosing cholangitis.

(Sleisenger, 9th edition, P-121)

78. **Ans. (D)** Precore mutation and core gene mutation have been associated with poor response to IFN therapy.

(Sleisenger, 9th edition, P-1298)

79. **Ans. (C)** With possible exception of autoimmune thyroiditis, all other side effects are reversible upon lowering or cessation of drug.

(Harrison, 17th edition, P-1847)

80. **Ans. (A)** 3' Thiacytidine=Lamivudine.

(Sleisenger, 9th edition, P-1302)

81. **Ans. (B)** HBV genome is partially double stranded with 4 ORF s/gene.

(Sleisenger, 9th edition, P-1289)

82. **Ans. (D)** Prevalence of upto 5 to 20% is found in person with Down syndrome lepromatous leprosy, Hodgkin's leukemia. PAN, CRF on hemodialysis and in injection drug users.

(Harrison, 17th edition, P-1830)

83. **Ans. (C)** Replicative phase is characterized by presence of HbeAg, HBV DNA, Intraheptocytic HBcAg, High infectivity, accompany liver injury and extrachromosomal HBV DNA.

(Harrison, 17th edition, P-1845)

84. **Ans. (A)** Blumberg discovered HBs Ag

(Schiff's, 4th edition, P-766)

85. **Ans. (E)** HBV genome is partially double stranded with 4 ORFs/genes.

(Sleisenger, 9th edition, P-1289)

86. **Ans. (D)** HBcAg is not found in serum as same is sequestered by IgM HBcAg Anti HBsAb is found in patients who have recovered from Hep B infection or in vaccinated individuals. Anti HBsAg Ab is the only protective antibody against Hep B vaccinated individuals. Anti HbsAg Ab is the only protective antibody against Hep B.

(Sleisenger, 9th edition, P-1291)

87. **Ans. (B)** HbeAg, Precore mutation results in stop codon at 1896–no HBeAg production.

(Sleisenger, 9th edition, P-1291)

88. **Ans. (D)** All other 3 are known risk factors.

(Sleisenger, 9th edition, Pp-1292-1294)

89. **Ans. (B)** Acute Hep B–Transient, symmetrical polyarthritis affecting mainly hands and knees may be additive or migratory.

Chronic active hepatitis–Transient, asymmetrical, arthritis or arthralgia.

PAN–Symmetrical poly arthritis in 50%.

Mixed cryoglobins–Chronic arthralgia, arthritis is rare.

(Source: Arthritis and Hepatitis West J med Jan 1979, Pubmed Arthropathy in Hep. B)

90. **Ans. (E)** All are manifestations of HBV.

(Sleisenger, 9th edition, Pp-1285-1290)

91. **Ans. (B)** Less than 5% of adults will not clear HBsAg HBs Ag clearance is delayed in females, elderly and those with chronic hepatitis and cirrhosis.

(Schiff's, 4th edition, Pp-771, 776)

92. **Ans. (D)** Surface mutants develop due to selection because of immune pressure created by HBIG infusion at birth and after liver transplantation HBeAg is product of core gene and has nothing to do with S mutation.

(Sleisenger, 9th edition, P-1291; Schiff's, 4th edition, P-783)

93. **Ans. (E)** Hepatitis B vaccination is indicated in high risk patient live health worker. Hemodialysis patient, injection drug user, homosexual man, patient with chronic liver disease.

(Sleisenger, 9th edition, P-1308)

94. **Ans. (D)** Protective antibody response rate after vaccination typically exceed 90%.

(Sleisenger, 9th edition, P-1308)

95. **Ans. (E)** Other factors are smoking, obesity, CLD, HLA, DR3, DR7, DQ2, Hemodialysis.

(Sleisenger, 9th edition, P-1308)

96. **Ans.** (A) Picornaviridae.

(Sleisenger, 9th edition, P-1279)

97. **Ans.** (D) 10-15% year convert from replicative to non replicative phase.

(Harrison, 17th edition, Pp-1845-1846)

98. **Ans.** (A) Sleisenger indications of HAV vaccination are: As part of UIP, endemic area exposure, exposure to infected person, HIV, drug abusers, CLD, homosexuals, clotting factor abnormality.

(Sleisenger, 9th edition, P-1283)

99. **Ans.** (D) HAV is hepatotropic virus. Once virus reaches hepatocytes it starts replicating in cytoplasm.

(Sleisenger, 9th edition, P-1279)

100. **Ans.** (A) Non-enveloped icosahedral 27-32 nm virus resistant to 60 C for 60 min, pH of 3, ether.

(Schiff's, 4th edition, P-729)

101. **Ans.** (E) Fulminant hepatitis is associated with HEV more often than any other viral hepatitis.

(Schiff's, 4th edition, P-741)

102. **Ans.** (D) Vaccine is appropriate management in such situation.

(Sleisenger, 9th edition, Pp-1308-1309)

103. **Ans.** (C) Median age of onset is 50 years, with a range of 21 to 91 years. PBC has not been documented in children or adolescents. HLA DR8 is most frequently observed, conversely the DQA 1*0102 haplotype seems to be strongly associated with resistance to the disease.

(Sleisenger, 9th edition, Pp-1477-1479)

104. **Ans.** (C) In PBC autoantibodies have been shown to be directed against the E2 component of the pyruvate dehydrogenase complex (PDC-E2) the E2 unit of the branched chain 2oxo-acid dehydrogenase complex (BCOADC-E2) and the E2 subunit of PDC and protein X.AMAs are predominately of the IgG_1 and IgG_3 classes, PBC specific autoantibodies like anti gP210 and anti P62 antibodies appear to be mutually exclusive in PBC patients.

(Sleisenger, 9th edition, P-1478)

105. **Ans.** (B) Fatigue is the most common symptom followed by pruritus. Pruritus is most troublesome in the evening and might often resolve as the disease progresses.

(Sleisenger, 9th edition, P-1479)

106. **Ans.** (D) Autoimmune disease associated with PBC are Sjögren's syndrome, scleroderma and its variant, rheumatoid arthritis, some cutaneous disorders, renal tubular acidosis and thyroiditis. Although HCC is uncommon occurring in 1% to 2% of patients, patients with PBC have a substantially higher risk of hepatocellular carcinoma than the general population. Associated disorders such as inflammatory bowel disease and interstitial pulmonary fibrosis are rare.

(Sleisenger, 9th edition, P-1480)

107. **Ans.** (A) In PBC aminotransferase are mildly elevated (usually less than three times normal). Marked elevation may suggest a PBC autoimmune hepatitis overlap syndrome or coexisting viral hepatitis. AMA are present in approximately 90% to 95% of patient with PBC. Other auto antibodies found in patients with PBC or rheumatoid factor (70%), anti smooth muscle antibody 66%, anti-thyroid (antimicrosomal, antithyloglobulin) antibody (41%) and anti nuclear antibody (35%). The florid duct lesion, with the formation of poorly defined, non caseating epitheloid granulomas, is nearly diagnostic of poorly defined, non caseating epitheloid granulomas, is nearly diagnostic of PBC but is found in a relatively small number of cases, mainly in the early stages.

(Sleisenger, 9th edition, P-1483)

108. **Ans.** (C) UDCA is the only medication approved by the USFDA for the treatment of PBC. Proposed mechanism of actions of UDCA are inhibition of intestinal absorption of toxic, hydrophobic, endogenous toxic bile acids and reduction of the expression of MHC antigens on the biliary epithelium. UDCA decreases the risk of gastroesophageal varies and delays progression to cirrhosis.

(Sleisenger, 9th edition, P-1483)

109. **Ans.** (C) PBC patients with osteopenia have underlying osteoporosis rather than osteomalacia. The cause of osteoporosis associated with PBC is poorly understood that seems to be related to the cholestasis itself. Surgical removal of xanthelasmas is seldom successful and should not be performed. In some PBC patients coexisting pancreatic exocrine insufficiency, celiac sprue, intestinal bacterial over growth can cause steatorrhea.

(Sleisenger, 9th edition, P-1484)

110. **Ans.** (A) Approximately 1500 ml of fluid be present before dullness is detected. Ultrasonography can detect as little as 100 ml of ascetic fluid.

(Sleisenger, 9th edition, P-1519)

111. **Ans. (B)** Even after multiple paracentesis, bloody ascites usually does not develop in patients with severe prolongation of prothrombin. Transfusion of FFP or platelets before paracentesis is not supported by data. Hematoma occurs in 1% of patients, approximately 100 to 200 units of FFP or platelets would have to be given to prevent the transfusion of approximately 2 units of red blood cells. Left lower quadrant is preferable than the right lower quadrant because the cecum may be distended with gas from Lactulose therapy.

(Sleisenger, 9th edition, P-1519)

112. **Ans. (B)** High SAAF (≥ 1.1 g/dl) ascites is seen in cirrhosis, alcoholic hepatitis, cardiac ascites, "Mixed" ascites, massive liver metastases, fulminant hepatic failure, Budd Chiari syndrome, Port vein thrombosis, veno occlusive disease, myxedema, fatty liver of pregnancy.

Low SAAG (<1.1 g/dl) ascites is seen in peritoneal carcinomatosis, tuberculous peritonitis, pancreatic ascites, bowel obstruction or infarction, biliary ascites, nephrotic syndrome, postoperative lymphatic leak, serositis in connective tissue diseases.

(Sleisenger, 9th edition, P-1523)

113. **Ans. (C)** The accuracy of the SAAG is about 97% even with ascites fluid infection, diuresis, therapeutic paracentesis, intravenous infusions of albumin and varying causes of liver disease. Arterial hypotension may result in a decrease in the portal pressure and a narrowing of the SAAG. Lipid interferes with the assay for albumin and chylous ascites may result in a falsely high SAAG. Serum hyperglobulinemia (>5 g/dl{50 g/1} leads to a high ascitic fluid globulin concentration and can narrow the albumin gradient by contributing to the oncotic forces.

(Sleisenger, 9th edition, Pp-1523-1524)

114. **Ans. (C)** Multiple prospective studies have demonstrated that bedside inoculation of ascitic fluid into blood culture bottles is superior. Also bedside inoculation is superior to delayed laboratory inoculation of blood culture bottles in the laboratory. In late SBP and in the setting of gut perforation into ascitic fluid, the ascitic glucose concentration usually drops to 0 mg/dl (0 mmol/L) because of large number of stimulated neutrophils and bacteria. The ascitic fluid concentration of LDH is usually less than half of the serum level uncomplicated cirrhotic ascites. In SBP, the ascitic fluid LDH level rises because of the release of LDH from neutrophils and the ascitic fluid concentration is greater than that of serum. In secondary peritonitis, the LDH level is even higher than that seen in SBP and may be several fold higher than the serum LDH level.

(Sleisenger, 9th edition, Pp-1524-1525)

115. **Ans. (A)** In patients of ascites a cause other than liver disease found in approximately 20% of patients. Mixed ascites is seen in 5% of patients. Rare cause of ascites are POEMS (Polyneurotherapy, organomegaly, endocrinopathy, M component and skin changes syndrome and chemotherapy with 5 fluorouracil for colon cancer.

(Sleisenger, 9th edition, P-1527)

116. **Ans. (C)** Polymicrobial bacteriascitis is diagnosed when (1) multiple organisms are seen on gram stain or cultured from the ascetic fluid; and (2) the PMN count is lower than 250 cells/mm^3, SBP occurs usually in chronic liver disease (cirrhosis) but may acute (fulminant hepatic failure) or subacute (alcoholic hepatitis).

(Sleisenger, 9th edition, Pp-1529-1530)

117. **Ans. (D)** Patients with detectable ascites fluid opsonin activity appear to be protected from SBP unless they are exposed to a particularly virulent organisms (e.g. salmonella). Although 87% of patients with SBP are symptomatic at the time of infection is diagnosed, the symptoms and signs of infection are often subtle, such as a slight change in mental status.

(Sleisenger, 9th edition, P-1529)

118. **Ans. (D)** In patients undergoing selective intestinal decontamination usually gram positive organisms cause SBP GI hemorrhage is an under recognized risk factor for the development of SBP. The cumulative probability of infection during a single hospitalization for bleeding is approximately 40%. This is probably mediated by a shock induced increase in the translocation of bacteria from the gut to extra intestinal sites.

(Sleisenger, 9th edition, Pp-1529-1530)

119. **Ans. (B)** In the setting of perforated virus, cultures of ascitic fluid nearly always disclose multiple organism, except gallbladder rupture, which is usually non-microbial.

(Sleisenger, 9th edition, Pp-1530-1531)

120. **Ans. (B)** In MNB asymptomatic patient may not need treatment. Only approximately 10% of gram stains demonstrates organism in SBP.

(Sleisenger, 9th edition, Pp-1529-1530)

121. Ans. (B) Sympathetic pleural effusion in cirrhotic ascites are usually unilateral and right sided, but occasionally may be bilateral and large on the right side than the left. A unilateral left sided effusion suggests tuberculosis.

(Sleisenger, 9th edition, P-1535)

122. Ans. (A) Patients with low SAAG ascites do not respond to salt restrictions and diuretics (except nephrotic syndrome). Conversely, patient with a high SAAG have portal hypertension and usually are responsive to these measures.

(Sleisenger, 9th editon, P-1536)

123. Ans. (C) Although 24-hour specimens are the gold standard, one study has demonstrated that when a random urine specimen has a sodium concentration that is greater than the potassium concentration, a 24- hour specimen will reveal sodium excretion greater than 78 mmol/L day in 95% cases. Patients who do not lose weight despite a random urine sodium/potassium ratio greater than 1 are probably not compliant with the diet. Once the edema has resolved a reasonable maximum weight loss is probably 0.5 kg/day.

(Sleisenger, 9th edition, Pp-1536-1537)

124. Ans. (D) Ulcerative colitis may run a milder course in patients with PSC than in those without PSC.

(Sleisenger, 9th edition, P-1156)

125. Ans. (A) The Median age of diagnosis is 39 years and there is preponderance of men. The majority of affected patients have both intrahepatic and extrahepatic disease, although in some patients, the disease is predominantly intrahepatic and extrahepatic disease, although in some patients, the disease is predominantly intrahepatic (27%) or extrahepatic (6%).

(Sleisenger, 9th edition, Pp-1155-1156)

126. Ans. (B) A small proportion of patients with inflammatory bowel disease and cholestatic liver tests abnormalities may show histologic lesion typical of PSC on needle biopsy of the liver, without characteristic abnormalities on radiologic studies and cholangio-graphy. Small duct PSC (sometimes referred to in the older literature as "pericholangitis") comprises less than 5% of the PSC disease spectrum.

(Sleisenger, 9th edition, P-1158)

127. Ans. (C) Extrahepatic duct involvement may be more common in PSC that occurs in the absence rather than the presence of inflammatory bowel disease.

(Sleisenger, 9th edition, P-1156)

128. Ans. (B) Remission in symptoms and signs attributed to biliary microlithiasis and sludge, which produces sporadic, self limiting obstruction within the diffusely strictured biliary tree. Another mechanism may be low grade, intermittent and self limiting bacterial cholangitis which produces an acute inflammatory reaction in the already narrowed ductal system. Patients with asymptomatic PSC constitute 20% to 44%. An estimated 6% of patients with PSC have normal serum alkaline phosphate levels, which may reflect hypophos-phatasia hypothyroidism, or zinc or magnesium deficiency.

(Sleisenger, 9th edition, P-1158)

129. Ans. (B) It is not possible to predict who will develop cholangiocarcinoma and as yet a good screening method for the tumor has not been developed. Difficulty stems in pat from the lack of an association between the occurrence of cholangiocarcinoma and the duration and severity of PSC or the duration or frequency of inflammatory bowel disease. Patients present at a more advanced stage (35%) and die from colorectal cancer (4.5%) than were those with ulcerative colitis alone.

(Sleisenger, 9th edition, Pp-1162-1163)

130. Ans. (C) The disease occurs with equal frequency in both genders.

(Sleisenger, 9th edition, P-1169)

131. Ans. (B) The majority of the intrahepatic duct stones are composed of calcium bilirubinate, although changing diets have been implicated in a shift toward greater cholesterol content in the stones.

(Sleisenger, 9th edition, Pp-1167-1168)

132. Ans. (A) Less than 10% of patients with cirrhotic ascites are refractory to standard medical therapy.

Paracentesis induced circulatory dysfunction can occur after large volume paracentesis due to increase in post paracentesis plasma rennin level and can be prevented by albumin, colloid and terlipressin infusion.

(Sleisenger, 9th edition, Pp-1538-1540)

Chapter 7

PANCREAS

1. **A 32-year-old man present to the emergency department with a 6 hours history of progressively increasing, diffuse abdominal pain that radiates to his back. Physical examination reveals echymosis involving the flanks. Each of the following statements concerning his physical finding is true *except:***
   A. It presents subcutaneous fatty necrosis
   B. It may be associated with a rise in methema-lbumin levels
   C. It is associated with hemorrhagic pancreatitis
   D. It may indicate a poor prognosis

2. **All are true regarding pancreatitis associated hypocalcemia *except:***
   A. It is associated with a poor prognosis
   B. It may reflect albumin loss
   C. It occurs as a result of an increased release of pancreatic glucagons
   D. It reflects a failure of calcium release from bone in response to calcium release from bone in response to circulating parathyroid harmone

3. **False statements concerning pain associated with chronic pancreatitis is true *except:***
   A. The onset of painful attacks coincides with the development of pancreatic exocrine insufficiency
   B. A reduction in intraductal pressure by decompre-ssive surgery may relieve pain in selected patients
   C. Alterations in the histology of peripancreatic nerves have been demonstrated in patients with chronic pancreatitis
   D. Celiac plexus blockade provides only limited relief of pain in most patients with chronic pancreatitis

4. **A 48-year-old man is admitted to the hospital with acute pancreatitis. His initial course is uncomplicated but 4 days after admission, he experiences an exacerbation of abdominal pain. An abdominal ultrasonographic examination reveals a pseudocyst involving the head of the pancreas. Each of the following statements regarding pancreatic pseudocysts is true *except:***
   A. Pseudocysts larger than 5 cm should be surgically repaired immediately because of the increased risk of rupture
   B. Hemorrhage casued by erosion of a pseudocyst into a vascular structure is the etiology of upto 40% of deaths associated with this complication
   C. Pseudocysts may be suspected clinically if serum amylase levels remain persistently elevated
   D. Pseudocysts that fail to resolve after 6 weeks should be evaluated for surgical drainage

5. **Regarding pancreatic abscesses all are true *except:***
   A. Adult respiratory distress syndrome is mainly due to the damaging effect of free fatty acid
   B. Recent prospective studies demonstrate a decreased incidence of infectious complications and improved survival in patients with extensive necrosis of the pancreas when given prophylactic antibiotics
   C. They can be diagnosed by percutaneous fine needle aspiration of peripancreatic fluid

6. **A 39-year-old woman hospitalized with acute pancreatitis with progressive dyspnea and aterial blood gas analysis demonstrates marked hypoxemia. This patient is at risk for each of the following *except:***
   A. Atelectasis caused by splinting to avoid pain
   B. Adult respiratory distress syndrome
   C. Development of a large pleural effusion
   D. Acute pulmonary hemorrhage

7. **All are true regarding pancreatic pseudocysts *except:***
   A. In the absence of complications, drainage of pseudocysts should be restricted to those that are larger than 6 cm in diameter and that have persisted for more than 6 weeks
   B. Pseudocysts associated with a normal pancreatic duct can be treated by percutaenous drainage
   C. Pseudocysts that are proximal to a pancreatic ductal stricture should be drained percutaneously
   D. Pseudocysts located at the head of the pancreas may be amenable to endoscopic drainage through the major or minor papilla

8. **Regarding malabsorption secondary to chronic pancreatitis all are true *except:***
   A. Steatorrhea due to pancreatic insufficiency does not develop until 90% of the pancreatic exocrine function is lost
   B. Fat, protein and starch absorption may be impaired in severe pancreatic disease
   C. There is a greater increase in fecal weight due to pancreatic insufficiency compared with other etiologies of steatorrhea
   D. Fat-soluble vitamin deficiency states are less common in association with steatorrhea of chronic pancreatitis compared with celiac sprue

9. **A 42-year-old man with chronic pancreatitis complicated by steatorrhea continues to have oily diarrhea despite taking 4 tablets of pancrelipase (4500 IU lipase/tablet) with each meal. Possible reasons for refractory steatorrhea include each of the following *except:***
   A. Insufficient lipase activity with present dosing
   B. Inactivation of lipase by acid in the stomach
   C. Presence of undiagnosed bacterial overgrowth
   D. Concurrent use of cimetidine

10. **A 63-year-old man with chronic diarrhea submits a 72-hour fecal collection while consuming a diet of 100 g/day of fat. Analysis reveals 15 g/day of fecal fat. Which of the following statements is most accurate?**
   A. This test is specific for the detection of pancreatic insufficiency
   B. A 72-hour fecal collection detects pancreatic exocrine insufficiency when 50% of lipase activity is lost
   C. A two-stage fecal fat collection (with and without exogenous pancreatic enzymes) can be used to assess the adequacy of pancreatic enzyme replacement
   D. Pancreatic disease typically leads to greater levels of steatorrhea than does small bowel disease

11. **Regarding pancreatic enzymes all are true *except:***
   A. The four major enzyme types are amylolytic, lipolytic, proteolytic and nucleolytic
   B. Pancreatic enzymes are synthesized within ductal cell and packaged into zymogen granules
   C. Trypsinogen is converted into the biologically active trypsin by duodenally secreted enterokinase
   D. All proteolytic enzymes are secreted as inactive proenzymes

12. **The ability of a given lipid to stimulate pancreatic enzyme secretion is dependent on each of the following factors *except:***
   A. Chain length of fatty acids
   B. Presence of acid in the stomach
   C. Saturation of the fatty acids
   D. Concentration of bile salts

13. **All are potent stimulus of pancreatic enzyme secretion *except:***
   A. Glucose
   B. Fatty acids
   C. Essential amino acids
   D. Distention of the gastric antrum

14. **All of the following statements about pancreatic anatomy are true *except:***
   A. The pancreas is a retroperitoneal organ that lies in an oblique orientation behind the peritoneum of the posterior abdominal wall
   B. The pancreatic head is covered by the first portion of the duodenum
   C. Disruption of the pancreatic duct as a result of blunt abdominal injury most commonly occurs in the tail
   D. Because the duodenum and the pancreatic head share a blood supply, a 95% pancreatectomy may compromise blood flow to the duodenum

15. **Pancreas divisum is characterized by all *except:***
   A. The condition results from non-communication between the main and accessory pancreatic ducts, caused by abnormal fusion of the dorsal and ventral pancreatic buds during fetal development
   B. Autopsy studies report an incidence of about 7% for this condition in the United States
   C. Patients with pain and chronic pancreatitis are most likely to respond to endoscopic therapy
   D. Endoscopic treatment generally includes sphincterotomy of the minor papilla

16. **True statements regarding the CA 19-9 tumor associated antigen and pancreatic cancer all *except:***
   A. It is the most sensitive and specific marker available
   B. The sensitivity and specificity of this marker are not affected by tumor size
   C. Serum levels of CA 19-9 may be elevated with other cancers and conditions
   D. It may be useful surveillance tool to assess response to an intervention or therapy

17. True statement regarding therapy for pancreatic cancer is:

A. Treatment with 5-fluorouracil and radiotherapy confers no survival benefit compared to radiotherapy alone for unresectable cancers
B. 5-fluorouracil and radio therapy provide no survival benefit following curative resection
C. Gemcitabine may decrease pain, increase weight and improve quality of life
D. Preoperatively, conditions warranting urgent biliary stenting are preferably treated with a wire mesh stent rather than a plastic stent

18. Studies for insulinoma includes all *except:*

A. Serum proinsulin levels
B. Serum C-peptide levels
C. Assessment for antibodies to insulin
D. Cosyntropin stimulation test

19. Regarding hereditary pancreatitis and its gene mutation, false statement is:

A. Hereditary pancreatitis involves a mutation in the cationic trypsinogen gene
B. Trypsinogen is activated exclusively by enterokinase in the small bowel under normal physiologic conditions
C. Autodigestion and acute pancreatitis may occur in hereditary pancreatitis from autoactivation of trypsin and/or failure to inactivate trypsin within the pancreas
D. It is not clear whether other forms of inherited pancreatitis share the gene mutation found in hereditary pancreatitis

20. All are true regarding pancreatic cancer and diabetes *except:*

A. Similar to type II diabetics, patients with pancreatic commonly develop hyperinsulinemia and marked peripheral insulin resistance
B. Pancreatic tumors may release a substance than stimulated the secretion of islet amyloid polypeptide, which causes insulin resistance and decreased glycogen synthesis
C. Islet amyloid polypeptide levels in patients with pancreatic cancer and type II diabetes are elevated compared to those with other cancers and insulin requiring diabetes
D. Following tumor resection, the diabetes frequently becomes more severe

21. Which of the following statements regarding less common exocrine pancreatic tumors is false?

A. Mucinous cystadenomas are premalignant and should be resected
B. Serous cystadenomas, or microcystic adenomas may undergo malignant transformation and should be removed if it can be done safely
C. Mucinous ductal ectasia commonly demonstrates papillary malignant changes in 50% of cases warranting resection
D. Solid and papillary epithelial neoplasms have a poor prognosis

22. The effects of vagotomy on pancreatic function are all *except:*

A. It reduces the bicarbonate-secretory response to secretin
B. It reduces the release of cholecystokinin and secretin
C. It reduces the sensitivity of the pancreas to enzyme release mediated by submaximal doses of cholecystokinin
D. It reduces pancreatic enzyme responses to intestinal stimulants and food

Explanation

1. **Ans. (A)** Ecchymosis of the flanks and periumbilical areas (Grey Turner and Cullen signs) result from retroperitoneal hemorrhage, which may occur with hemorrhagic pancreatitis. These signs often are indicative of a poor prognosis. Elevations of serum methemalbumin levels have been demonstrated to occur in this clinical setting.

   (Sleisenger, 9th edition, P-969)

2. **Ans. (C)** Hypocalcemia with acute pancreatitis is a poor prognostic sign. Significant loss of albumin as a result of severe exudative inflammation in the peripancreatic region will cause a decline in total serum calcium. However in severe pancreatitis the fall in serum calcium exceeds that predicted for the level of hypoalbuminemia. Although hypocalcemia was initially felt to be secondary to fat necrosis with calcium sequestration, more recent studies suggest the decline is the result of diminished end-organ responsiveness to parathyroid hormone. There is no evidence suggesting that hypocalcemia observed in acute pancreatitis is due to hyperglucagonemia.

   (Sleisenger, 9th edition, Pp-965-970)

3. **Ans. (A)** The onset of pancreatic insufficiency in patients with chronic pancreatitis has been associated with the resolution of abdominal pain in studies of patients with alcohol-induced pancreatitis.

   (Sleisenger, 9th edition, Pp-995-996)

4. **Ans. (A)** Pseudocysts result from disruption of the pancreatic duct, resulting in a collection of pancreatic fluid encased in a simple fibrous membrane. Pseudocysts are capable of expanding and may erode into vascular structures in 5% of cases, resulting in massive hemorrhage with a resultant mortality of 40%. Although pseudocysts larger than 5 cm in size and lasting longer than 6 months seldom resolve spontaneously, in the absence of immediate complication, surgery is usually deferred until the fibrous membrane matures a process that generally requires approximately.

   (Sleisenger, 9th edition, Pp-1010-1011)

5. **Ans. (C)** Most pancreatic abscesses are polymicrobial, and although there have been a few reports of successful management with large percutaneous drains; prompt surgical debridement of necrosis remains the standard of care.

   (Sleisenger, 9th edition, P-981)

6. **Ans. (D)** Acute pancreatitis may produce hypoxemia by several mechanisms. Most commonly, patients develop atelectasis as a result of poor respiratory effort and splinting in the setting of abdominal pain. Pleural effusions may result from diaphragmatic inflammation, transdiaphragmatic spread of pancreatic ascites or extension of a pancreatic pseudocyst. The most serious complication is the development of adult respiratory distress syndrome, which results in an extended clinical course and frequently death. Pulmonary hemorrhage does not commonly result from acute pancreatitis.

   (Sleisenger, 9th edition, P-970)

7. **Ans. (C)** Pancreatic pseudocysts are most frequently encountered after pancreatic inflammation resulting from alcohol- or gallstone-induced injury. Those pseudocysts that are larger than 6 cm and persist for more than 6 weeks should be considered for drainage. If the pancreatic duct is intact and does not communicate with the pseudocyst, percutaneous drainage may be attempted. However, if the pseudocyst is in continuity with the pancreatic duct, percutaneous drainage may result in the development of a pancreatic fistula. Recent advances in endoscopic methods have afforded the ability to endoscopically drain appropriately located pseudocysts into the stomach or small intestine.

   (Sleisenger, 9th edition, Pp-1010-1011)

8. **Ans. (C)** As a rule, the degree of fecal weight increase due to pancreatic malabsorption is less than in other conditions with comparable steatorrhea. This relatively low weight reflects a lesser quantity of fecal water. Patients may pass bulky formed stool as apposed to the frank watery diarrhea observed in other conditions.

   (Sleisenger, 9th edition, Pp-996-997)

9. **Ans. (D)** The failure of enzyme replacements to correct pancreatic steatorrhea in chronic pancreatitis may be caused by an inadequate delivery of lipase to the small intestine. Inadequate dosing, peptic acid inactivation of lipase, and delayed entry of coated tablets into the lipase and delayed entry of coated tables into the duodenum in relation to the meal all may cause insufficiency enzyme activity. In addition a concomitant malabsorptive condition such as bacterial overgrowth may result in lipid maldigestion independent of pancreatic insufficiency. The use of an H_2-receptor antagonist can reduce the likelihood of acid induced degradation of lipase and may enhance the response to a given dose of enzyme supplementation.

(Sleisenger, 9th edition, Pp-1009-1010)

10. **Ans. (C)** 72-hour fecal collection is the gold standard for the detection of lipid maldigestion. The presence of 15 g/day of fecal fat (normal, 7 g/day), confirms lipid maldigestion as a cause for this patient's diarrhea. This test is not specific for pancreatic insufficiency and cannot provide a diagnosis in the absence of additional studies. Because of a significant reserve in the production of lipase by the normal pancreas, lipid digestion remains intact until more than 90% of pancreatic exocrine function is lost. A repeat 72-hour fecal collection taken while the patient consumes pancreatic enzyme replacement.

(Sleisenger, 9th edition, P-1009)

11. **Ans. (B)** Pancreatic enzymes are synthesized within acinar cells, not ductal cells.

(Sleisenger, 9th edition, P-923)

12. **Ans. (B)** Fat in the intestine stimulates pancreatic secretion by way of cholecystokinin (CCK) release. The potency of a given lipid to induce CCK release varies according to the chain length, the degree of saturation, and the concentration of bile salts relative to fatty acids in the intestinal lumen. Gastric acid is not required for lipid-evoked CCK release and pancreatic enzyme secretion.

(Sleisenger, 9th edition, P-926)

13. **Ans. (A)** Both essential amino acids and fatty acids are potent stimuli or pancreatic enzyme secretion. Antral distention also leads to pancreatic enzyme secretion. In contrast, glucose causes little or no pancreatic secretion in humans.

(Sleisenger, 9th edition, Pp-927-928)

14. **Ans. (C)** The body of the pancreas lies across and is pushed anteriorly by the first and second lumbar verterbrae. This position, couple with the fixed nature of the gland in this region, make the body portion of the pancreatic duct more susceptible to disruption from blunt abdominal injury.

(Sleisenger, 9th edition, Pp-909-910)

15. **Ans. (C)** Patients with pancreas divisum and otherwise unexplained recurrent acute pancreatitis are most likely to respond to endoscopic therapy. Patients with chronic pancreatitis respond poorly to both surgical and endoscopic therapies. Only about 30% of patients with pancreas divisum and chronic pancreatitis experience symptomatic improvement following minor sphinctero-tomy.

(Sleisenger, 9th edition, P-918)

16. **Ans. (B)** A variety of tumor-associated antigens have been studied; however all are of limited value in detaching lesions smaller than 1 cm. Although the CA19-p tumor maker is most sensitive (80%) and most specific (90%), levels in patients with small lesions are almost never significantly elevated.

(Sleisenger, 9th edition, P-1023)

17. **Ans. (C)** Combination therapy using 5-fluorouracil (5-FU) and super voltage radiation appears to improve survival in patients with both locally advance and surgically respectable pancreatic cancer. In a study of patients with unrespectable disease, 5-FU plus radiation resulted in a median survival of 10.4 months, compared to 6.3 months for patients receiving radiation alone. Gemcitabine is a newer chemotherapeutic agent with radio sensitizing properties. In several studies, only a small subpopulation of patients received a slight survival benefit with 5-FU alone. However, for about 25% of patients, gemcitabine reduced pain, increased weight and improved the quality of life. Wire mesh stents should never to be placed in potential candidates for pancreatic resection.These stents incite a severe inflammatory reaction and eventually may be incorporated into the bile duct wall. Potentially complicating or even preventing surgical intervention.

(Sleisenger, 9th edition, Pp-1025-1027)

18. **Ans. (D)** This patient has the classic findings of insulinoma. She is a woman between age 40 and 50 and her symptoms are associated with fasting. Symptoms suggest catecholamine-excess with diaphoresis as well as neuroglycopenia as evidenced by emotional irritability, headache and confusion. The most reliable test to document hypoglycemia is a 72-hour fast done during an inpatient stay. During this exercise, patients are allowed free access to water.

Most patients with insulinoma become symptomatic within 24 hours. During fasting, the diagnosis of insulinoma is suspected if serial insulin levels remain stable or increase in the face of serial glucose level less than 50 mg/dL or if the insulin-glucose ratio is greater than 0.3. The differential diagnosis of fasting hypoglycemia includes insulinoma, B cell hyperplasia, surreptitious administration of insulin or oral hypoglycemic agents and auto antibodies to insulin or the insulin receptor. In patients with insulinomas, the proinsulin and C-peptide levels are usually elevated, no autoantibodies to insulin or the insulin receptor are detected, and there are no oral hypoglycemic agents in the blood. Adrenal insufficiency receptors are detected and there are no oral hypoglycemic agents in the blood. Adrenal insufficiency would not cause the test results described.

(Sleisenger, 9th edition, P-982)

19. **Ans. (B)** Trypsinogen is normally secreted into pancreatic juice and is converted to trypsin upon reaching the duodenum, where it is exposed to enterokinase. However small amounts of trypsinogen undergo auto activation with the pancreas even under normal condition. Pancreas trypsin inhibitor produced by pancreatic acinar cells prevents intrapancreatic trypsin from damaging the host tissues. Alteration in this balance in favor of the activation of intrapancreatic trypsinogen has remained a central hypothesis for the development of acute pancreatitis. The identification of a mutation in the cationic trypsinogen gene in hereditary pancreatitis suggests that intrapancreatic trypsin activation likely plays a pathophysiologic role in this disease and possibly in other forms of acute pancreatitis.

(Sleisenger, 9th edition, Pp-949-951)

20. **Ans. (D)** Patients with insulin- or noninsulin-requiring diabetes resulting from pancreatic cancer have elevated levels or islet amyloid polypeptide (IAPP). The diabetes and high IAPP levels disappear in some patients after surgical resection of pancreatic cancer.

(Sleisenger, 9th edition, P-997)

21. **Ans. (D)** Solid and papillary epithelial neoplasms have favorable prognosis and most patients are cured by resection. However, some tumors may recur locally or metastasize to the liver.

(Sleisenger, 9th edition, P-1033)

22. **Ans. (B)** Cholinergic stimuli acting through vagal efferents primarily modulate the action of gut peptides on pancreatic secretion. Acetylcholine has no physiologically relevant effect on the release of peptides that stimulate the pancreas–neither CCK nor secretin.

(Sleisenger, 9th edition, Pp-925-926)

Chapter 8

LIVER AND BILIARY TRACT

LIVER

1. **Match the type of gallstone with its usual gross or microscopic description:**
   1. Cholesterol
   2. Mixed
   3. Black pigment
   4. Brown pigment
   A. Small, crumble easily, abundant mucin glycoproteins
   B. Multiple, generally faceted
   C. Contain bacterial skeletons
   D. Large, often solitary

2. **Regarding cholangiocarcinoma, each of the following contraindicates resection for possible cure *except*:**
   A. Vascular invasion of the portal vein
   B. Perihilar adenopathy
   C. Tumor invading the underside of the liver
   D. Tumor extending into the intrahepatic ducts

3. **Each of the following statements regarding ursodeoxycholate treatment of gallstones is true *except*:**
   A. Unlike chenodeoxycholate, ursodeoxycholate can dissolve stones irrespective of their composition
   B. Dissolution with ursodeoxycholate is achieved in up to 70% of selected patients
   C. Ursodeoxycholate is much more expensive than chenodeoxycholate
   D. Ursodeoxycholate, unlike chenodeoxycholate, causes neither diarrhea or hepatotoxicity

4. **An autosomal dominant disorder characterized by a decreased number of interlobular bile ducts, chronic cholestasis, and dysmorphic facies is:**
   A. Primary biliary cirrhosis
   B. Alagille's syndrome
   C. Caroli's disease
   D. Biliary atresia

5. **Which of the following statements regarding acquired immunodeficiency syndrome (AIDS) cholangiography (infectious sclerosing cholangitis) are TRUE?**
   A. Patients generally present with pain, elevated alkaline phosphates level and jaundice
   B. Endoscopic sphincterotomy is warranted if a bile duct stone is present
   C. Endoscopic sphincterotomy with placement of an endoprosthesis is warranted to relieve persistent right upper quadrant pain
   D. Cholangiographic findings resemble those of primary sclerosing cholangitis

6. **Each of the following statements regarding the anatomy of the biliary tract is true *except*:**
   A. The common bile duct and common hepatic duct possess a mucosa, submucosa, and muscularis
   B. The arterial supply of the bile ducts comes mainly from the right hepatic artery
   C. The right and left hepatic duct merge inside the liver in the majority of cases
   D. The cystic duct may run a variable course before joining the medial aspect of the common bile duct

7. **Regarding the placement of a biliary endoprosthesis for the treatment of bile duct obstruction (either benign or malignant), which of the following statements are TRUE?**
   A. Stent occlusion is to be expected, with the mean time to occlusion ranging from 1 to 12 months
   B. The most frequent early complications after stent placement are due to accompanying sphincterotomy
   C. Proximal bile duct lesions are more effectively drained than periampullary lesions
   D. Occluded stents usually become manifest by mild signs and symptoms rather than by frank cholangitis

8. **Each of the following is a common complication of percutaneous transhepatic biliary drainage *except*:**
   A. Cholangitis B. Sepsis
   C. Pancreatitis D. Bleeding

9. **Which of the following is a specific physical finding in alcoholic cirrhosis?**
   A. Dupuytren's contracture

B. Parotid gland enlargement
C. Muckrakers lines
D. None of the above

10. **Each of the following statement about secondary bacterial peritonitis is true *except*:**
A. A low ascitic fluid glucose concentration is a clue to diagnosis
B. Empirical antibiotic coverage should include an agent effective against anaerobes
C. Peritoneal fluid cultures remain positive after 48 hours of antibiotics
D. A high serum ascites/albumin gradient argues against the diagnosis

11. **In developed countries the cause of ascites in order from the most to least frequent are:**
A. Tuberculosis B. Malignancy
C. Cirrhosis D. Pancreatitis

12. **Which antibody confers the greatest resistance to reinfection by hepatitis B?**
A. Anti-HBc IgM B. Anti-HBc IgG
C. Anti-HBs D. Anti-Hbe

13. **A 45-year-old Chinese man with chronic hepatitis B and cirrhosis presents with hepatomegaly. An abdominal ultrasonogram shows a mass in the right lobe of the liver without evidence of cirrhosis. An α-fetoprotein value is normal. What is the MOST likely diagnosis?**
A. Hepatic adenoma
B. Hepatocellular carcinoma
C. Cystadenocarcinoma
D. Hemangioma

14. **Although medical management was initially successful, ascites has now worsened and the patient require therapeutic paracentesis every two weeks. She has been evaluated for liver transplantation but was rejected owing to an unstable social situation. Placement of a peritoneovenous shunt is considered. With regard to peritoneovenous shunting, which of the following is FALSE?**
A. It will permit discontinuation of diuretics in most patients
B. It does not reduce the incidence of infections
C. It does not improve survival
D. It will prolong the interval between hospitalizations

15. **Which of the following causes of chronic liver disease also pose an increased risk of hepatocellular carcinoma? (More than one answer may be correct):**
A. Wilson's disease
B. Chronic hepatitis C
C. Chronic hepatitis B
D. Genetic hemachromatosis

16. **Which of the following are TRUE statements about pyogenic hepatic abscesses?**
A. The most common cause is biliary tract infection
B. Radiologic differentiation from amebic abscess is difficult
C. Right upper quadrant tenderness is common
D. Treatment with percutaneous drainage plus antibiotics is usually effective

17. **A 42-year-old man with a long-standing history of ethanol dependence presents with new-onset ascites. A diagnostic paracentesis reveals a polymorphonuclear leukocyte count of 75 cells/mm. The following day an ascitic fluid culture is growing gram-negative rods. Under which conditions should empirical antibiotic treatment be started?**
A. If abdominal pain or fever is present
B. If the organism is identified as pseudomonas
C. If the ascitic fluid protein concentration is low
D. Under all circumstances

18. **Which of the following test of peritoneal fluid has the greatest sensitivity for detecting spontaneous bacterial peritonitis?**
A. White blood cell count
B. Gram's stain
C. pH
D. Lactate

19. **The primary toxic metabolite of ethanol is:**
A. Ethyl aldehyde
B. Acetaldehyde
C. Formaldehyde
D. None of the above

20. **Which of the following represents a contraindication to abdominal paracentesis?**
A. Obesity
B. Extensive prior abdominal surgery
C. Abdominal aortic aneurysm
D. Disseminated intravascular coagulation

21. **Which of the following countries has the lowest incidence of hepatocellular carcinoma?**
A. China
B. Japan
C. Mexico
D. Italy
E. South Africa

22. **A 25-year-old homosexual man is admitted to your service with fatigue, arthralgia, abdominal pain and dark urine. He was well until 3 days ago but now has difficulty staying awake during the evaluation. Physical examination reveals mild scleral Icterus, mild right upper quadrant abdominal tenderness on palpation and asterixis. Initial laboratory study reveals an alanine aminotransferase level of more than 2000 IU/L and negative HbsAg determination. A screen for toxins and urine copper is normal, and there is no history of mushroom ingestion. He requires mechanical ventilation. Which of the following is MOST likely to cause the death of this patient?**
   A. Acute renal failure
   B. Sepsis
   C. Gastrointestinal hemorrhage
   D. Cerebral edema

23. **Each of the following laboratory abnormalities is suggestive of alcoholic liver disease *except*:**
   A. Hypoalbuminemia
   B. Parallel elevation of the aspartate and alanine
   C. Erythrocyte macrocytosis
   D. Leukocytosis

24. **Acute infection with hepatotrophic viruses HAV, HBV or HCV may rarely result in fulminant hepatic failure. In western countries, the rank order for the probability of acute infection progression to fulminant hepatic failure is:**
   A. HCV - HBV - HAV
   B. HAV - HBV - HCV
   C. HBV - HAV - HCV
   D. HBV - HCV - HAV

25. **Regarding the decision of whether to treat autoimmune hepatitis, all of the following are considered to be absolute indications for treatment *except*:**
   A. Incapacitating symptoms
   B. Severe cytopenia
   C. Aspartate aminotransferase greater than ten times normal
   D. Aspartate aminotransferase greater than five times normal and gammaglobulin greater than two times normal
   E. Bridging necrosis on liver biopsy

26. **Each of the following hepatobiliary disorders is associated with a renal lesion *except*:**
   A. Choledochal cyst
   B. Congenital hepatic fibrosis
   C. Caroli's disease
   D. Adult polycystic disease

27. **Which physical sign has the highest diagnostic accuracy for detection of ascites?**
   A. Bulging flanks
   B. Shifting dullness
   C. Fluid wave
   D. Puddle sign

28. **Which of the following is the most effective long term therapy for hepatic hydrothorax?**
   A. Chest tube drainage
   B. Salt restriction and diuretics
   C. Liver transplantation
   D. Peritoneovenous shunting

29. **The single best imaging test in evaluating a hepatic cyst is:**
   A. Abdominal ultrasonography
   B. Abdominal computed tomography
   C. Radionuclide scanning
   D. Abdominal magnetic resonance imaging

30. **Each of the following may cause fulminant hepatic failure *except*:**
   A. Lassa fever
   B. Yellow fever
   C. Cytomegalovirus infection
   D. Hepatitis D

31. **Which of the following is MOST common in spontaneous bacterial peritonitis?**
   A. Encephalopathy
   B. Abdominal pain
   C. Rebound tenderness
   D. Fever

32. **Each of the following agents has been shown to be cholestatic *except*:**
   A. Estrogens
   B. Flucloxacillin
   C. Chlorpromazine
   D. Ursodeoxycholic acid
   E. Anabolic steroids

33. **Each of the following cause of ascites is associated with a high serum ascites/albumin gradient *except*:**
   A. Nephrotic syndrome
   B. Fatty liver of pregnancy
   C. Constrictive pericarditis
   D. Hepatic vein thrombosis

34. **Which of the following laboratory finding in an alcoholic with fulminant hepatic failure would MOST suggest acetaminophen overdosage?**
   A. Disproportionately elevated prothrombin time in comparison to aminotransferase levels

B. Markedly elevated alanine aminotransferase level of 8000 IU/L
C. Hyperammonemia
D. Hyperbilirubinemia

35. Congenital hepatic fibrosis is associated with each of the following *except*:
A. Berry aneurysms
B. Deformity of the gallbladder
C. Pancreatic insufficiency
D. Congenital heart disease

36. Common paraneoplastic finding in hepatocellular carcinoma include each of the following *except*:
A. Hypercalcemia
B. Erythrocytosis
C. Dermatomyositis
D. Hypoglycemia

37. Each of the following biopsy findings is consistent with alcoholic hepatitis *except*:
A. Councilman bodies
B. Mallory bodies
C. Microvesicular and macrovesicular fat
D. Hepatocyte degeneration

38. Which of the following is LEAST likely to be the cause of ascites formation?
A. Spontaneous bacterial peritonitis
B. Peritonitis carcinomatosis
C. Nephrotic syndrome
D. Congestive heart failure
E. Peritoneal tuberculosis

39. Which of the following methods can be used for the prenatal diagnosis of cystic fibrosis?
A. Monoclonal antibodies to measure microvillous enzyme levels in amniotic fluid
B. DNA probes linked to the cystic fibrosis gene
C. Direct mutation analysis
D. All of the above

40. The absorption of which of the following vitamins is LEAST dependent on intact hepatic function?
A. Vitamin A
B. Cobalamin
C. Vitamin K
D. Tocopherol (Vitamin E)
E. Vitamin D

41. With which of the following conditions are patients LEAST likely to present with complaints of odynophagis?
A. Caustic ingestion
B. Herpetic esophagitis
C. Severe peptic esophagitis
D. Esophageal carcinoma

42. A 66-year-old woman presents complaining of frequent soiling to the point she must wear dipers. Her past medical history is significant for diabetes mellitus controlled with oral hypoglycemics for the past 15 years. Which of the following statements are TRUE?
A. Her incontinence is probably due to reduced anal sphincter pressure and impaired sensation
B. Incontinence occurs in approximately 20% of patients with long-standing diabetes mellitus
C. Her incontinence may improve with biofeedback training
D. Her incontinence is most likely caused by her diabetic diarrhea
1. A and C
2. B and D
3. A, B and C
4. All of the above

43. Which of the following radiologic studies is of LEAST practical value in the diagnosis of abdominal abscess?
A. Chest radiograph with abdominal films
B. Abdominal ultrasonography
C. Computed resonance imaging of the abdomen

44. Administering fat-free parenteral nutrition can cause biochemical evidence of essential fatty acid deficiency within:
A. Two days
B. Two weeks
C. Two months
D. Six months

45. All of the following are true statements about peritoneal mesothelioma *except*:
A. Most cases are benign
B. Diagnosis usually requires laparoscopy or laparotomy
C. Spouses of asbestos workers are at risk
D. Optimal treatment for malignancy is chemotherapy and radiation

46. Obesity is properly defined as:
A. Body mass index (wt/ht^2) greater than 27.8 kg/m^2
B. Body mass index (wt/ht^2) greater than 27.8 lbs/ft^2

C. 1.4 times UBW (usual body weight)
D. 1.4 times IBW (ideal body weight)

47. **Which of the following statements concerning caustic ingestion are TRUE?**
I. The lower esophageal sphincter is the most common site of esophageal stricture formation
II. Oropharyngeal lesions are more frequent after solid lye ingestion
III. A careful visual examination of the oropharynx generally predicts the extent of esophageal injury
IV. Hoarseness and stridor after casustic ingestion should be evaluated with direct laryngoscopy
A. I and III
B. II and IV
C. I, II and III
D. All of the above

48. **The incidence of hiatal hernia among the elderly of North America approximates:**
A. 10%
B. 25%
C. 60%
D. 90%

49. **Medical options for treating cholestatic liver disease include:**
I. Naloxone
II Rifampin
III Ursodiol
IV Omeprazole
A. I and III
B. II and IV
C. I, II and III
D. All of the above

50. **Which of the following abdominal abscess locations is LEAST favorable for catheter drainage?**
A. Between the duodenum and vena cava
B. Within the pelvis
C. Between the liver and diaphragm
D. Periappendicular

51. **Which of the following can be determined by rectal manometry?**
I. The threshold for sensation of rectal distention
II. The competence of the rectoanal inhibitory reflex
III. The rectoanal contractile response
IV. Rectal compliance
A. I and III
B. II and IV
C. I, II and III
D. All of the above

52. **Lavage of the peritoneum with 1 L of the normal saline can be diagnostically useful in the setting of suspected peritonitis when clinical, biochemical and radiographic information is non-diagnostic. Each of the following findings in the lavage fluid supports the diagnosis of peritonitis *except*:**
A. White blood cell count greater than 500 cells/mm^3
B. Albumin less than 0.5 g/dL
C. Bilirubin greater than serum bilirubin
D. Bacteria on gram stain

53. **In person of normal weight, death from starvation usually occurs when what percentage or body weight has been lost?**
A. 20
B. 30
C. 40
D. 50

54. **In patients with fecal incontinence, anal manometry can directly measure which of the following?**
A. Rectal sensation and compliance
B. Motor nerve supply and skeletal muscle responses
C. Basal and squeeze pressures in the anal canal
D. Rectal compliance

55. **Which of the following have been shown to be of value in treating patients with fecal incontinence?**
A. Metamucil
B. Lomotil
C. Loperamide
D. Tincture of opium

56. **Each of the following statement about peritoneal tuberculosis is true *except*:**
A. The lymphocyte count in the peritoneal fluid is usually elevated
B. Laparoscopy is virtually always diagnostic
C. Fever is uncommon
D. Ascites may resolve with diuretics if cirrhosis is present

BILIARY TRACT

57. An 85-year-old man presents with a history of three discreet episodes of severe epigastric pain. The pain occurs suddenly, increases gradually to a peak within 15 minutes of onset and lasts 1 to 2 hours without fluctuation before slowly resolving. Radiation to the upper back is noted; however, no participating events can be recalled. Ultrasonography of the right upper quadrant reveals seven small (<1 cm diameter), buoyant, high-amplitude echoes with postacoustic shadowing within the gallbladder a normal gallbladder wall and a non-dilated biliary tree. The patient requests that all treatment alternatives be discussed. Reasonable option include all of the following *except*:

A. Ursodeoxycholic acid (UDCA)
B. Extracorporeal shock-wave lithotripsy (ESWL)
C. Laparoscopic cholecystectomy
D. Contact dissolution with methyl-tert-butyl ether (MTBE)

58. Each of the following statement regarding gallstones is true *except*:

A. Pure cholesterol stones are common (approximately 85% of gallstones)
B. Most gallstones are found incidentally and are not associated with symptoms
C. Biliary colic develops in gallstone carriers at a rate of 1% to 2% per year
D. Complications of gallstone disease (e.g. pancreatitis cholangitis) are usually preceded by episodic pain

59. In addition to medical management with fluids antibiotics and insulin, what treatment would you recommend for gallstone ileus?

A. Surgery after medical stabilization
B. Endoscopic retrograde cholangiopancreatography with sphincterectomy
C. Urgent decompressive colonoscopy after medical stabilization
D. Medical management alone will suffice

60. Choledochal cysts may be complicated by any of the following *except*:

A. Pancreatitis
B. Biliary cirrhosis
C. Cholecystitis
D. Hepatitis

61. A 65-year-old man presents with a history of epigastric pain and progressive weight loss over the past 4 months. The pain is constant and interferes with sleep. He also reports the onset of jaundice and clay-colored stools about 1 month ago. The physical examination is notable for jaundice and palpable epigastric fullness. Laboratory evaluation disclosed the following data: a total bilirubin level of 14 mg/dL, an aspartate aminotransferase level of 80 U/L, an alanine aminotransferase level of 75 U/L and an alkaline phosphatase level of 400 U/L. Considering the most likely diagnosis, which of the following statements is most accurate?

A. Stent placement into the common bile duct will significantly reduce the risk of ascending cholangitis and improve survival
B. Stent placement into the common bile duct is efficacious in the management of pruritus and in relieving jaundice
C. Biliary drainage will improve the associated abnormalities of gastric emptying
D. Stent placement into the pancreatic duct will assist in pain control

62. Which feature characterizes the most common type of choledochal cyst?

A. Dilation of the common bile duct without hepatic duct involvement
B. True diverticula of the common bile duct
C. Dilation of the distal intraduodenal segment of the common bile duct
D. Multiple extra and intrahepatic cysts
E. Intrahepatic cysts only

63. A 49-year-old man underwent open cholecystectomy for symptomatic gallstones. An intraoperative cholangiogram suggested two common bile duct (CBD) stones; these were removed after exploration of the CBD. His recovery was uneventful and he returned several weeks later for a T-tube cholangiogram in preparation for removal of the T-tube. Although the patient was asymptomatic, an 8 mm stone was identified in the CBD during cholangiography. What would be the best course of action?

A. Repeat laparotomy and CBD exploration to remove the stone
B. Endoscopic retrograde cholangiopancreatography with sphincterotomy and stone extraction
C. Stone extraction through the T tube
D. Remove the T tube as planned and because he is asymptomatic, no further intervention recommended

64. **Which of the following statements is false?**
   A. A moderate rise in serum amylase is rare following diagnostic endoscopic retrograde cholangiopancreatography (ERCP) and indicates the presence of a complication
   B. Acute pancreatitis following ERCP may occur even when the pancreatic ducts has not been cannulated
   C. Addition of sphincter of Oddi manometry increases further risk of ERCP pancreatitis
   D. ERCP in patients with known pancreatic pseudocysts can be dangerous and should be coordinated with either a surgical or endoscopic drainage procedure in the event of complications

65. **True statements regarding primary sclerosing cholangitis (PSC) in patients with ulcerative colitis include all of the following *except*:**
   A. Proctocolectomy will not reverse the course of PSC
   B. Proctocolectomy prevents the development of the duct cancer
   C. Endoscopic retrograde cholangiopancreatography cannot exclude underlying cholangiocarcinoma in this patient
   D. The patient should be referred for consideration of liver transplantation

66. **Which of the following findings is the best predictor of pain relief after endoscopic sphincterotomy in patients with suspected sphincter of Oddi dysfunction?**
   A. A dilated common bile duct on endoscopic retrograde cholangiopancreatography (ERCP)
   B. Delayed drainage of contrast after filling the biliary system during ERCP
   C. An elevated sphincter of Oddi basal pressure during manometry
   D. The presence of a juxtapapillary diverticulum

67. **In patients with sphincter of Oddi dysfunction, all of the following findings can be observed *except*:**
   A. Transient elevations in liver chemistries
   B. A dilated common bile duct
   C. Rapid biliary drainage during endoscopic retrograde cholangiopancreatography
   D. Increased sphincter of Oddi basal pressure during manometry

68. **A 50-year-old woman is referred for evaluation of an asymptomatic elevation of her serum alkaline phosphatase level. Additional laboratory data reveal detectable titers of anti-mitochondrial antibody and an elevated serum IgM level, other associated medical problems may include each of the following:**
   A. Thyroiditis
   B. Renal tubular acidosis
   C. Sjögren syndrome
   D. Diabetes mellitus

69. **A 67-year-old man presents with a 2 months history of progressive weight loss, decreased appetite, jaundice and a 2-week history of alcoholic stools. The patient denies having abdominal pain. Physical examination reveals a soft, palpable mass in the right upper quadrant of the abdomen. Laboratory studies disclose the following values:**
   Total bilirubin: 7.0 mg/dL (normal, 0.0-0.9 mg/dL)
   Alkaline phosphatase:738 U/L
   Aspartate aminotransferase: 34 U/L
   Alanine aminotransferase: 42 U/L
   Total protein: 6.0 g/dL
   Albumin: 3.2 g/dL (normal, 3.5-5.0 g/dL)
   Leukocyte count: 7000/mm^3
   Platelets: 237,000/mm^3
   Electrolytes: Normal
   Creatinine: 1.0 mg/dL (normal, 1.4 mg/dL)
   Blood urea nitrogen: 8 mg/dL (normal, 8-20 mg/dL)
   Chest and abdominal radiographs: Normal

70. **What is the most likely diagnosis?**
   A. Chronic pancreatitis with stricture
   B. Enlarged gallbladder as a result of a tumor of the pancreas or bile duct
   C. Cholelithiasis
   D. Choledocholithiasis

71. **What is the best initial diagnostic imaging technique?**
   A. Endoscopic retrograde cholangiopancreatography
   B. Endoscopic ultrasonography
   C. Abdominal ultrasonography
   D. Abdominal computed tomography scan

72. **All but one of the following characteristics predict successful dissolution of gallstones:**
   A. Smaller than 1.5 cm diameter
   B. Large surface area in relation to mass
   C. Pigment stones
   D. Mobile and buoyant gallstones

73. **All *except* one of the following conditions may be associated with primary sclerosing cholangitis:**

A. Ulcerative colitis
B. Acquired immunodeficiency syndrome
C. Recurrent pancreatitis
D. Hepatitis B

74. A 52-year-old immigrant from Thailand presents with abdominal pain, mild hepatomegaly, diarrhea and icterus. The presence of which one of the following parasites would be most consistent with this presentation?
A. Clonorchis sinensis
B. Diphyllobothrium latum
C. Taenia saginata
D. Enterobius vermicularis

75. Statements pertaining to human infection with liver flukes include each of the following *except*:
A. Adult flukes reside in the lumen of the human gastrointestinal tract
B. Fluke lifespan of 10 to 30 years are common
C. Bile duct strictures and fibrosis frequently occur
D. Ingestion of watercress is associated with human

76. What percentage of cases of acute cholecystitis are associated with cholelithiasis?
A. 10% B. 50%
C. 75% D. 90%

77. Risk factors for the development of gallbladder carcinoma include all of the following *except*:
A. Porcelain gallbladder
B. Salmonella typhi
C. Alcoholism
D. Chronic cholelithiasis (i.e. lasting longer than 40 years)

78. The following are typical features of AIDS associate cholangiopathy *except*:
A. Abdominal pain
B. Fever
C. Elevations of total bilirubin (>5 mg/dL)
D. Marked elevations of alkaline phosphate (>500 U/L)

79. Which of the following statements concerning gallbladder cancer is false?
A. Metastasis occurs early: More than 50% of patients have lymph node involvement at the time of diagnosis
B. Less than 10% of patients with liver metastases have cancer confined to the gallbladder wall
C. Jaundice develops in 30% to 60% of patients as result of obstruction of intrahepatic ducts
D. Jaundice is a favorable prognostic sign, because more than 50% of these patients will be diagnosed earlier in the course of the disease allowing resection of the tumor

80. Hepatic conditions associated with AIDS include each of the following *except*:
A. Granulomatous hepatitis
B. An illness similar to primary biliary cirrhosis
C. Microvesicular or macrovesicular hepatosteatosis
D. Nodular regenerative hyperplasia

81. Laboratory evaluations of persons with primary sclerosing cholangitis disclose all of the following findings *except*:
A. Antimitochondrial antibody (AMA)
B. Alkaline phosphatase elevation
C. Increased levels of circulating immune complexes
D. Perinulcear antineutrophilic cytoplasmic antibody (pANCA)

82. All of the following statements regarding laparoscopic cholecystectomy complications are true *except*:
A. Bile duct injuries are usually recognized within the first week after surgery
B. Duct injury requires either endoscopic stentingor urgent exploratory laparotomy and repair
C. Nauseas on the first postoperative day is an indication for emergent biliary scintigraphic scanning
D. Ileus is rarely scan on the second postoperative day unless there is a complication

83. The treatment of choice for the majority of patients with this disorder is:
A. Endoscopic retrograde cholangiopancreato-graphy
B. Surgery
C. Percutaneous transhepatic drainage
D. Steroids

84. In normal bile, the ratio of glycine to taurine conjugates is:
A. 3:1 B. 1:3
C. 2:1 D. 4:1

85. The anomalous position of the gallbladder, which predisposes to acute torsion, is:
A. Left sided GB
B. Retrodisplacement of GB
C. Floating GB
D. Intra-hepatic GB

86. Most important mechanism of gall stone formation is:
A. Increased biliary secretion of cholesterol
B. Defective vesicle formation

C. Nucleation of cholesterol crystals
D. Biliary sludge formation

87. All of following are predisposing factors for pigment stones in GB *except:*
A. Alcoholic cirrhosis
B. Chronic biliary tract
C. Octreotide treatment
D. Increasing age

88. On ultrasound, biliary sludge has following characters *except:*
A. Presence of acoustic shadows
B. Low echogenicity layer
C. Shift of this layer with posture
D. No acoustic shadows

89. All are indications for prophylactic cholecystectomy *except:*
A. Presence of prior biliary complication
B. Very large stones (>2 cm)
C. Young age with silent stones
D. Stones in a congenitally anomalous GB

90. Bacterial infection implicated in acute acalculous cholecystitis is:
A. Leptospira
B. E. coli
C. Klebsiella
D. Clostridium

91. All the following characterize acalculous cholecystopathy *except:*
A. Recurrent right upper quadrant biliary tract pain
B. Abnormal GB ejection fraction >40% at 45 minutes
C. Large GB on ultrasound
D. Reappearance of pain on CCK infusion

92. Most common fistula complicating cholecystitis open into:
A. Duodenum B. Hepatic flexure
C. Stomach D. Jejunum

93. Most common site of obstruction in gall stone ileus:
A. Ileocecal valve B. Duodenum
C. Jejunum D. Proximal ileum

94. Triad of choledochal cyst includes all *except:*
A. Fever B. Abdominal pain
C. Abdominal mass D. Jaundice

95. Following the relief of obstruction in choledocholithiasis, the parameter(s) that rapidly normalizes is:
A. Serum alkaline phosphatase
B. Serum bilirubin
C. Aminotransferases
D. A+C

96. The first bile channel to be accompanied by portal vein and hepatitis artery:
A. Canals of Hering
B. Inter lobular bile ducts
C. Bile canaliculi
D. Septal bile ducts

97. Total bile flow in man per day is:
A. 400 ml B. 600 ml
C. 800 ml D. 1000 ml

98. Bile is normally secreted at a pressure of:
A. 5-10 cms of water
B. 10-15 cms of water
C. 15-25 cms of water
D. 25-50 cms of water

99. Cyclosporine A inhibits:
A. Canalicular bile acid transporter
B. Multispecifc organic ion transporter
C. Na+ K+ ATPase
D. ATP dependent phopholipid transporter (Flippase)

100. Cytochalasin B and androgens disrupt:
A. Micro tubules
B. Microfilaments
C. Na+ K+ ATPase activity
D. Cytokeratins

101. 'Bile lakes' represent:
A. Accumulation of bile in canaliculi
B. Accumulation of bile in interlobular ducts
C. Ductular proliferation
D. Ruptured interlobular ducts

102. After bile duct obstruction the earliest period when cholestasis features develop is:
A. 12 hours B. 24 hours
C. 36 hours D. 72 hours

103. Xanthomas in cholestasis develop if lipids deposits in:
A. Tendon sheaths
B. Peripheral nerves
C. Liver (focally)
D. Bone

104. Xanthomas in cholestasis develop if serum cholesterol is more than:
A. 250 mg% for 6 months
B. 350 mg% for > 6 months

C. 450 mg% for 6 months
D. 450 mg% for 3 months

105. All are extrahepatic effects of cholestasis *except:*
A. Impaired cerebral metabolism
B. Increased susceptibility of kidneys to hypoxia and hypotension
C. Platelet dysfunction
D. Impaired wound healing

106. False statement regarding Byler's disease:
A. Cholestatic disorder
B. Autosomal recessive
C. Defect in microfilament function
D. Liver transplant not useful

107. LP-X in cholestasis is:
A. LDL B. VLDL
C. HDL D. Chylomicrons

108. All are prognostic indicators in PBC *except:*
A. Age
B. Serum bilirubin
C. Serum alkaline phosphatase
D. Oedema

109. In PBC if serum bilirubin >6 mg%, the expected survival is less than:
A. 1 year B. 2 years
C. 4 years D. 3.5 years

110. The drug that affects survival in PSC:
A. UDCA B. Methotrexate
C. Colchicine D. Cyclosporine A

111. PSC and AIDS cholangiopathy can be distinguished:
A. Clinically
B. Biochemically
C. Histopathologically
D. Radiographically

112. Wrong statement regarding CBD is:
A. It is approximately 7 cms long
B. Diameter varies between 0.5 and 1.5 cm
C. Lies posterior to portal vein and right of hepatic artery
D. In 10-15% of patients CBD and PD open separately

113. Most common cause of extrinsic compression of extrahepatic bile ducts is:
A. Carcinoma head of pancreas
B. Chronic pancreatitis
C. Lymph nodes at porta
D. Acute pancreatitis

114. All are pronucleating factor in gall stone formation *except:*
A. Mucin
B. IgA
C. Phospholipase C
D. Apo-Lipoprotein A2

115. One of the following is not an anti-nucleating factor for formation of gall stones:
A. Aspirin
B. Aminopeptidase
C. α_1 acid glycoprotein
D. Mucin

116. Loxiglide is a:
A. Selective antagonist of CCK
B. Selective agonist of secretin
C. Selective antagonist of secretin
D. Selective agonist of CCK

117. Chronic rejection following liver transplantation is defined as bile duct loss involving:
A. 50% of portal triads
B. 30% of portal triads
C. 60% of portal triads
D. 75% of portal triads

118. UDCA is not effective in:
A. PSC
B. PBC
C. Gall stone dissolution
D. GVHD

119. Cytokine implicating in sepsis related cholestasis is:
A. IL-2
B. IL-4
C. IL-6
D. IL-10

120. Most sensitive imaging modality for evaluation of obstructive jaundice is:
A. CT scan
B. Ultrasound
C. ERCP
D. PTC

121. Histological findings strongly suggestive of extra hepatic biliary obstruction include all *except:*
A. Bile infarct
B. Bile lakes
C. Neutorphils in interlobular ducts
D. Canalicular bile plugs

122. Cholestasis associated pruritus is best treated by:
A. Anti histamines
B. UDCA
C. Cholestyramine
D. Phenobarbitol

123. All are true regarding AIDS cholangiopathy *except:*
A. Includes both sclerosing cholangitis and papillary stenosis
B. Most commonly caused by opportunistic infection
C. Papillary stenosis responds to endoscopic sphincterotomy
D. Associated with shortened survival

124. GB is patent in-utero by:
A. 4 weeks
B. 8 weeks
C. 12 weeks
D. 16 weeks

125. Part of the biliary tract that proliferates in chronic extrahepatic obstruction is:
A. Bile canaliculus
B. Canals of Hering
C. Terminal bile ducts
D. Interlobular ducts

126. Portion of CBD most liable to develop post-operative strictures is:
A. Supra-duodenal
B. Intra-duodenal
C. Intra-pancreatic
D. None

127. The part of sphinchter of Oddi that promotes bile flow is:
A. Fasiculi longitudinales
B. Pancreatic sphincter
C. Sphincter ampullae
D. Sphincter choledochus

128. Contraction of which part of sphincter of Oddi prevents reflex of intestinal contents?
A. Fasiculi longitudinales
B. Pancreatic sphincter
C. Sphincter ampullae
D. Sphincter choledochus

129. The part of GB that presents at the level of ninth costal cartilage at right lateral border of rectus abdominus for clinical palpation is:
A. Neck
B. Body
C. Fundus
D. Infundibulum

130. Spiral valves of Heister are formed by:
A. Mucous membrane
B. Lamina propria
C. Smooth muscle layer
D. Serosa

131. The most common cause of neonatal cholestasis is:
A. EHBA
B. α_1 AT deficiency
C. Choledochal cyst
D. Idiopathic neonatal hepatitis

132. The most common Kasai type of EHBA:
A. Type I
B. Type II a
C. Type II b
D. Type III

133. The most frequent abnormal renal function test in Caroli's disease:
A. Elevated BUN
B. Elevated creatinine
C. Decreased GFR
D. Inability to concentrate urine

134. False statement regarding Alagille's syndrome is:
A. Most common familial intrahepatic cholestasis
B. Most common associated congenital heart disease is peripheral pulmonic stenosis
C. Transmitted as autosomal recessive trait
D. Predisposes to HCC

135. For a histological definition of ductular paucity the ratio of interlobular ducts to portal areas should be less than:
A. 0.4
B. 0.2
C. 0.6
D. 1

136. Most common cause of cholelithiasis in infancy is:
A. TPN
B. Sepis
C. Hemolytic anemias
D. Hepatobiliary disorders

137. The most common cause of cholelithiasis in the age group of 1-5 years is:
A. TPN
B. Sepsis
C. Hemolytic anemias
D. Hepatobiliary disorders

138. The most common cause of cholelithiasis in the age group of 6-21 years is:
A. Obesity
B. Abdominal surgery
C. Pregnancy
D. Hemolytic anemias

139. Acute hydrops of GB is associated with:
A. PAN
B. Kawasaki disease
C. SLE
D. RA

140. In sphincter of Oddi dysfunction (SOD) histology is abnormal in:
A. 20% B. 40%
C. 60% D. 80%

141. All the following values indicate asymptomatic sphincter of Oddi dysfunction manometrically *except:*
A. Basal pressure >35 mm
B. Basal ductal pressure >13 mm
C. Amplitude of phasic contractions >120 mm
D. Duration of contraction >8 sec

142. Triad of acute cholecystitis includes all *except:*
A. Leucocytosis
B. Jaundice
C. Right upper quadrant pain
D. Fever

143. During pregnancy cholecystectomy is best preferred during following trimester:
A. I B. II
C. III D. None

144. The most common site of post-operative biliary stricture:
A. Mild-CHD
B. Hilar region
C. Low CHD
D. Hilar with confluence

145. The segments between which GB overlies the liver
A. III and IV B. IV and V
C. VII and VI D. VI and IV

146. The false statement regarding acute hydrops of GB is:
A. It is a non-calculus, non-inflammatory distention of GB
B. It may be associated with Kawasaki's disease
C. Cholecystectomy is the treatment of choice
D. Never predisposes to GB carcinoma

147. All the following relax sphincter of Oddi *except:*
A. Nitrates B. Bethenacol
C. Glucagon D. Secretin

148. The drug which has no effect on sphincter of Oddi is:
A. Diazepam B. Morphine
C. Calcium blockers D. Meperdine

149. Normal CBD pressure is:
A. 2-5 cm of water B. 5-10 cm of water
C. 10-15 cm of water D. 5-10 mm of Hg

150. All the following are indication for cholecystectomy in asymptomatic cholelithiasis *except:*
A. Diabetes
B. Sickle cell disease
C. Prior to organ transplant
D. Prolonged space travel

151. Surgically correctable type of EHBA includes:
A. Type I B. Type II a
C. Type II b D. B+C

152. The most common biliary cause of post-cholecystectomy symptoms is:
A. Biliary stricture
B. Choledocholithiasis
C. Cystic duct remnant syndrome
D. SOD

153. Bile acid implicated in pathogenesis of gall stone is:
A. Deoxycholate B. Cholate
C. UDCA D. Lithocolic acid

154. Risk factor of carcinoma GB include all *except:*
A. Large gall stones
B. Typhoid carries
C. Long common channel
D. Adenomyoma of GB

155. Selection criteria for bile acid dissolution therapy include all *except:*
A. Uncomplicated symptomatic gall stones
B. Radiolucent stones
C. GB emptying of more than 60% of fasting volume
D. Opacification of GB on oral cholecystography

156. The false statement regarding UDCA therapy of gall stones:
A. It is administered in the dose of 8-12 mg/kg/day
B. Produces mild transaminase elevation and diarrhea
C. Bedtime dosage is preferred
D. Spontaneous gall stone calcification warrants withdrawal

157. Median rate of decrease in size of gall stone with UDCA treatment is:
A. 0.2 mm per month
B. 0.4 mm per month
C. 0.7 mm per month
D. 1 mm per month

158. Proportion of IBD patients having PSC is:
A. 7% B. 10%
C. 15% D. 30%

159. 'Obliterating fibrosis cholangitis' the histological pathognomic lesion of PSC is seen in:
A. 5% B. 10%
C. 15% D. 40%

160. The most common site of dominant stricture in PSC is:
A. Bifurcation of common hepatic duct
B. Distal common hepatic duct
C. Distal common bile duct
D. Junction of cystic duct and common hepatic duct

161. Immunological associations of PSC include all *except:*
A. Elevated IgM
B. Anti-colon antibodies
C. Elevated circulating immune complexes
D. AMA

162. PSC with normal serum alkaline phosphates is due to all the following *except:*
A. Zinc deficiency
B. Hypothyroidism
C. Calcium deficiency
D. Hypophosphatasia

163. The most common cause of death in PSC is:
A. Variceal hemorrhage
B. Refractory ascites
C. Liver cell failure
D. HCC

164. GB and cystic duct involvement in PSC is around:
A. 5% B. 10%
C. 15% D. Absent

165. Medium survival of patient with PSC from the time of diagnosis:
A. 5 months
B. 5 years
C. 11 months
D. 11 years

166. The most common cause of death following ERCP is:
A. Cholangitis
B. Acute pancreatitis
C. Hemorrhage
D. Perforation

167. One of the following is not a determinant of gall stone risk:
A. Low HDL levels
B. High triglyceride level
C. High serum cholesterol
D. None

168. Highest known prevalence of gall stone is seen in following population:
A. American Indians B. Egyptians/Greece
C. Japan D. U.S.A whites

169. Lowest prevalence of gall stones is seen in the following population:
A. American Indians B. Egyptians/Greeks
C. Japanese D. U.S whites

170. Least vascularized part of GB:
A. Body B. Infundibulum
C. Fundus D. Neck

171. Somatostatin receptors are expressed on the malignant cells of:
A. Periampullary tumors
B. Carcinoma GB
C. Pancreatic carcinoma
D. Cholangiocarcinoma

172. Following liver transplantation, the cause of PSC-like biliary strictures include all *except:*
A. ABO incompatibility
B. Hyperacute rejection
C. Hepatic artery thrombosis
D. Preservation related ischemia

173. One of the following is not a metallic stent used for draining biliary tract:
A. Palmaz stent B. Gianturco-Rosch
C. Carey-coons D. Wall stent

174. Highest frequency of cholangitis is seen with the following clinical setting:
A. Post-traumatic bile duct stricture
B. Choledocholithiasis
C. Neoplastic obstruction
D. Congenital biliary disease

175. In acalculous biliary pain the GB ejection fraction is abnormal in:
A. 10% B. 25%
C. 50% D. 75%

176. The true statement regarding acute acalculous cholecystitis is:
A. It occurs predominantly in elderly females
B. It is commonly seen in ambulatory patients
C. Factor XII activation is implicated in the pathogenesis
D. Total WBC count and amylase level are usually normal

177. Sump syndrome occurs after:
A. Billorth II
B. Hepatico jejunostomy
C. Choledochoduodenostomy
D. Choledochojejunostomy

178. All the following types are included as primary sclerosing cholangitis *except:*

A. IBD associated
B. Autoimmune
C. Immunodeficiency
D. Infiltrative

179. One of the following is not a secondary cause for sclerosing cholangitis:
A. Pancreatic carcinoma
B. Cholangiocarcinoma
C. Hepatocellular carcinoma
D. Lymphoma

180. Crohn's disease in PSC is seen in:
A. 15% B. 20%
C. 25% D. 60%

181. What proportion of PSC is constituted by 'small duct' type?
A. 1% B. 5%
C. 12% (5%-20%) D. 25%

182. The true statement regarding histology of PSC is:
A. Onion skin fibrosis is virtually diagnostic
B. Obliterating fibrosis cholangitis is seen in 50% of patients
C. Pathologic involvement of blood vessels is uncommon
D. Hepatic copper is not usually elevated

183. True statement regarding cholangiographic pattern in PSC is:
A. Gallbladder is affected in 20% of cases
B. Extraheptic ducts are involved more often than intrahepatic ducts
C. Extraheptic ducts are involved less commonly in the absence of IBD
D. Dominant strictures usually involve distal CBD

Explanation

LIVER

1. **Ans. (1-D, 2-B, 3-A, 4-C)** The type of gallstone can generally be identified by inspection. Large, pale, yellow-white stones are often referred to as pure cholesterol stones because they contain more than 90% cholesterol. The core of these stones is usually dark and composed of the calcium salt of un-conjugated bilirubin. Mixed cholesterol stones, containing more than 50% cholesterol are common and tend to be smaller and multiple. Their contiguous surfaces are usually faceted. Pigment stones are either black of brown. Black stones are composed mostly of the calcium salt of unconjugated bilirubin are small and crumble easily. Brown pigment stones are larger and firmer than black stones and contain a mixture of unconjgated bilirubin, cholesterol and calcium soaps of fatty acids. They often contain bacterial cytoskeletons, suggesting that their formation is triggered by infection.

   (Sleisenger, 9th edition, P-1093)

2. **Ans. (B)** Perihilar adenopathy is not considered a contraindication for surgical resection of cholangiocarcinoma.

   (Sleisenger, 9th edition, P-1176)

3. **Ans. (A)**

   Ursodeoxycholate has greater safety and efficacy than chenodeoxycholate and is now the preferred agent for clinical cholesterol stones. Unlike chenodeoxycholate, it does not inhibit the synthesis of normal bile salts. Because normal cholesterol catabolism and excretion are maintained, serum cholesterol and low-density lipoproteins do not rise while the patient is under treatment, as is true for chenodeoxychoferase levels are uncommon. The rate of stone dissolution with small (<20 mm), radiolucent, floating stones made eased (e.g. unable to concentrate dye as assessed by an oral recurrence of stones occurs in 50% of responding patients laparoscopic cholecystectomy, the final role of bile salts in the treatment of gallstones is uncertain.

   (Sleisenger, 9th edition, P-1122)

4. **Ans. (B)** Syndromic paucity of interlobular bile ducts (Alagille's syndrome, or arteriohepatic dysplasia) is the most common form of amilial intraheptic cholestasis. This number interlobular bile ducts and a variety of other congenital malformations. An autosomal dominant mode of transmission with reduced penetrance and variable expressivity has been suggested from familiar pedigrees.

   (Sleisenger, 9th edition, Pp-1060-1061)

5. **Ans. (B, D)** Acquired immunodeficiency syndrome cholangiography (infectious sclerosing cholangitis) typically presents as pain and an elevated alkaline phosphatase level but not with jaundice. The cholangiographic appearance is similar to that seen in primary sclerosing cholangitis, namely beading and ulceration along the intrahepatic and extrahepatic bile ducts. These immunocompromised patients are extremely susceptible to bacterial cholangitis as a complication of an indwelling stent; therefore, stents should be placed across high-grade strictures only to relieve severe pruritus or acute bacterial infection not just to relieve pain.

   (Sleisenger, 9th edition, P-534)

6. **Ans. (C)** The right and left hepatic ducts join outside the liver in most cases. It is uncommon for the ducts to merge inside the liver or for the cystic duct to join the right hepatic duct proximal to the hilum.

   (Sleisenger, 9th edition, P-1047)

7. **Ans. (A, B, D)** Early complications from stent placement are indeed most likely due to the sphincterotomy and include hemorrhage, pancreatitis, perforation and cholangitis. Stent patency average 6 months, but occlusion may occur immediately or be delayed for up to 12 months. Therefore when a malignant obstruction, many investigators will not routinely replace stents but rather will wait until sign or symptoms suggests an occlusion. These include alkaline phosphatase level elevation and low-grade fever or chills. It is uncommon for an occluded stent to present as fullblown cholangitis and sepsis. Distal bile

ducts lesions are more effectively stented than are lesions occurring proximally at the hilum.

(Sleisenger, 9th edition, Pp-1006-1007)

8. **Ans. (C)** Unlike endoscopic retrograde cholangiopancreatography, pancreatitis is unlikely after percutaneous biliary drainage because there is no direct injection of contrast into the pancreatic duct.

(Sleisenger, 9th edition, P-1187)

9. **Ans. (D)** There are no physical findings that are pathognomonic for alcoholic cirrhosis. Dupuytren's contracture is more commonly found in alcoholics but can be seen in other individuals, as is true for the other conditions.

(Sleisenger, 9th edition, P-1394)

10. **Ans. (D)** Clues to the diagnosis of secondary bacterial peritonitis include a low ascitic fluid glucose concentration, a high protein concentration and an elevated lactate dehydrogenase level (LDH). Anaerobic organisms are often present and peritoneal fluid cultures usually remain positive after 48 hours of antibiotic treatment. In the setting or portal hypertension, the serum ascites/albumin gradient is usually high whether or not a superimposed complications is present.

(Sleisenger, 9th edition, P-1529)

11. **Ans. (C, B, A, D)** Cirrhosis is the most common cause of ascites in the United States. In one series, it was present in 85% of patients. Malignancy accounted for 10% of patients in this series. Although tuberculosis is a common cause of ascites cause in more developed countries. Pancreatic ascites is relatively unusual.

(Sleisenger, 9th edition, P-1842)

12. **Ans. (C)** Anti-HBS in the serum of convalescent patients confers almost complete resistance to reinfection with hepatitis B virus of either the same or a different subtype. This is the basis for vaccination with purified HbsAg preparations. In contrast, anti-HBc and anti-Hbe do not appear to be protective.

(Sleisenger, 9th edition, Pp-1308-1309)

13. **Ans. (B)** The most likely diagnosis is a hepatocellular carcinoma even with a normal á-fetoprotein level. Up to 20% of hepatocellular carcinomas in high-risk populations are associated with normal levels of this tumor marker. This man is at very high risk because he has presumably had chronic hepatitis B since birth. á-fetoprotein levels can be normal in up to 50% of low-risk persons with hepatocellular carcinoma.

(Sleisenger, 9th edition, P-1571)

14. **Ans. (A)** Although placement of a peritoneovenous shunt may permit a decrease in the dosage of diuretics, most patients continue to require diuretics for management of ascites. Bacterial infection is a major complication of peritoneous shunting. In large randomized trial (the Veterans Administration Cooperative Study), shunted patients actually had a higher incidence of infections than medically managed patients and survival was not altered. Although there was an increased interval between hospitalizations, shunting did not reduce the total days spent in hospital.

(Sleisenger, 9th edition, P-1540)

15. **Ans. (A, B, C, D)** The risk of hepatocellular carcinoma is dramatically increased in all forms of chronic viral hepatitis and is also particularly high in genetic hemochromatosis, patients with Wilson's disease are also at some risk, although only if they have cirrhosis.

(Sleisenger, 9th edition, P-1575)

16. **Ans. (A, B, D)** Biliary tract infections account for 40% to 50% of all pyogenic absceses of the liver. It is difficult to differentiate amebic from non-amebic abscesses by abdominal computed tomography of ultrasonography. Serologic test, such as the indirect hemagglutination test are helpful in distinguishing these conditions. Although hepatomegaly may be found in half of patients with pyogenic liver abscesses, right upper quadrant tenderness is unusual.The mainstay of therapy for a pyogenic liver abscess is percutaneous drainage and broad-spectrum intravenous antibiotics, followed electively by correction of the underlying disease.

(Sleisenger, 9th edition, Pp-1368-1369)

17. **Ans. (A)** This probably a case of bacterial ascites in which a substantial proportion of cases resolve spontaneously. However the rate spontaneous resolution is significantly lower among patients with signs or symptoms compatible with peritonitis. Symptomatic patients should be treated with antibiotics.

(Sleisenger, 9th edition, P-1532)

18. **Ans. (A)** There is not true gold standard in the diagnosis of spontaneous bacterial peritonitis. If the white blood cell count is more than 250 cells/mm^3, there is a greater than 95% chance that bacterial peritonitis is present. The sensitivities of ascitic fluid lactate and pH are less than 50%, whereas that of the Gram stain is less than 10%.

(Sleisenger, 9th edition, P-1531)

19. **Ans. (B)** Acetaldehyde is the immediate metabolic by-product of the oxidation of ethanol. Acetaldehyde is a vasoactive substance and account for many of the physiologic effects of ethanol consumption (i.e. flushing, tachycardia). Subjects with low activity of aldehyde dehydrogenase (approximately half of Japanese and Chinese people) are particularly prone to flushing and tachycardia and accordingly usually avoid alcohol.

(Internet source)

20. **Ans. (D)** There are few contraindications to abdominal paracentesis. The most important is the presence of severe uncontrollable coagulopathy. If there are concerns about localizing site for aspiration of peritoneal fluid in obese patients or those with a history of extensive abdominal surgery, ascitic fluid collections can be localized by ultrasonography.

(Sleisenger, 9th edition, P-1531)

21. **Ans. (C)** The primary risk factor for hepatocellular carcinoma is hepatitis B, especially when acquired as an infant. Within high-risk countries, the risk is not evenly distributed throughout the population. People who emigrate from a low-risk country to one with high risk retain the low risk of their country of origin.

(Sleisenger, 9th edition, Pp-1569-1570)

22. **Ans. (D)** This patient has fulminant hepatitis B, probably acquired through sexual activity. The surface antigen is already negative, owing to an intense immune response. On admission he had evidence of stage II hepatic encephalopathy and rapidly deteriorated to stage IV coma. In a large series of patients with fulminant hepatic failure from a variety of causes, cerebral edema was the most common immediate cause of death, followed by major gastrointestinal hemorrhage, hepatocellular failure and sepsis. Virtually all organ systems may be affected.

(Sleisenger, 9th edition, P-1565)

23. **Ans. (B)** Chronic alcoholism is characterized by a number of laboratory abnormalities, including hyperuricemia, hypomagnesemia and erythrocyte macrocytosis. Alcoholic liver disease is characterized by leukocytosis, hypoalbuminemia, hyperbilirubinemia, and a disproportionate elevation in the aspartate aminotransferase level when compared with the alanine aminotransferase level.

(Sleisenger, 9th edition, Pp-1390-1391)

24. **Ans. (C)** Infection with both hepatitis A virus (HAV) and hepatitis B virus (HBV) is major cause of fulminant hepatic failure (FHF) in western countries. Although the incidence of HAV infection is higher than that of HBV infection, the likelihood of progression to FHF is greater for patients infected with HBV. Acute infection with hepatitis C virus (HCV) is a rare cause of FHF in western countries but may play a significant role in FHF in Japan.

(Sleisenger, 9th edition, P-560)

25. **Ans. (B)** The therapy prednisone or azathioprine, is directed against and hence is effective only against the manifestations of inflammation. Incapacitating symptoms, usually extreme fatigue, along with biochemical or histologic evidence of inflammation, always warrant treatment whereas severe cytopenia and other measures of hepatic dysfunction such as hyperbilirubinemia or hypoprothrombinemia in the absence of inflammation do not warrant therapy.

(Sleisenger, 9th edition, P-1472)

26. **Ans. (A)** Congenital hepatic fibrosis and adult polycystic disease are both associated with cystic disease of the kidney. Many patients with Caroli's disease also have renal lesions. Although choledochal cysts are congenital, there is not associated renal lesion.

(Sleisenger, 9th edition, Pp-1058-1059)

27. **Ans. (B)** Clinical diagnosis of early ascites is notoriously difficult and ultrasound is much more sensitive and specific for diagnosis than any of the sign listed. Shifting dullness has a much higher sensitivity and specificity for detecting ascites than the puddle sign (dependent dullness detected with the patients on hand and knees). Or the presence of a fluid wave. If not flank dullness is present there is less than a 10% chance that ascites is present. However, flank dullness is often present without ascites.

(Sleisenger, 9th edition, Pp-1518-1519)

28. **Ans. (C)** All of the listed treatment have used for hepatic hydrothorax. Salt restriction and diuretics represent the mainstay of therapy. By contrast, placement of a chest tube should be reserved for severe respiratory compromise because it can lead to profound intravascular volume depletion and protein loss. Peritoneovenous shunting has been successfully used but it is associated with inherent complications. Poorly controlled hepatic hydrothorax is an indication for liver transplantation which has the best long-term result.

(Sleisenger, 9th edition, Pp-1538-1540)

29. **Ans. (A)** Abdominal ultrasonography is the least expensive, single most valuable test in evaluating a hepatic cyst. It can reliably differentiate between solid and cystic lesions, definitively diagnose certain types of cystic lesions such as congenital and hydatid cyst and with aspiration make a microbiologic diagnosis of abscesses. Computed tomography and magnetic resonance imaging may provide additional information in specific circumstance, but at substantially greater cost.

(Sleisenger, 9th edition, Pp-1589-1590)

30. **Ans. (C)** A wide variety of infections cause fulminant hepatic failure as part of a systemic hemorrhagic fever. These include Lassa and yellow fevers. Hepatitis D superinfection of a patients with hepatitis B may precipitate fulminant hepatic failure. On the other hand, cytomegalovirus infection generally causes only mild hepatic inflammation.

(Sleisenger, 9th edition, P-1558)

31. **Ans. (D)** Fever, abdominal pain, and encephalopathy are all common manifestations of spontaneous bacterial peritonitis, with fever present in over two thirds of patients. By contrast rebound tenderness of the abdomen is present in only 10% of patients.

(Sleisenger, 9th edition, Pp-1528-1532)

32. **Ans. (D)** All are associated with cholestasis, with the exception of ursodeoxycholic acid. This hydrophilic bile acid promotes bile flow and tends to relieve many of the symptoms associated with profound cholestatic states.

(Sleisenger, 9th edition, P-1423)

33. **Ans. (A)** Portal hypertension results in an abnormally high hydrostatic pressure gradient between the portal bed and the ascitic fluid. To balance, there must be a similarly large difference in oncotic forces between plasma and ascitic fluid, resulting in a large albumin gradient. All of the conditions listed cause ascites through portal hypertension except nephrotic syndrome, which is associated with a normal serum ascites/albumin gradient.

(Sleisenger, 9th edition, P-1523)

34. **Ans. (B)** In comparison to other forms of fulminant hepatic failure, acetaminophen-related hepatic failure in alcoholics is characterized by very high level of alanine aminotransferase (ALT) usually in the range of 2000 to 10000 IU/L. In contrast, ALT rarely rises above 600 IU/L in patients with alcoholic hepatitis.

(Sleisenger, 9th edition, Pp-1558-1560)

35. **Ans. (C)** Cerebal artery aneurysms, congenital heart disease, bile duct and gallbladder anomalies, renal collection duct defects and intestinal lymphangiectasia are all seen in association with congenital hepatic fibrosis. Pancreatitis is not.

(Sleisenger, 9th edition, Pp-1059-1060)

36. **Ans. (C)** Hypercalcemia, erythrocytosis and hypoglycemia are common paraneoplastic complications of hepatocellular carcinoma, owing to production by the tumor of parathyroid hormone-related protein, erythropoietin and precursor of insulin-like growth factor, respectively. Dematomyositis is sometimes seen but is rare.

(Sleisenger, 9th edition, P-1571)

37. **Ans. (A)** Alcoholic hepatitis is a histopathologic diagnosis characterized by fatty change, necrosis of hepatocytes and an inflammatory infiltrate. Mallory bodies (condensed cytoskeletal elements) are often present. Councilman bodies are found in viral hepatitis.

(Sleisenger, 9th edition, P-1390)

38. **Ans. (A)** Spontaneous bacterial peritonitis occurs in pre-existing ascitic fluid (usually in low protein ascitic fluid due to portal hypertension) but is not the cause of ascites per se. All of the other conditions listed actually cause ascites, albeit through different mechanisms.

(Sleisenger, 9th edition, P-1523)

39. **Ans. (D)** The least reliable method for in utero diagnosis of cystic fibrosis is measurement of microvillous enzyme levels in amniotic fluid using monoclonal antibodies, with a flase positive rate of 1% and a false-negative rate of 17%. DNA probes linked to the cystic fibrosis gene can be used in over 80% of gestation. Direct mutation analysis is the most reliable and specific test. However the most common mutation (F508) is present in only about 70% of all affected chromosomes.

(Sleisenger, 9th edition, Pp-935-936)

40. **Ans. (B)** The fat-soluble vitamins include vitamins A,D,E and K and all are dependent on adequate fatty acid micellization in the intestine by sufficient bile acids. Vitamin A occurs in nature in three forms. All trans-retinol (Vitamin A_1) and 3-dehydroretinol (Vitamin A_2) are found in mammals, whereas in plants Vitamin A occurs as the water soluble precursor beta-carotene. Vitamin D, produced by the action of ultraviolet light on 7-dehydrocholesterol in the skin of human subjects, is called cholealciferol (Vitamin D_3). The plant form of vitamin D is ergocalciferol or Vitamin D_2. Vitamin D is hydroxylated in the liver to 25 hydroxy D and in the

kidney to 1.25-dihydroxy D, the active form. Vitamin E (tocopherol) is an antioxidant that protects against lipid per oxidation in membranes. Vitamin K (phylloquinone) is necessary for normal coagulation and is inhibited by warfarin. Cobalamin, or Vitamin B_{12}, is not a fat-soluble Vitamin, although Vitamin B_{12}/intrinsic factor complex is absorbed in the ileum.

(Sleisenger, 9th edition, P-1078)

41. **Ans. (D)** Common causes of odynophagia include pill esophagitis, caustic ingestion and inftious esophagitis. Gastroesophageal reflux complicated by severe ulcerative esophagitis may present as odynophagia, whereas it is rare for esophageal carcinoma to present in this fashion.

(Sleisenger, 9th edition, Pp-735-742)

42. **Ans. (C)** Fecal incontinence complicates the course of the diabetes in approximately one in five diabetics. It seems to reflect reduced anal sphincter pressure and impaired sensation. Coexisting diarrhea may complicate the incontinence but is not usually the cause. Biofeedback training may sometimes be helpful in regaining control of sphincter.

(Sleisenger, 9th edition, Pp-241-258)

43. **Ans. (A)** Although chest radiography and abdominal films will not definitively demonstrate the presence of an abscess, they provide valuable clues with respect to the presence of fluid collections and extraluminal gas. Both abdominal ultrasonography and computed tomography are quite useful because they permit image-guided aspiration of suspicious fluid collection. In contrast, magnetic resonance imaging is significantly more expensive and cannot be used for directing fine-needle aspiration.

(Sleisenger, 9th edition, Pp-411-416)

44. **Ans. (B)** Administering fat-free parenteral nutrition can cause biochemical evidence of essential fatty acid deficiency within two weeks. The optimal percentage of calories that should be infused as fat is not known. A minimum of about 5% of total calories as a lipid emulsion is necessary to prevent essential fatty acid deficiency. Parenteral nutrition can cause biochemical evidence of essential fatty acid deficiency within two weeks because the resulting increase in plasma insulin suppresses release of essential fatty acids from endogenous fat stores. Complications are more common when intravenous lipid emulsions are provided in excess of 1.0 kcal/kg/hr. Thus 25% to 50% of daily caloric intake should be in the form of lipid emulsions unless contraindicated and the infusion rate should not exceed 0.7 kcal/kg/hr.

(Internet source)

45. **Ans. (A)** Most cases of mesothelioma are malignant. Asbestos workers and members of their households are at risk, but the interval between exposures and diagnosis is long. Although surgical resection has been advocated by some, the best results are obtained by radiation therapy in combination with systemic and intraperitoneal chemotherapy.

(Internet source)

46. **Ans. (A)** The term obesity means the excessive accumulation of body fat. In general, men in whom more than 25% and women in whom more than 35% of body weight is fat are considered obese. In contrast the term overweight refers to persons whose body weight is greater than an ideal standard. Because it ignores the composition of the body, nonobese persons with muscular bodies may be classified as overweight. The National Center for Health Statistics defines obesity as a body mass index of 27.8 or more determined by weight in kilograms divided by estimated surface areas in metres squared. Defining obesity in terms of usual or ideal body weight for a given height incorrectly assumes a strong correlation between weight and adiposity. Other problems with widespread use of height-weight tables include variations in skeletal mass, bone density and the definition of ideal body weight.

(Sleisenger, 9th edition, Pp-99-103)

47. **Ans. (B)** Solid agents are difficult to swallow, adhering to mucus membranes in the oropharynx; however the absence of oropharyngeal injury does not exclude severe esophageal or gastric injury. The most common site of esophageal stricture after caustic ingestion is in the proximal esophagus at the level of the cricopharyngeus or the aortic arch. Stridor and hoarseness suggest airway injury and should be evaluated before endoscopic examination of the gastrointestinal tract to ensure airway safety.

(Sleisenger, 9th edition, Pp-406-409)

48. **Ans. (C)** Routine radiographic studies demonstrate a 60% incidence of hiatal hernia in unselected elderly patients the most common type being a sliding hiatal hernia.

(Internet source)

49. Ans. (C) In patients with biliary obstruction, therapy is typically directed at mechanical relief of obstruction. In cholestatic liver disease, treatment is directed toward reversing the underlying metabolic defect. Pruritus is a potentially disabling symptom of cholestatic hepatobiliary disease. Bile acid-binding resins such a cholestyramine have been of some benefit in treating this disorder. Naloxone, Rifampin and ursodiol have also been used with some success. Omerprazole has not known value in cholestasis.

(Sleisenger, 9th edition, P-1486)

50. Ans. (A) Percutaneous abscess drainage requires that a safe access route be available that avoids traversing bowel and is not adjacent to major vascular structures, owing to risk of perforation or hemorrhage.

(Sleisenger, 9th edition, Pp-411-416)

51. Ans. (D) Rectal balloon manometry can provide information about several physiologic functions. By inflating the rectal balloon with increasing volumes of air or water the threshold for conscious sensation of rectal distention can be estimated normally, as little as 10 mL of rectal distention can be detected. By monitoring pressure in the upper anal canal during rectal distention, on can evaluate the rectoanal inhibitory reflex. The threshold amount of rectal distention required to elicit reflex relaxation of the internal and sphincter averages about 20 mL in normal subjects. It is usually higher than the threshold for conscious sensation. The increase in pressure in the lower anal canal after rectal distention reflects contractile activity in the external and sphincter and is called the rectoanal contractile response. Absence of this response can be due to interruption of the afferent or efferent extrinsic nerves, weakness of the external anal sphincter, or forgetting this learned response. Finally, rectal balloon manometry can be used to estimate rectal compliance.

(Sleisenger, 9th edition, Pp-241-258)

52. Ans. (B) The presence on peritoneal lavage of a white blood cell count greater than 500 cells/mm^3, a bilirubin or amylase level greater than serum value, or bacteria on Gram stain is associated with a more than 90% chance that peritonitis is present. Albumin levels no value in this setting.

(Sleisenger, 9th edition, Pp-614-615)

53. Ans. (D) The duration of survival during starvation depends on the stores of body fuels available. People of normal weight can survive for about two months when ingesting only water. Death in Irish hunger strikers generally occurred after they had lost about 35% of their body weight and is common after loss of 40%. In contrast, obese people have undergone therapeutic fasts for more than one year without adverse consequences, surviving only on water, vitamins and minerals.

(Internet source)

54. Ans. (C) Anal manometry can provide a direct measure of the pressure sensation in the anal canal under basal conditions and with squeezing. As a group patients, with fecal incontinence have significantly lower basal squeeze pressures than age and sex-matched controls. Manometry is most valuable when it demonstrates abnormally low pressures and thus confirms the presence of a sphincter defect.

(Sleisenger, 9th edition, P-247)

55. Ans. (B & C) The only two drugs that have been systematically studies for an effect on fecal continence are Lomotil (a combined product of diphenoxylate and atropine) and loperamide. Lomotil reduced stool frequency and weight. It had no effect on sphincter pressure or on tests for incontinence for solids or rectally infused saline. Loperamide at a dose of 4 mg three times a day significantly reduced the frequency of incontinence episodes and urgency, increased basal anal sphincter pressure slightly, and improved continence for rectally infused saline.

(Sleisenger, 9th edition, P-252)

56. Ans. (D) The diagnosis of peritoneal tuberculosis is suggested by an elevated lymphocyte count in the peritoneal fluid and negative cytology. Fever is present in the majority of patients. Peritoneal fluid smears stained for acid fast bacilli are rarely positive. By contrast histology and culture of the peritoneum obtained by laparoscopic biopsy are virtually always diagnostic.

(Sleisenger, 9th edition, P-1684)

BILIARY TRACT

57. Ans. (B) This patient has symptomatic gallstone disease, bile acid therapy is more successful for cholesterol stones that are small (i.e.<1.5 cm diameter) and buoyant. Extracorporeal shock wave lithotripsy can be successful with single, small stones, however, it is less effective with multiple, larger stones. Contact dissolution (therapy than involves infusion of the gallbladder with methyl-tert-butyl ether (MTBE) can be performed within a few hours of the patient's attack and is successful in upto 90% of selected cases (i.e. if cholesterol stones are small, without calcified rims).

Elective cholecystectomy remains the standard care for the majority of eligible patients, because recurrence rates are high after non-surgical therapy.

(Sleisenger, 9th edition, Pp-1122-1124)

58. Ans. (A) Although 85% of gall stones contain cholesterol, only 20% are relatively pure cholesterol stones.

(Sleisenger, 9th edition, Pp-1102-1104)

59. Ans. (A) This patient has gallstone ileus, inflammation and necrosis of the gallbladder resulted in a fistula between the bowel and the gallbladder. After the stone passed into the bowel, the patients' symptoms subsided and the acute cholecystits resolved. However, the stone caused bowel obstruction, which can occur with stones larger than 2.5 cm in diameter. The most common site of obstruction is the distal ileum (65% to 85% of cases) followed by the jejunum. Surgery is required to relieve the obstruction.

(Sleisenger, 9th edition, P-1133)

60. Ans. (D) Choledochal cysts may be complicated by pancreatitis, cholangitis, cholecystitis, cyst rupture, biliary cirrhosis, portal hypertension, and cholangiocarcinoma.

(Sleisenger, 9th edition, Pp-1058-1060)

61. Ans. (B) The most likely diagnosis is pancreatic carcinoma. Stent placement into the common bile duct is an effective as surgery for achieving biliary drainage: however, for palliation of nausea and pain it has not been compared in a controlled fashion with no intervention.

(Sleisenger, 9th edition, P-1025)

62. Ans. (A) Seventy percent to 90% of reported choledochal cysts are type I. Characterized by fusiform or saccular dilation of the common bile duct, without hepatic duct involvement. Type II choledochal cysts, true diverticula of the common bile duct, comprise less than 3% of all cases. Type III choledochal cysts, also known as choledocholceles are located in the distal intraduodenal segment of the common bile duct and represent 2% to 20% of all cases. Type IV is the classification for multiple extra hepatic or mixed intra and extra hepatic cyst whereas type V represents intra hepatic cysts only – the condition known as Caroli disease.

(Sleisenger, 9th edition, P-1058)

63. Ans. (C) The best management plan in this situation is to remove the stones though the existing T tube when the tract is mature, usually 4 to 6 weeks postoperatively. If this fails, endoscopic retrograde cholangiopancreatography with sphincterotomy and stone extraction is indicated. Repeat laparotomy usually is unnecessary; however, if the other options fails it should be performed because common bile duct stones should not be left in situ.

(Sleisenger, 9th edition, P-1134)

64. Ans. (A) A moderate rise in serum amylase is observed following 35% to 70% of pancreatograms. Typically the hyperamylasemia is not accompanied by clinical symptoms and subsides in 1 to 2 days. Although overfilling of the pancreatic duct is claimed to be the main causative factor in the development of acute pancreatitis, acute pancreatitis has been observed in some patients after unsuccessful cannulation of the pancreatic duct. This may in part be the result of repeated trauma and subsequent development of edema of the papilla. The addition of sphincter of Oddi manometry increase the risk of procedure-related pancreatitis and patients should be advised of this risk. Infection of a pseudocyst and subsequent abscess formation can occur if the pseudocyst communicates with the pancreatic duct; therefore, endoscopic retrograde cholangiopancratography should not been performed unless drainage of the pseudocyst is anticipated.

(Sleisenger, 9th edition, P-967)

65. Ans. (B) There is no evidence that proctocolectomy has any beneficial effect on the course of primary sclerosing cholangitis (PSC) nor that it will prevent the development of cholagiocarcinoma in patients with chronic ulcerative colitis. PSC may obscure the diagnosis of cholangiocarcinoma. The incidence of cholangiocarcinoma ranges from 7% to 15% in patients with PSC. About 10% of patients undergoing liver transplantation for PSC are found to have cholangiocarcinoma. Secondary biliary cirrhosis is found in 30% of patients at the time of diagnosis of PSC; therefore, liver transplantation should be considered for those with deterioration of hepatic synthetic function.

(Sleisenger, 9th edition, Pp-1158-1160)

66. Ans. (C) An elevated basal pressure in the sphincter of Oddi is a better predictor of pain relief after endoscopic sphincterotomy than are cholangiographic findings of a dilated common bile duct or delayed drainage of contrast from the bile duct.

(Sleisenger, 9th edition, P-1072)

67. Ans. (C) Delayed drainage of injected contrast material (i.e. >45 minutes) has been documented in many patients with sphincter of Oddi dysfunction.

(Sleisenger, 9th edition, P-1069)

68. Ans. (D) Primary biliary cirrhosis may be associated with other autoimmune disorders, such as Sjögren syndrome and thyroidits. An association between primary biliary cirrhosis and diabetes mellitus has not been reported.

(Sleisenger, 9th edition, Pp-1020-1021)

69. Ans. (B) Ultrasonography is the best imaging technique for the detection of cholelithiasis; conversely, in the typical patient with painless jaundice, a computed tomography (CT) scan may be the best initial investigative tool. If a pancreatic mass is noted without evidence of metastatic spread on the CT scan, further investigation is not needed before proceeding to surgery. If there is no mass visible on the CT scan, diagnostic endoscopic retrograde cholangiopancreatography may be performed to determine the site and type of obstruction.

(Sleisenger, 9th edition, P-1344)

70. Ans. (C) For explanation see Ans. no. 69.

(Sleisenger, 9th edition, P-1344)

71. Ans. (C) Ultrasonography of abdomen is the best initial imaging for suspected gall stone disease.

(Sleisenger, 9th edition, P-1106)

72. Ans. (C) The proper selection of patients is a key factor affecting the success of bile acid dissolution therapy. Favorable criteria include the following characteristic: gallstones composed chiefly of cholesterol, small stones (<1.5 cm diameter), stones with a large surface area in relation to mass, and stones that are mobile within the gallbladder. Pigment stones or calcified stones cannot be dissolved with bile acids.

(Sleisenger, 9th edition, P-1022)

73. Ans. (D) Primary sclerosing cholangitis (PSC) may be associated with many disorders. The most common is ulcerative colitis, which occurs in 50% of 75% of patients with PSC. Other associated disorder includes AIDS, pancreatitis, Riedel thyroiditis, celiac disease and sarcoidosis. Hepatitis A and B do not cause PSC.

(Sleisenger, 9th edition, Pp-1156-1157)

74. Ans. (A) Liver flukes such as Clonorchis sinensis can infect persons in Japan, China, Indochina, South Korea and Taiwan who eat uncooked fish. The major pathologic changes induced by chronic infection occur in the bile ducts.

(Sleisenger, 9th edition, Pp-1934-1936)

75. Ans. (A) Adult liver flukes (e.g. Clonorchis sinensis, Opisthorchis viverrini and Fasciola hepatica) live in the distal portion of biliary tract.

(Sleisenger, 9th edition, Pp-1934-1936)

76. Ans. (D) The most common cause of acute cholecystitis is obstruction of the cystic duct by gallstones, resulting in acute inflammation of the gallbladder. Approximately 90% of cases are associated with cholelithiasis.

(Sleisenger, 9th edition, P-1105)

77. Ans. (C) Alcohol abuse is not a risk factor for gallbladder carcinoma.

(Sleisenger, 9th edition, P-1178)

78. Ans. (C) Clinically, patients with AIDS associated cholangiopathy present with right upper quadrant or epigastric abdominal pain (64% to 88%), fever (20% to 65%) and cholestasis (75% to 80%). The serum bilirubin level is usually normal or minimally elevated, whereas the alkaline phosphatase level is typically elevated to values in the rage of 700 U/L.

(Sleisenger, 9th edition, P-534)

79. Ans. (D) Jaundice is a poor prognostic sign in gall-bladder cancer; more that 85% of these patients having unresettable tumors.

(Sleisenger, 9th edition, Pp-1178-1180)

80. Ans. (D) Hepatobiliary disease associated with AIDS include diffuse hepatocellular injury, granulomatous hepatitis and sclerosing cholangitis. Fatty infiltration of the liver is common in patients with AIDS who have abnormal liver chemistries. A primary biliary cirrhosis like syndrome has also been reported. Nodular regenerative hyperplasia is not reported to be associated with AIDS.

(Sleisenger, 9th edition, P-532)

81. Ans. (A) In primary sclerosing cholangitis, the alkaline phosphatase level is elevated in more than 90% of cases; increased circulating immune complexes are measurable in 80% of cases, and the test for perinuclear anti-neutrophilic cytoplasmic antibody is positive in 80% to 85% of cases. Anti-mitochondrial antibody, rheumatoid factor and smooth muscle antibody are absent in more than 90% of cases.

(Sleisenger, 9th edition, P-1160)

82. Ans. (A) Only 10% of ductal injuries, such as a bile leak, are recognized in the first postoperative week. Patients with bile leaks usually present with acute bile peritonitis. Two-thirds of patients with ductal injury present with strictures as late as 1 year after the operation. The outcome is better if the repair of the ductal injury is immediate either by endoscopic stent placement or by laparotomy, than if the repair is delayed for several days. Most patients have virtually not symptoms after laparoscopic cholecystectomy. Therefore, the presence of any symptoms such as nausea or pain, on the first postoperative day, even if vague, is justification for emergent biliary scintigraphy. Development of an ileus on the second post-operative days is an indication of a complication that must be evaluated.

(Sleisenger, 9th edition, P-1128)

83. **Ans. (A)** Bile duct injury-defected in immediate postoperative period best increased with by endoscopic stent placement or by laparotomy.

(Sleisenger, 9th edition, Pp-1134-1135)

84. **Ans. (A)** In healthy subjects, the ratio of glycine to taurine conjugates in bile is ~3:1.

(Harrison, 17th edition, P-1991)

85. **Ans. (C)** A caudal bud that advances further than the cranial bud may become buried within the cranial structure, creating an intrahepatic gallbladder. If the caudal bud lags behind the movement of the cranial bud, a floating gallbladder results. In this setting, the gallbladder is covered completely with peritoneum and suspended from the undersurface of the liver by mesentery to the gallbladder or cystic duct. In this anomaly, the gallbladder is abnormally mobile and prone to torsion.

(Sleisenger, 8th edition, P-1338)

86. **Ans. (A)** Cholesterol, phospholipids, and bile acids are the major lipid components in bile. In humans, the extent of cholesterol saturation in gallbladder bile is the most important single determinant of crystal formation.

(Sleisenger, 8th edition, P-1096)

87. **Ans. (C)** As with cholesterol gallstones, the prevalence of pigment stones increases with age and is generally higher in women than men. Black pigment stone formation is typically associated with chronic hemolysis (as in α-thalassemia, hereditary spherocytosis, and sickle cell hemoglobinopathy), cirrhosis, and pancreatitis. In patients with cirrhosis, the higher risk of pigment stones is associated with advanced stages of disease, although the reported frequency rates vary widely. Whether alcoholic cirrhosis carries a higher risk of stone formation than other forms of cirrhosis is controversial.

* Octreotide therapy associated with formation of cholesterol stress.

(Sleisenger, 9th edition, P-1092)

88. **Ans. (A)** Smaller stones may be missed or may be confused with biliary sludge (layering echogenic material that does not cast acoustic shadows).

(Sleisenger, 8th edition, P-1398)

89. **Ans. (C)** Cholecystectomy should be performed in asymptomatic patient if patient (a) Morbid obese (b) Size 72.5 cm (c) Porcelain gallbladder (d) Hemolytic anemia with pigment stone (e) Patient anxiety for heart, lung transplantation (f) History of prior biliary complication (g) Stones in congenitally anomalous gall-bladder.

(Sleisenger, 9th edition, P-1129)

90. **Ans. (A)** "Unusual" bacterial infections of the gallbladder (e.g., *Leptospira*, *Streptococcus*, *Salmonella*, or *Vibrio cholerae*), and parasitic infestation of the gallbladder. Acalculous cholecystitis may also be seen with a variety of other systemic disease processes (sarcoidosis, cardiovascular disease, tuberculosis, syphilis, actinomycosis, etc.).

(Harrison, 17th edition, P-1996)

91. **Ans. (B)** The following criteria can be used to identify patients with acalculous cholecystopathy: (1) recurrent episodes of typical RUQ pain characteristic of biliary tract pain, (2) abnormal CCK cholescintigraphy demonstrating a gallbladder ejection fraction of <40%, and (3) infusion of CCK reproduces the patient's pain. An additional clue would be the identification of a large gallbladder on ultrasound examination.

(Harrison, 17th edition, P-1996)

92. **Ans. (A)** Fistulas into the duodenum are most common, followed in frequency by those involving the hepatic flexure of the colon, stomach or jejunum, abdominal wall, and renal pelvis.

(Harrison, 17th edition, P-1997)

93. **Ans. (A)** The site of obstruction by the impacted gallstone is usually at the ileocecal valve, provided that the more proximal small bowel is of normal caliber.

(Harrison, 17th edition, P-1997)

94. **Ans. (A)** Only one-third of patients show the classic triad of abdominal pain, jaundice and an abdominal mass.

(Harrison, 17th edition, P-1998)

95. Ans. (C) Following relief of the obstructing process, serum aminotransferase elevations usually return rapidly to normal, while the serum bilirubin level may take 1-2 weeks to return to normal. The alkaline phosphatase level usually falls slowly, lagging behind the decrease in serum bilirubin.

(Harrison, 17th edition, P-1999)

96. Ans. (B) The interlobular bile ducts form a richly anastomosing network that closely surrounds the branches of the portal vein. These bile ducts are initially 30 to 40 mm in diameter and are lined by a layer of cuboidal or columnar epithelium that demonstrates a microvillous architecture on its luminal surface.

(Sleisenger, 8th edition, P-1335)

97. Ans. (B) The total daily basal secretion of hepatic bile is ~500–600 mL.

(Harrison, 17th edition, P-1991)

98. Ans. (C) Bile is normally secreted at a pressure of about 15-25 cm arise to about 35 cm water result in suspension of bile flow and jaundice.

(Sheila Sherlock, 8th edition, P-223)

99. Ans. (A) Many drugs used after HCT have been associated with cholestatic liver disease. Cyclosporine (CSP) inhibits canalicular bile transport and commonly causes mild increases in serum bilirubin.

(Sleisenger, 8th edition, P-693)

100. Ans. (B) *Anabolic steroids* can produce a syndrome that is clinically indistinguishable from estrogen-induced cholestasis. The anabolic steroids methyl-testosterone and norethandrolone may impair the integrity of hepatocellular *microfilaments,* thereby increasing the permeability of tight junctions and resulting in back diffusion of biliary solutes intoserum.

(Sleisenger, 8th edition, P-307)

101. Ans. (D) Following bile duct obstruction, the hepatic changes develop very rapidly. Cholestasis is seen within 36 hours. Bile duct proliferation is early; portal fibrosis develops later. Bile lakes represent ruptured interlobular ducts.

(Sheila Sherlock, 8th edition, P-225)

102. Ans. (C) Following bile duct obstruction, the hepatic changes develop very rapidly. Cholestasis is seen within 36 hours.

(Sheila Sherlock, 8th edition, P-225)

103. Ans. (A) Xanthoma usually developed when lipid depostis in tendon sheath

(Sleisenger, 9th edition, Pp-1086-1087)

104. Ans. (D) X usually develops when serum cholesterol level exceeds 450 mg% and persists for more than 3 months.

(Sleisenger, 9th edition, Pp-1086-1087)

105. Ans. (A) Extrahepatic effects: The kidneys have an increased susceptibility to hypotension and hypoxic damage. The processes involved in responding to sepsis and in wound healing is impaired. The prolonged PT is correctable with Vit K but coagulation may still be abnormal due to platelet dysfunction.

(Sheila Sherlock, 8th edition, P-230)

106. Ans. (D) PFIC type 1 (Byler's disease) is autosomal recessive disease. Recurrent episodes of intrahepatic cholestastis lead to permanent cholestasis, fibrosis, cirrhosis and liver failure. Liver transplantation may be necessary in the first decades of life.

(Sleisenger, 9th edition, P-1085)

107. Ans. (A) Lipoprotein -X (LP-X) is a spherical particle, 70 mm in diameter, associated with low density lipoprotein fraction. It is increased in both intra and extra hepatic cholestasis but is of no practical diagnostic value.

(Sheila Sherlock, 8th edition, P-231)

108. Ans. (C) Table 86.4: Independent predictors of survival in patients with primary biliary cirrhosis (Mayo Clinic) Age, Bilirubin, Albumin, Prothrombin Time, Edema.

(Sleisenger, 8th edition, P-1891)

109. Ans. (B) In patients with a serum bilirubin level greater than 10 mg/dL, however, the average life expectancy is reduced to 2 years. In order to predict survival in patients with PBC, prognostic models, some of which rely on Cox's proportional hazard analysis, have been developed.

(Sleisenger, 8th edition, P-1891)

110. Ans. (A) The Mayo risk score, a cross-validated index of survival in PBC, decreases significantly during UDCA therapy.

(Sleisenger, 8th edition, P-1893)

111. Ans. (C) Further, biliary tract lesions in AIDS include infection and cholangiopancreatographic changes similar to those of PSC. Changes noted include: (1)

diffuse involvement of intrahepatic bile ducts alone, (2) involvement of both intra- and extrahepatic bile ducts, (3) ampullary stenosis, (4) stricture of the intrapancreatic portion of the common bile duct, and (5) pancreatic duct involvement.

(Harrison, 17th edition, P-2000)

112. Ans. (C) The common bile duct is approximately 7 cm long, runs between layers of the lesser omentum, and lies anterior to the portal vein and to the right of the hepatic artery. The common bile duct normally is 0.5 to 1.5 cm in diameter.

(Sleisenger, 8th edition, P-1337)

113. Ans. (A) The most common cause of this form of obstructive jaundice is carcinoma of the head of the pancreas. Biliary obstruction may also occur as a complication of either acute or chronic pancreatitis or involvement of lymph nodes in the portahepatis by lymphoma or metastatic carcinoma.

(Harrison, 17th edition, P-2000)

114. Ans. (D) *Mucin glycoprotein* is the most important pronuclear to be identified. The core of mucin glycoproteins contains hydrophobic regions that can bind cholesterol, phospholipids and bilirubin.

Secretion of mucin is mediated, at least in part, by prostaglandins, and may be inhibited by nonsteroidal anti-inflammatory drugs (NSAIDs). Administration of aspirin prevents gallstone formation in prairie dogs and reduces mucin secretion in humans.

Other pronucleators in model bile systems isolated through lecithin chromatography using concanavalin A sepharose are immunoglobulin (Ig)G and IgM, aminopeptidase N, haptoglobin and α_1-acid glycoprotein, *Antinucleating proteins* that have been identified in model bile systems include apoA-I and apoA-II, and a biliary glycoprotein. The physiologic role of these factors requires further study.

(Sleisenger, 8th edition, P-1394)

115. Ans. (D) *Mucin glycoprotein* is the most important pronuclear to be identified. The core of mucin glycoproteins contains hydrophobic regions that can bind cholesterol, phospholipids and bilirubin.

Secretion of mucin is mediated, at least in part, by prostaglandins, and may be inhibited by nonsteroidal anti-inflammatory drugs (NSAIDs). Administration of aspirin prevents gallstone formation in prairie dogs and reduces mucin secretion in humans.

Other pronucleators in model bile systems isolated through lecithin chromatography using concanavalin A sepharose are immunoglobulin (Ig)G and IgM, aminopeptidase N, haptoglobin and α_1-acid glycoprotein, *Antinucleating proteins* that have been identified in model bile systems include apoA-I and apoA-II, and a biliary glycoprotein. The physiologic role of these factors requires further study.

(Sleisenger, 8th edition, P-1394)

116. Ans. (A) Lonigluide is a selective antagonist of CCK.

(Sleisenger, 8th edition, P-1474)

117. Ans. (A) Dutopenia rejection is defined as loss of interlobular and septal bile ducts in 50% of portal tracts. Duct loss is calculated from the ratio of number of hepatic arteries to bile ducts within a portal tract (normal greater than 0.7). Preferably 20 portal tracts should be studied.

(Sheila Sherlock, 8th edition, P-672)

118. Ans. (A) Small studies suggest that high-dose UDCA may influence the progression of disease favorably. Larger randomized studies of high-dose UDCA are currently in progress.

(Sleisenger, 9th edition, P-743)

119. Ans. (C) IL-6–responsible for sepsis related cholestasis.

(Sleisenger, 9th edition, P-1130)

120. Ans. (C) MRCP/ERCP are the most sensitive investigation for obstructive jaundice.

(Sleisenger, 9th edition, P-1115)

121. Ans. (D) Histological findings strongly suggestive of extra hepatic biliary obstruction are bile infarct, bile lakes and neutrophils in interlobular ducts.

(Sleisenger, 9th edition, Pp-1480-1496)

122. Ans. (C) Pruritus associated with cholestasis are best treated with cholestyramine.

(Sleisenger, 9th edition, P-1487)

123. Ans. (D) The outcome (mean survival 7.5 months) is similar to that and matched AIDS controls. Only

14% survive 1 year prognosis depends on the stage of immunosuppression. Treatment is primarily endoscopic sphincterotomy gives striking relief of pain and cholangitis.

(Sleisenger, 9th edition, P-530)

124. Ans. (C) Gallbladder is patent by third month of gestation.

(Sleisenger, 9th edition, P-1047)

125. Ans. (B) Canal of hering is proliferated in response to extrahepatic biliary obstruction.

(Sleisenger, 9th edition, P-1284)

126. Ans. (A) Supraduodenal portion of CBD is more susceptible to postoperative stricture.

(Sleisenger, 9th edition, P-1136)

127. Ans. (A) Fasiculi longitudinales of sphinchter of Oddi that promotes bile flow.

(Sleisenger, 9th edition, P-1067)

128. Ans. (C) Sphincter ampullae contraction prevents reflex of intestinal contents.

(Sleisenger, 9th edition, P-1067)

129. Ans. (C) Fundus lies at the level of right ninth costal cartilage.

(Sleisenger, 9th edition, P-1049)

130. Ans. (A) Spiral valve of heister is formed by mucous membrane.

(Sleisenger, 9th edition, P-1049)

131. Ans. (D) Idiopathic neonatal hepatitis is the most common cause of neonatal cholestasis accounting for 30-35% of cases.

(Sleisenger, 9th edition, P-1051)

132. Ans. (D) Type III is the most common type of extrahepatic biliary atresia.

(Sleisenger, 9th edition, P-1053)

133. Ans. (D) Inability to concentrate is the most common renal manifestation of caroli disease.

(Sleisenger, 9th edition, P-1051)

134. Ans. (C) Syndromic paucity of interlobular bile ducts (Alagille's syndrome or arteriohepatic dysplasia) is the most common form of familial intrahepatic cholestasis. It is characterized by chronic cholestasis, a decreased no. of interlobular bile ducts and a variety of other congenital malformations. Congenital heart disease occurs in most patients and peripheral pulmonic stenosis is observed in approximately 90%. Autosomal dominant mode of transmission with incomplete penetrance and varying expression has been established mutation in JAGI gene has been identified in 70% of affected patients. Progression to cirrhosis and liver failure was infrequent hepatocelluar carcinoma was an occasional complication.

(Sleisenger, 9th edition, P-1060)

135. Ans. (A) Paucity is defined as ratio of number of interlobular bile duct to no. of portal tract less than 0.4:1.

(Sleisenger, 9th edition, P-1061)

136. Ans. (A) Pigmented gall stone predominate in infants and children higher frequency of calculous cholecystitis (29.1%) is reported in sick premature infants who undergo a period of prolonged fasting without frequent stimulation of gallbladder contraction and who require period of prolonged parenteral nutrition. Many of these patients have complicated medical course that involve frequent blood transfusion, episodes of sepsis, abdominal surgery and use of diuretics and narcotic analgesic.

(Sleisenger, 9th edition, P-1063)

137. Ans. (D) In age group of 1-5 years, hepatobiliary disease attributes to be most common course of cholelithiasis followed by abdominal surgery, artificial heart valve, malabsorption.

(Sleisenger, 9th edition, P-1063)

138. Ans. (C) In age group of 6-21 years, most common cause of cholelithiasis appears to be pregnancy (37.2) followed by obesity (8.1), hemolytic anemia abdominal surgery.

(Sleisenger, 9th edition, P-1063)

139. Ans. (B) Acute non-calculus, non-inflammatory distension of the gallbladder may be observed in infant and children. Absence of GB inflammation and generally benign prognosis distinguish acute hydrops from acute acalculous cholelithiasis. Association with generalized merenteric adenitis, scarlet fever, leptospirosis, Kawasaki disease and Henöch purpura has been observed and also with prolonged nutrition.

(Sleisenger, 9th edition, P-1065)

140. Ans. (C) Upto 60% of cases of SOD-dysfunction, may have history of abdominal pain.

(Sleisenger, 9th edition, P-1070)

141. Ans. (C) Amplitude of phasic contraction >120 usually associated with recurrent pancreatitis.

(Sleisenger, 9th edition, P-1070)

142. Ans. (B) Triad of sudden onset of RUQ tenderness, fever and leukocytosis is highly suggestive of acute cholecystitis.

(Harrison, 17th edition, P-1996)

143. Ans. (B) In case of gall stone during pregnancy, surgery is probably safest when performed during the second trimester thereby avoiding the risk of fetal loss and teratogenicity in the first trimester and the risk of preterm labor in third trimester.

(Sleisenger, 9th edition, P-1132)

144. Ans. (B) Most common site of stricture is around Hilar region.

(Sleisenger, 9th edition, P-1134)

145. Ans. (B) Gallbladder overlies-segment IV and V of liver.

(Sleisenger, 9th edition, Pp-1046-1047)

146. Ans. (C) Cholecystectomy is required if GB appears gangrenous, however, the treatment of GB hydrops is commonly non-surgical with focus on supportive care and management of intercurrent illness.

(Sleisenger, 9th edition, P-1065)

147. Ans. (B) All drugs that releax sphincter of oddi are nitrate, calcium channel blockers and anticholinergic or stimulate it (narcotic and cholinergics) should be avoided for 12 hours prior to manometry. Diazepam and meperidine do not affect basal sphincter pressure, although mepirdine does increase phasic wave's frequency. Midazolam may lower basal pressure in hypertensive sphincters and is best avoided. Glucagon should be avoided although some use it to achieve canulation if necessary.

(Sleisenger, 9th edition, Pp-1070-1071)

148. Ans. (D) Diazepam, meperidine and fentanyl.

(Sleisenger, 9th edition, P-1070)

149. Ans. (C) Pressure in CBD is normally 10 to 15 cm H_2O and rises to 25-40 cm H_2O with complete obstruction. When pressure exceeds 15 cm H_2O, bile flow, at 30 cm H_2O, bile flow stops.

(Sleisenger, 9th edition, P-1068)

150. Ans. (A) Diabetics are prone to development of both gall stones and complications from the stones. Morbidity and mortality rates for diabetic patients who undergo emergency operations for complications of gall stone disease have been thought to be excessive. These perceptions have not been borne out when confounding variables such as hyperlipidemia, obesity, cardiovascular disease and chronic kidney disease are taken into account. Hence prophylactic cholecystectomy in an asymptomatic diabetic patient with gall stones does not appear to be warranted.

(Sleisenger, 9th edition, Pp-1126-1128)

151. Ans. (D) Three main types of atresia have been defined. Type-I – atresia of CBD with patent proximal duct; type-II – atresia of hepatic duct with cystically dilated bile ducts at portahepatis. In II a, cystic and common ducts are patent, in II b these are obliterated. These two types have been referred as surgically correctable.

(Sleisenger, 9th edition, Pp-1054-1055)

152. Ans. (B) CBD stones are the most common cause of postcholecystectomy symptoms. They may be residual stones overlooked at the time of cholecystectomy or less frequently, stones that have formed primarily in the duct.

(Sleisenger, 9th edition, P-1436)

153. Ans. (A) Composition of bile acid pool is an important determinant of bile lithogenicity. The more hydrophobic the bile acid, the greater its ability to induce cholesterol secretion and suppress bile acid synthesis. Patient with gall stones have smaller pools of cholic acid and larger pools of its metabolic deoxycholic acid. Latter is hydrophobic and raises CSI (cholesterol saturation index). It also produces arachidonic acid and which stimulate mucin secretion a proposed pronucleator.

(Sleisenger, 9th edition, P-1893)

154. Ans. (C) Elderly (age >50), female sex gall stones, calcified gallbladder (porcelain gallbladder) long common channel formed by union of pancreatic and CBD chronic typhoid carrier state are considered risk factor of CA gallbladder.

(Sleisenger, 9th edition, Pp-1178-1187)

155. Ans. (C) Criteria for oral bile acid dissolution therapy. Stage of gall stone disease–Symptomatic (biliary pain without complication). Gallbladder function–Opacification of GB on OCG (patent cystic duct)–Normal result of stimulated cholescintigraphy (normal gallbladder emptying). Normal result of functional USG (normal gallbladder emptying after a test meal). Stone characteristic–Radiolucent on X-ray, isodense or hypodense to bile and absence of calcification on CT, Diameter <6 mm (Optimal) or 6-10 mm acceptable.

(Sleisenger, 9th edition, P-1122)

156. **Ans. (B)** UDCA is preferred drug for oral dissolution treatment. It is taken in a dose of 8 to 10 mg/kg/day night time dosing is more effective and associate with better patient compliance than meal time dosing. Unlike chenodeoxycholic acid, UDCA is well tolerated and has no important side effects. Treatment should continue until stone dissolution is documented by two consecutive negative USG performed at least 1 month apart. Treatment should be stopped if the patient does not tolerate or experiences a complication of gallstone during treatment if the stones fail to dissolve after 6 months or if partial gallstones dissolution after 6 months fail to progress to complicate dissolution by 2 years.

(Sleisenger, 9th edition, P-1122)

157. **Ans. (C)** The time of dissolution varies among patients with a median rate of 0.7 mm per month.

(Sleisenger, 9th edition, P-1122)

158. **Ans. (D)** PSC is present in 2.4 to 4.0% with chronic UC and 1.4% to 3.4% patients with Crohn's disease.

(Sleisenger, 9th edition, P-1156)

159. **Ans. (B)** Obliterating cholangitis fibrosis cholangitis in only 5-10% of biopsy specimen.

(Sleisenger, 9th edition, P-1161)

160. **Ans. (A)** Major area of focal narrowing, known as dominant stricture, may be seen in PSC and often involve hepatic duct bifurcation.

(Sleisenger, 9th edition, P-1162)

161. **Ans. (D)** Several immunologic markers and auto antibodies are found in majority of patient with PSC, although none is specific hyperglobulinemia is common with elevation of IgM in upto 50% patient ANA, in low titer may be present in 24% to 83% smooth muscle antibodies in 13 to 20% but AMA are found is less than 10%. Auto antibodies against colonic and biliary epithelium have been demonstrated. Atypical P-ANCA most commonly found.

(Sleisenger, 9th edition, P-1160)

162. **Ans. (C)** PSC with normal, serum alkaline phosphate are found in zinc deficiency hypothyroidism, hereditary, hypophosphatasia and associated Wilson's disease.

163. **Ans. (C)** Cholangiocarcinoma remains the leading cause of death in PSC patient.

(Sleisenger, 9th edition, P-1162)

164. **Ans. (C)** Cystic duct and gallbaldder may be involved in upto 15% of cases but may not be visualized well on routine cholangiography.

(Sleisenger, 9th edition, P-1162)

165. **Ans. (C)** The Kaplan meir estimate of median survival for the entire cohort of patient with PSC both symptomatic and asymptomatic was 11.9 for symptomatic cohort, estimated survival was between 8 and 9 years. Similar observation was made in other studies also.

(Sleisenger, 8th edition, P-1446)

166. **Ans. (A)** Most common complication is pancreatitis but most common cause of death is infection cholangitis.

(Sleisenger, 9th edition, P-1197)

167. **Ans. (C)** High serum cholesterol does not seen to be a risk factor for gall stone formation. In fact, some studies have shown an inverse relationship between serum cholesterol levels and risk of gall stone. Hypertriglyceridemia is associated with a higher frequency of gall stone disease. HDL chol level have correlated inversely with gall stones in some studies.

(Sleisenger, 9th edition, P-1093)

168. **Ans. (A)** High risk group population for gall stone includes: Indians, Scandinavian and American Indian.

(Sleisenger, 9th edition, P-1093)

169. **Ans. (B)** Population with lowest risk reside in Africa and Asia.

(Sleisenger, 9th edition, P-1434)

170. **Ans. (C)** The portions of GB are fundus, body infundibulum and neck. GB is supplied by cystic artery, artery from R hepatic artery. It divides into two branches of GB. Cystic artery is an end artery therefore GB is particularly susceptible to ischemic injury and necrosis.

(Sleisenger, 8th edition, P-1337)

171. **Ans. (D)** Cholangiocarcinoma express somatostatin receptors.

(Sleisenger, 9th edition, Pp-1172-1174)

172. **Ans. (B)** Biliary strictures commonly occur after liver transplantation for PSC. In addition, potential course of post strictures are ABO old group incompatibility, hepatic artery thrombosis chronic ductopenic rejection, Rouxeny related cholangitis and preservation injury related graft ischemia.

(Sleisenger, 9th edition, P-1166)

173. Ans. (C) Palinaz stent is balloon expandable metal biliary stent. Wall stent is self expanding covered stainless metallic stent. Gianturco is self expanding stainless steel metallic stent.

(Sleisenger, 9th edition, P-117)

174. Ans. (A) Bile duct obstruction is necessary to cause cholangitis. Cholangitis is relatively common in patient with choledocholithiasis and nearly universal in patient with post traumatic bile duct stricture but seen in only 15% of patients with neoplastic obstruction of the CBD.

(Sleisenger, 9th edition, P-1117)

175. Ans. (C) GBEF is calculated using cholescintigraphy.

- I/V administrated radiolabeled hepatobiliary urgent is concentrated in GB and gamma camera mercury activity before and after stimulation with CCK over 30 min.
- It is defined as change in activity divided by baseline activity. It always exceeds 35% much less than one half has depressed GBEF.

(Sleisenger, 9th edition, P-1143)

176. Ans. (C) Common postoperative or hospitalized patients recovering from trauma or burns. Patients are more likely to be men and old. Most cases occur in setting of prolonged fasting and hemodynamic instability specific mediator implicated in tissue injury of factor XII and local release of prostaglandins right upper quadrant pain, fever, local tenderness and leukocytosis may be evident in classic presentation some or all of these are lacking in elderly postoperative patient's often unexplained fever or hyperamyalesia is the only clue.

(Sleisenger, 9th edition, P-1141)

177. Ans. (C) C sump syndrome usually occurs after choledochoduodenostomy.

(Sleisenger, 9th edition, P-1384)

178. Ans. (C) Disease association with PSC include IBD commonly, followed by systemic disease with fibrosis autoimmune disorders alloimmune disease, infiltrative disease like histiocytosis sarcoidosis and some immunodeficiency states. In patient with AIDS a disorder with cholangiographic appearance identical to that of PSC termed AIDS cholangiopathy can develop.

(Sleisenger, 9th edition, P-1157)

179. Ans. (A) Neoplastic condition causing is secondary sclerosing cholangitis cholangiocarcinoma include HCC, metastatic cancer and lymphoma.

(Sleisenger, 9th edition, P-1158)

180. Ans. (A) Approximately 80% of all patient with PSC have concomitant IBD. Of these patients, approximate 85% to 90% have UC and remainder have Crohn's colitis or ileocolitis.

(Sleisenger, 9th edition, P-1158)

181. Ans. (C) (P) Small duct PSC–account for 5%-20% of cases. 12%15% progressed to classic large duct PSC. Cholangiography study–normal no risk of cholangiocarcinoma.

(Sleisenger, 9th edition, P-1158)

182. Ans. (C) A wide range of liver biopsy finding may be seen in patient with PSC. Histologic findings typically are not diagnostic for PSC. Characteristic lesion is fibro obliterative process around median size bile duct with onion skin appearance seen in less than one half of patients. Fibrous obliterative cholangitis including small septal bile duct branches is present in only 5-10% of biopsy specimen virtually pathognomonic of PSC.

(Sleisenger, 9th edition, P-1161)

183. Ans. (B) Characteristic cholangiographic findings include multifocal stricturing and ectasia of biliary tree. Dominant strictures may be seen often involve hepatic duct bifurcation. Both extrahepatic and intrahepatic bile duct are abnormal in approximate only 75% of cases. Intrahepatic ducts alone are involved in 15 to 20% of cases. Cystic duct and gallbladder may be involved in upto 15% of cases.

PSC without IBD are predominantly female, isolated to extrahepatic duct only and always symptomatic.

(Sleisenger, 9th edition, P-1156)

Chapter 9

ENDOSCOPIC PROCEDURES

1. **The best treatment modality for primary hemostasis from gastric varices is:**
   A. Endoscopic variceal ligation
   B. Endoscopic variceal sclerotherapy
   C. Endoscopic variceal obliteration
   D. Balloon tamponade

2. **Which of the following is the most common finding in enteroscopy?**
   A. Gastrointestinal stromal tumor
   B. Stricture
   C. Meckel's Diverticulum
   D. Arteriovenous malformation

3. **Which of the following is/are used in chromoendoscopy?**
   A. Methylene blue dye
   B. Lugol's iodine + Indigo carmine dye
   C. Methylene blue + Indigo carmine dye
   D. Lugol's iodine

4. **Epinephrine produces hemostasis in active GI bleed by:**
   A. Promoting vessel constriction
   B. Producing vessel thrombosis
   C. Producing tissue necrosis
   D. None of the above

5. **The best procedure among the following to diagnose GIST is:**
   A. EUS + biopsy
   B. CECT + FNAC
   C. PET
   D. Surgical excision biopsy

6. **Role of endoscopy in patients with Crohn's disease are all *except*:**
   A. Biopsy from terminal ileum
   B. Detection of gastroduodenal involvement
   C. Dilatation of ileal stricture
   D. Confirm clinical remission

7. **Serpiginous ulcers in esophagoscopy are characteristic of:**
   A. Herpes simplex type I
   B. Herpes simplex type II
   C. Varicella zoster virus
   D. Cytomegalovirus

8. **Which of the following is not a risk factor for variceal bleeding?**
   A. Size of the varix
   B. Red signs
   C. Severity of liver disease
   D. Degree of portal pressure elevation above 12 mm Hg

9. **All of the following are indications for TIPS *except:***
   A. Refractory hepatic hydrothorax
   B. Refractory ascites
   C. Hepatopulmonary syndrome
   D. Budd Chiari syndrome

10. **Maximum risk for bacteremia is seen with which of the following?**
    A. Esophageal dilatation
    B. Sigmoidoscopy
    C. Variceal sclerotherapy
    D. Colonoscopy

11. **All of the following are complications of colonoscopy *except:***
    A. Acute colitis B. Splenic rupture
    C. Colonic stricture D. Volvulus

12. **Upper GI endoscopy showed a 5 mm diameter button battery is lodged in the lower esophagus. What is the most appropriate next step?**
    A. Observe the patient
    B. Chest X-ray in 48 hours
    C. Immediate endoscopic removal
    D. Push it into the stomach

13. **On upper GI endoscopy, an adherent clot was seen over an ulcer at D1. To which Forrest grade does this ulcer belong?**
    A. Grade IIa B. Grade IIb
    C. Grade III D. Grade IV

14. **The proportion of adenomatous polyps and cancers that can be detected by a 60 cms flexible sigmoidoscope is:**
    A. 35% B. 45%
    C. 55% D. 65%

15. **Upper GI endoscopy in a 45 years old female reveals three mucosal breaks < 5 mm and confined to the folds. Which Los Angeles grade is this?**
A. LA grade A
B. LA grade B
C. LA grade C
D. LA grade D

16. **The most common complication of endoscopic sphincterotomy is:**
A. Cholangitis
B. Pancreatitis
C. Perforation
D. Bleeding

17. **Best procedure for bleeding gastric ulcers:**
A. Epinephrine injection
B. Bipolar electrocoagulation
C. Endoscopic haemoclip application
D. Adrenaline injection+ Electrocoagulation

18. **Absolute contraindication for capsule endoscopy is:**
A. Cardiac pacemaker
B. Crohn's disease
C. Small bowel stricture
D. Slow transit constipation

19. **Virtual colonoscopy is indicated for:**
A. Evalution of colon proximal to colonic structure
B. Carcinoma colon
C. Lower GI bleed
D. Colonic polyps

20. **Preferred method for diagnosis of ileo-caecal tuberculosis is:**
A. Double contrast barium study
B. CT scan
C. Colonoscopy
D. Detection of AFB in stool

21. **All of the following are complications of endoscopic ultrasound guided celiac plexus block *except:***
A. Diarrhoea
B. Hemiplegia
C. Plain abdomen
D. Intestinal perforation

22. **Prophylactic antibiotic is necessary before UGIE in all of the following *except:***
A. PDA
B. Patient with vascular graft
C. Patient with artificial heart valve
D. Patient with history of infective endocarditis 1 year back

Explanation

1. **Ans. (C)** Gastric variceal obliteration by cyanoacrylate injection has been found superior to both variceal band ligation and sclerotherapy using alcohol.

(Sleisenger, 9th edition, P-1512)

2. **Ans. (D)** Arteriovenous malformation is the most common finding in double balloon enteroscopy.

(Sleisenger, 9th edition, P-634)

3. **Ans. (B)** Chromoendoscopy uses either indigo carmine dye or Lugol's iodine. This is helpful for detection of early gastric cancer.

(Sleisenger, 9th edition, P-899)

4. **Ans. (A)** Endoscopic epinephrine injection therapy for initial control of active bleeding followed by more definite therapy like–thermal probe or hemoclip–are most effective treatment options for actively bleeding ulcers epinephrine controls bleeding through vessels constriction.

(Sleisenger, 9th edition, P-296)

5. **Ans. (B)** CECT is essential to stage the extent of disease and FNAC can be taken from tumor.

(Sleisenger, 9th edition, P-466)

6. **Ans. (D)** Endoscopy in patients with Crohn's disease and useful in taking biopsy, detection of gastroduodine involvement and dilation of stricture. Histological remission may lag behind clinical remission.

(Sleisenger, 9th edition, Pp-1956-1957)

7. **Ans. (C)** VZV characteristically produces serpiginous ucler.

(Sleisenger, 9th edition, P-728)

8. **Ans. (D)** Risk factor for variceal bleed depends upon site and grade of varix associated with red wale sign, severe liver dysfunction (MELD score >20), coagulopathy and HPVG (Hepatic portal vein pressure gradient >12 mm.

(Sleisenger, 9th edition, P-1508)

9. **Ans. (C)** TIPS function as a side to side portacaval shunt and has been used to treat complication of portal hypertension mainly variceal bleeding, refractory ascites Budd-Chiari syndrome, hepatic hydrothorax and hepatorenal syndrome.

(Sleisenger, 9th editon, P-1504)

10. **Ans. (A)** Esophageal dilation is complicated by high risk of perforation (upto 10%) and high risk of bacteremia.

(Sleisenger, 9th edition, P-765)

11. **Ans. (D)** Colonoscopy used as a therapeutic mortality for treatment of volvulus.

(Sleisenger, 9th edition, P-658)

12. **Ans. (C)** Disc batteries ingestrin is particular concern because batteries an alkaline solution can cause rapid liquefactive necrosis in oesophagus so, any disc battery in oesophagus prompt emergency endoscopy and removal but once batteries in stomach and small intestine rarely cause clinical problem and observed radiographically for 72 hours.

(Sleisenger, 9th edition, P-403)

13. **Ans. (B)** Forrest grade classification Type-I. Active bleeding-Ia-spurting hemorrhage Ib-hemorrhage.

Type-II-stigmata of recent hemorrhage, Type-IIa-Non-bleeding visible vessels.

IIb-Adherent clot IIc-Flat pigmentation, Type-III-clean based ulcers.

(Sleisenger, 9th edition, P-879)

14. **Ans. (C)** Upto 55% of adenomatous polyps and cancers can be detected by a 60 cm flexible sigmoid scope.

(Sleisenger, 9th edition, P-2224)

15. **Ans. (A)** Los Angeles classification

Grade A-One or more mucosal, break, confined to <5 mm.

Grade B-One or more mucosal break >5 mm confined to fold.

Grade C-Mucosal breaks continuous between folds but not circumferential.

Grade D-Circumferential breaks.

(Sleisenger, 9th edition, P-716)

16. **Ans. (B)** The most common complication of ERCP is pancreatitis, occurs in 2%-25% of all cases. Hemorrhage, perforation, cholangitis are other rare complication.

(Sleisenger, 9th edition, P-660)

17. **Ans. (D)** Initial endoscopic hemastasis with epinephrine followed by the thermal or electrocoagulation–significantly decrease the rate of ulcer re-bleeding, urgent surgery and morality.

(Sleisenger, 9th edition, P-296)

18. **Ans. (C)** The primary complication of capsule endoscopy is retention due to unsuspected small intestinal stricture. This occurs in 1%-2% of capsule procedure. So small intestinal stricture is an absolute contraindication to capsule endoscopy.

(Sleisenger, 9th edition, P-658)

19. **Ans. (A)** Virtual colonoscopy -3D image construction using CT scan-helpful delineating the lesion. Virtual colonoscopy is also helpful in visualising the colon proximal to stricture, which cannot be assessed by conventional colonoscope. Rest other condition conventional colonoscopy is superior.

(Sleisenger, 9th edition, P-1877)

20. **Ans. (C)** Colonoscopic finding although non-specific, but definite diagnosis, usually, established by demonstration of AFB bacilli by biopsied specimen.

(Sleisenger, 9th edition, P-1374)

21. **Ans. (B)** Pain abdomen, intestinal perforation, diarrhea, bleeding may complicate EUS-guided celiac axis block but no hemiplegia noticed.

(Sleisenger, 9th edition, P-661)

22. **Ans. (A)** Prophylactic antibiotic is necessary before UGIE in the following condition.

Prosthetic heart valves, endocarditis.

Unrepaired cyanotic congenital heart disease including palliative shunt or conduits.

Completely congenital heart defects within 6 months of repair after cardiac transplant.

(Harrison, 17th edition, P-797)

Chapter 10

ABDOMINAL CAVITY

1. **Diarrhea is a common complaint in patients with AIDS. Which of the following statements about diarrhea associated with AIDS is not true?**
   A. A potential pathogen is more likely to be identified in a patient with weight loss and a CD4 count of fewer than 100 cells/mm than in a patient with 'no weight loss' and a CD4 count of 500 cells/mm
   B. A specific pathogen is identified in 0% to 85% of AIDS patients with diarrhea
   C. Cryptosporidium parvum and isospora belli are more common in AIDS patients living in developed countries than in AIDS patients living in developing countries
   D. Diagnostic evaluation of diarrhea in AIDS patients should begin with a stool culture for salmonella, shigella, and campylobacter species. If microscopy does not reveal a potential pathogen, an endoscopic examination with biopsy should be performed

2. **A 45-year-old man is referred for an opinion regarding the following liver chemistries: Bilirubin-2 mg%, ALT-124 IU/L, AST-299 IU/L, ALP-1944 IU/L:**
   A. Viral hepatitis
   B. Alcoholic hepatitis
   C. PBC
   D. PSC

3. **Which of the following statements regarding high output gastrointestinal fistulas is most accurate?**
   A. They are defined by fluid losses greater than 500 mL/day
   B. They are associated with metabolic alkalosis when they involve the duodenum
   C. They are associated with a high incidence of spontaneous closure
   D. They never result in clinically significant dehydration

4. **A 52-year-old man is referred because of abdominal swelling. He has a tattoo and gives a history of drinking six cans of beer per night–more on the weekends for the past 25 years. He works in an office and his hobby is bowling. His physical examination is remarkable for moderate ascites and two small spider angiomas on the face. Laboratory studies disclose the following values: serum bilirubin, 1.0 mg/dL; aspartate amino-transferase, alanine amino-transferase, and alkaline phosphatase levels between 1 and 2 times the upper limit of normal; serum albumin, 3.3 g/dL; and total protein, 6.8 g/dL. To deal with his ascites, which of the following options would you not select?**
   A. Diagnosis paracentesis
   B. Ascitic fluid white blood cell count and differential
   C. Ascitic fluid albumin level
   D. Ascitic fluid lactate dehydrogenase and bilirubin levels

5. **Each of the following autoimmune disease exhibits associated gastrointestinal manifestations *except*:**
   A. Systemic lupus erythematosus
   B. Graves' disease
   C. Psoriasis
   D. Rheumatoid arthritis
   E. Addison's disease (i.e. hypoadrenalism)

6. **Each of the following statements regarding the etiology of non-malignant ascites is true *except*:**
   A. In most cases, the ascites largely results from fluid weeping from the liver, not from the portal venous bed
   B. Portal vein thrombosis alone usually does not result in the development of clinically significant ascites
   C. Urinary secretion of sodium over a 24-hour period is typically less than 10 mEq
   D. Chylous ascites often develops with fulminant hepatic failure

7. **Each of the following statements concerning malignant ascitis is true *except*:**
   A. Peritoneal carcinomatosis is a relatively infrequent cause of malignant ascites
   B. In patient with intraabdominal lymphoma or ovarian cancer, malignant ascites may respond

to surgical or medical treatment of the primary tumors
C. In peritoneal carcinomatosis, ascites appears to result from the secretion of fluid and protein by malignant cells
D. The formation of ascites in patients with advanced liver metastases may be the result of portal hypertension

8. **The serum ascites albumin concentration gradient:**
A. Is calculated by dividing the difference between the serum albumin and the ascetic albumin by the volume of fluid removed
B. Is calculated by dividing the difference between the serum albumin and the ascetic albumin by the total blood volume
C. Will generally discriminate between alcoholic and non-alcoholic chronic liver disease
D. Will generally discriminate between ascites due to liver disease and ascites from other causes

9. **Each of the following statements regarding spontaneous bacterial peritonitis (SBP) is correct *except*:**
A. Patients with ascites as a result of heart failure rarely develop SBP
B. SBP most likely results from microperforation of colon with direct contamination of the ascetic fluid
C. Patients with malignant ascites resulting from peritoneal carcinomatosis rarely develop SBP
D. SBP usually results from infection with a single organism

10. **Each of the following statement regarding the ascetic fluid leukocyte count is correct *except*:**
A. As a patient undergoes diuresis, the total leukocyte count in ascetic fluid may rise significantly
B. As a patient undergoes diuresis, the neutrophil count in ascetic fluid may rise significantly
C. A neutrophil count greater than $250/mm^3$ in ascetic fluid strongly suggests peritonitis
D. In a traumatic paracentesis, the ratio of neutrophils to red blood cells should not exceed 1:250 in uninfected ascetic fluid

11. **Which statement about intestinal ischemia is incorrect?**
A. The majority of patients with intestinal ischemia are elderly and they have associated cardiovascular disease such as congestive heart failure or atrial fibrillation
B. When mesenteric venous thrombosis is diagnosed in a young person, evaluation for an underlying hypercoagulable state should be initiated
C. If there is strong evidence for small bowel ischemia, abdominal computed tomography and Doppler ultrasonography should be performed immediately. If these procedures do not reveal an occlusion, mensenteric arteriography should be performed
D. In patients with severe vascular disease and no exclusive lesion, intraarterial vasodilators may be successful and may prevent surgical intervention

12. **Correct statements concerning splenic vein occlusion include all of the following *except*:**
A. The incidence of gastric variceal bleeding is 11% to 65%
B. Esophageal varices are a common finding
C. Splenectomy is the treatment of choice
D. Venous collaterals involve the short gastric coronary and the gastroepiploic venis

13. **A 60-year-old man is admitted with a gradual onset of right upper quadrant abdominal pain associated with increased liver enzymes and hepatomegaly, documented by physical exami-nation. A radionuclide scan of the liver reveals inhomogeneous uptake in the liver with enhanced uptake in the caudate lobe, all the following statements regarding this condition are true *except*:**
A. Computed tomography often reveals diffusely hypodense hepatic parenchyma with preservation of a normal density in the caudate lobe
B. Ultrasonography with color flow Doppler imaging is the preferred diagnostic study
C. Portal vein occlusion is found in 10% to 20% of patients
D. Venography often reveals a 'spider-web' pattern

14. **Which of the following statements about endoscopic ultrasonography imaging is most accurate?**
A. Leiomyomas can be reliably distinguished from leiomyosarcomas
B. Malignant lymph nodes usually have poorly defined margins
C. Benign lymph nodes are usually hypercholic
D. The normal wall thickness of the gastrointestinal tract is 5 to 7 mm

15. **At the end of a 3-week course of radiation therapy directed at the chest wall, a patient presents with dysphasia and odynophagia. You suggest the most likely diagnosis is:**

A. Radiation-induced esophagitis
B. Radiation-induced mortality disorder
C. Radiation-induced stricture
D. None of the above

16. **All of the following are common symptoms of acute graft-versus-host disease *except*:**
A. Watery diarrhea
B. Skin rash
C. Jaundice
D. Arthritis

17. **Each of the following is a common manifestation of acute graft-versus-host disease *except*:**
A. Pancreatitis
B. Cholestasis
C. Diarrhea
D. Gastrointestinal bleeding

18. **Each of the following is a common manifestation of chronic graft-versus-host disease *except*:**
A. Cholestasis
B. Small bowel bacterial overgrowth
C. Typhilitis
D. Esophageal stricture

19. **Which of the following statements about spontaneous bacterial peritonitis is correct?**
A. More than 10% of patients with spontaneous bacterial peritonitis have not clinical evidence of infection
B. The complication rate of abdominal paracentesis is about 5%
C. Anaerobes rarely cause spontaneous bacterial peritonitis
D. Patients with ascites due to causes other than cirrhosis may have an elevated polymorphonulear leukocyte count

20. **Chronic graft-versus-host disease is best described by which of the following statements?**
A. It most commonly affects person who have no prior history of acute graft-versus-host disease
B. It is not associated with mucositis
C. It typically occurs within 10 weeks of bone marrow transplantation
D. It has clinical features than resemble scleroderma

21. **Which one of the following therapies is a thermal contact method of tissue destruction?**
A. Nd:YAG laser therapy
B. Chemical injection
C. Bipolar electrocoagulation
D. Argon plasma coagulation

Explanation

1. **Ans. (C)** Most diarrheal illnesses in patients infected with HIV-1 are caused by infectious agents, and using the current improved diagnostic techniques, a specific pathogen is identified in 50% to 85% of cases. Patients with low CD4 counts and systemic symptoms such as weight loss are more likely to be diagnosed with a specific causative pathogen. Some physicians advocate a three-phase work-up for these patients. Beginning with stool cultures for routine bacterial pathogens, clostridium difficile, and ova and parasites. Phase 2 involves esophagogastroduodenoscopy and colonoscopy to obtain biopsy specimens that are then stained specifically for mycobacteria, viruses and fungi. Step 3 includes electrone microscopy for microsporidia and adenovirus. Cryptosporidium species and isospora belli are more commonly found in patients in developing countries.

(Sleisenger, 9th edition, Pp-526-530)

2. **Ans. (B)** The aspartate aminotransferase-alanine aminotransferase ratio in serum is a useful indicator of alcoholic liver disease; a ratio greater than 2 is highly suggestive of alcohol-induced liver injury. Lesser elevations in serum aminotransferases (an aspartate aminotransferase level of 300 U/L) are usually observed in alcoholic hepatitis, whereas higher elevations (often 1000 U/L) occur with viral, toxin-induced, or ischemic hepatitis.

(Sleisenger, 9th edition, Pp-1389-1390)

3. **Ans. (A)** High output fistulas, when they involve the duodenum or proximal small bowel are associated with metabolic acidosis as a result of alkaline fluid loss and can produce significant dehydration in rare cases. Gastric fistulas typically produce an alkalosis. Low-output fistulas (<500 ML/day) are associated with a high incidence of spontaneous closure; however, high output fistulas rarely resolve without intervention.

(Sleisenger, 9th edition, Pp-419-422)

4. **Ans. (D)** Spider angioma are increased by exposure to sunlight and may therefore not be prominent in all cirrhotics. The clinical diagnosis is ascites, which is the presenting complaint and the only major physical sign. Diagnosis paracentesis is indicated to confirm this impression and to better understand the etiology of the ascites. Determination of the serum ascites albumin gradient can help in this regard. There is little merit in measuring lactate dehydrogenase or bilirubin levels in the ascetic fluid.

(Sleisenger, 9th edition, Pp-1521-1524)

5. **Ans. (C)** Psoriasis is not associated with gastrointestinal disease. Methotrexate a therapy for refractory psoriasis is associated with gastrointestinal complications such as nausea and vomiting, fatty liver, hepatic fibrosis, cirrhosis and rarely, colitis.

(Sleisenger, 9th edition, Pp-557-561)

6. **Ans. (D)** Chylous ascites is more suggestive of lymphatic obstruction and is not usually associated with fulminant hepatic failure.

(Sleisenger, 9th edition, Pp-1521-1524)

7. **Ans. (A)** Although peritoneal carcinomatosis is the leading cause of malignant ascites, not all malignancy-related ascites are caused by this condition. Ascites associated with malignancy may result from massive liver metastases, tumor-induced portal hypertension, or tumor-induced chylous ascites.

(Sleisenger, 9th edition, Pp-1517-1518)

8. **Ans. (D)** The utility of the serum ascites albumin concentration gradient is based on the concept of oncotic-hydrostatic balance. A high oncotic gradient will match a high portal pressure, and of the serum proteins, albumin has the most effect on the oncotic pressure of serum. In patients with portal hypertension. There are large differences between serum and ascetic fluid albumin concentration. The albumin gradient is approximately 97% accurate in grouping patients with ascites into those with and those without portal hypertension. Patients with peritoneal carcinomatosis, tuberculosis. Pancreatic ascites, or nephritic syndrome. A high albumin gradient ($\geq$1.1 g/dL) is seen in patients with portal hypertension, including those with cirrhosis,

alcoholic hepatitis, cardiac ascites, Budd-Chiari syndrome or portal vein thrombosis.

(Sleisenger, 9th edition, Pp-1522-1523)

9. **Ans. (B)** Spontaneous bacterial peritonitis (SBP) usually occurs in patients with severe liver disease and low-protein ascites. SBP rarely occurs in patients with ascites caused by heart failure or in patients with peritoneal carcinomatosis, both of whom have high-protein ascites. SBP is believed to result from the seeding of ascites after transient bacteremia. As a result, most cases of SBP result from contamination with a single organism.

(Sleisenger, 9th edition, Pp-1528-1532)

10. **Ans. (B)** Although the total leukocyte count may rise during clinically significant diuresis, neutorphil counts remain stable, presumably because of the short half-life of neutrophils. The usual cutoff value for the diagnosis of spontaneous bacterial peritonitis is a neutrophil concentration in ascetic fluid of $250/mm^3$, even with rapid diuresis.

(Sleisenger, 9th edition, Pp-1530-1533)

11. **Ans. (C)** Mesenteric arteriography should be performed promptly if small bowel ischemia is suspected. There are no laboratory tests that are sufficiently specific to be helpful in the initial diagnosis; therefore, the physicians must persist with other diagnostic procedures to confirm or exclude ischemia. The patient should be stabilized prior to angiographic study. Computed tomography and ultrasonography are appropriate initial tests for patients with a history of deep vein thrombosis or a family history of coagulation disorders, who are likely to have mesenteric vein thrombosis.

(Sleisenger, 9th edition, Pp-2031-2037)

12. **Ans. (B)** Splenic vein occlusion is a common cause of the development of isolated gastric varices, which present a significant risk for spontaneous hemorrhage. This condition is best treated by surgical resection of the spleen. Esophageal varices are rare in patients with splenic vein occlusion.

(Sleisenger, 9th edition, P-1377)

13. **Ans. (B)** This presentation is characteristic of hepatic vein occlusion, also known as Budd-Chiari syndrome. Hepatic venography is the diagnostic test of choice. Because the results of ultrasonography with Doppler examination are associated with a high false-negative rate. The venous drainage of the caudate lobe is distinct from the other hepatic regions and thus may not be in volved in Budd-Chiari syndrome.

(Sleisenger, 9th edition, Pp-1373-1374)

14. **Ans. (C)** Benign lymph nodes are usually hyperechoic with an irregular shape and poorly defined margins. Malignant nodes are more commonly hypoechoic and round with sharply defined borders. Endoscopic ultrasonography cannot distinguish between leiomyoma and leiomyosarcoma without needle aspiration. The normal gastrointestinal wall thickness is 3 to 5 mm.

(Sleisenger, 9th edition, P-739)

15. **Ans. (A)** The timing of the onset of symptom as following the induction of radiation therapy suggests radiation induced esophagitis. Endoscopic evaluation is the diagnostic test of choice, although radiologic and endoscopic findings can mimic opportunistic infections, in particular candidiasis, so biopsies may be helpful. The motility disorder induced by radiation therapy usually does not appear for 4 to 12 weeks after the induction of radiation therapy and stricture formation may take 6 to 8 months. Opportunistic infections, such as candidiasis, herpes simplex or cytomegalovirus infection, particularly if accompanied by severe ulcerative esophagitis, must be excluded. Following long-term radiation therapy, it is possible to see radiation-induced fibrosis and progressive nerve loss that can mimic disease such as scleroderma or achalasia.

(Sleisenger, 9th edition, Pp-640-641)

16. **Ans. (D)** Acute graft-versus-host disease is a common complication of bone marrow transplantation. Classically patients develop watery diarrhea, mucositis, and hepatic abnormalities including hyperbilirubinemia beginning 3 weeks after bone marrow transplantation. Arthritis is not typically reported in acute disease.

(Sleisenger, 9th edition, Pp-553-554)

17. **Ans. (A)** Acute graft-versus-host disease develops in 20% to 50% of bone marrow transplant patients, typically occurring 20 to 80 days following transplantation, and may produce jaundice, diarrhea, and gastrointestinal blood loss. Other clinical manifestations commonly include dermatitis, protein-losing enteropathy, vomiting, abdominal pain and ileus, but pancreatitis is rarely observed.

(Sleisenger, 9th edition, Pp-551-552)

18. **Ans. (C)** Chronic graft-versus-host disease (GVHD) commonly develops 3 to 9 months after bone marrow transplantation and may be associated with esophageal

desquamation and stricture formation, small bowel bacterial overgrowth and chronic cholestasis. Typhlitis (i.e. neutropenic enterocolitis) may occur with acute GVHD, but it is not a common manifestation of GVHD.

(Sleisenger, 9th edition, Pp-551-552)

19. **Ans. (C)** Clinical evidence of infection in patients with spontaneous bacterial peritonitis (SBP) can be subtle or absent. In one study, more than 10% of patients with SBP had no signs or symptoms. However most patients present with fever, abdominal pain, or mental status change. There are very few contraindications to paracentesis. Even in the patient with coagulopathy paracentesis causes minimal complication; and cirrhotic do not bleed seriously from needle sticks, unless conditions such as fibrinolysis or disseminated intravascular coagulation are concurrent. Ascites fluid analysis from culture-negative neutrocytic ascites, secondary bacterial peritonitis, and SBP will show more than 250 polymorphonuclear leukocytes per mm^3. Tuberculosis peritonitis and peritoneal carcinomatosis cause an elevated white cell count, but the differential is primarily lymphocytic.

(Sleisenger, 9th edition, Pp-1522-1527)

20. **Ans. (D)** Chronic graft-versus-host disease typically presents with clinical features similar to scleroderma and includes the sicca complex among its manifestations.

(Sleisenger, 9th edition, P-547)

21. **Ans. (C)** Bipolar electrocoagulation is the only thermal contact method of tissue destruction mentioned in this list. The argon plasma coagulator and the Nd:YAG laser are non-contact methods of tissue destruction and injection therapy has no thermal component.

(Sleisenger, 9th edition, Pp-291-292)

Chapter 11

HIV AND GUT

1. **All of the following are true regarding gastro-intestinal consequences of AIDS *except*:**
   A. CD4 count of less than 300/ul is the threshold for the development of most opportunistic infections (OIS)
   B. Some OIS may resolve with highly active antiretroviral therapy (HAART) alone
   C. Antiretroviral drugs are associated with GI and hepatic side effects that in short studies
   D. Drug induces side effects and other non opportunistic disease are among the most common causes of GI symptoms during HAART therapy
2. **All of the following are true regarding gastro-intestinal and hepatobiliary infections in AIDS *except:***
   A. Clinical sign and symptoms frequently suggests a specific diagnosis
   B. In AIDS, GI pathogens are usually part of a systemic infection
   C. Multiple infections are common
   D. Evidence of tissue invasion indicates pathogenicity
3. **All of the following are true regarding cryptosporidium in AIDS patients *except:***
   A. Cryptosporidium is the most frequent protozoa that causes diarrhea
   B. Small bowel is the most common site of infection
   C. Diagnosis made by acid fast stain of the stool
   D. Metronidazole is the drug of choice
4. **All of the following are true regarding microsporidium in AIDS patients *except:***
   A. Causes bloody diarrhea
   B. Brown Bernn, gram stain, or modified trichrome stains are superior to hematoxylin and eosin staining
   C. Enterocytozoon bienusi is smaller than encephalitozoon intestinalis
   D. Albendazole is effective for E-intestinalis
5. **All of the following are true regarding diarrhea in AIDS patients *except:***
   A. Giardia lamblia and entamoeba histolytica are seen with increased frequency
   B. Entamoeba dispar is morphologically similar to entamoeba histolytica
   C. Blastocytis homins, endolimax nana and entamoeba coli are common in homosexual men
   D. Enteric leishmaniasis can cause small or large bowel infiltration
6. **All of the following are true regarding cytomegalovirus (CMV) in AIDS patients *except:***
   A. Most common viral cause of diarrhea
   B. Symptoms include abdominal pain, peritonitis, watery non-bloody diarrhea or hematochezia
   C. Cultures are more sensitive and specific than histopathologic identification
   D. Cidofovir can be given once weekly
7. **All of the following are true regarding idiopathic AIDS enteropathy *except:***
   A. Lack an identifiable pathogen
   B. Mucosal hypoproliferation seen
   C. Diminished numbers of activated lymphocytes expressing the interleukin-2 receptor (CD25 cells) cell seen
   D. AIDS enteropathy may be via the effects of enteric HIV on autonomic nerves
8. **All of the following are true regarding bacterial infections in AIDS patients with diarrhea *except:***
   A. Salmonella, shigella and campylobacter are common
   B. Campylobacter found only by culturing tissue biopsy specimens
   C. Clostridium difficile can occur as opportunistic infection
   D. Small bowel bacterial overgrowth is uncommon
9. **All of the following are true regarding mycobacterial infection in AIDS patients with diarrhea *except:***
   A. In mycobacterium avium complex (MAC) duodenal involvement is most common
   B. In biopsy granulomas are rarely present
   C. MAC eradication is commonly achieved
   D. Mycobacterium tuberculosis usually involves ileoceal region of colon
10. **All of the following are true regarding drug induces diarrhea during HAART therapy *except:***
    A. Associated with protease inhibitors, with nelfinavir

B. Occurs in 20%
C. Associated with weight loss
D. Symptomatic therapies are generally effective

11. All of the following are true in the evaluation of diarrhea in AIDS patients *except:*
A. Hematochezia usually implies colonic infection by CMV, Shigella or campylobacter
B. One time stool examination is sufficient in the initial evaluation
C. Isolated right sided colitis with CMV has been variably reported in 0% to 30%
D. Jejunal biopsies are superior to duodenal biopsies for identifying microspordia

12. All of the following are true regarding esophageal disorders in AIDS patients *except*:
A. In CMV esophagitis odynophagia or substernal chest pain are more common than dysphagia
B. Herpes simplex virus esophagitis is infrequent in AIDS
C. Herpes simplex esophagitis ulcers are large and deep
D. Idiopathic ulcers response in more 90% of patient on oral corticosteroids

13. All of the following are true regarding abdominal pain in AIDS patients *except*:
A. Perforation results most often from CMV infection
B. Obstruction is most likely to develop from an intestinal neoplasm
C. Infections are most common causes for pancreatitis in AIDS patients
D. Infiltration by lymphoma or Kaposi's sarcoma can cause pancreatitis

14. All of the following are true regarding anorectal disease in AIDS patients *except*:
A. Lymphoma can occur in anorectal region
B. Anorectal carcinoma are more common in homosexual men with HIV
C. Human papilloma virus (HPV) types 16 and 18 are implicated
D. Cytologic specimens of the anal canal are not useful

15. All of the following are true regarding gastrointestinal bleeding in AIDS patients *except:*
A. Upper GI bleeding is most frequently cause by peptic ulcer
B. Most common cause of lower GI bleeding is CMV colitis
C. Bleeding from herpes simplex virus esophagitis is less common than CMV esophagitis
D. MAC, microsporidia and cryptosporidia cause severe bleeding

16. All of the following are true regarding drug induced liver injury in AIDS patients *except:*
A. Before HAART hepatotoxicity was most commonly due to sulfonamides
B. Presently protease inhibitors are the most common cause of abnormal liver tests
C. Liver biopsy shows evidence of granulomatous containing eosionophils in hepatotoxicity from protease inhibitors
D. Jaundice is most frequently observed with indinavir

17. All of the following are true regarding syndrome characterized by marked hepatomegaly, steatosis, lactic acidosis and liver failure that occurs during HAART therapy are true *except:*
A. Due to impaired mitochondrial DNA synthesis
B. Usually from nucleoside reverse transcriptase inhibitors such as zidovudine, DDL and stavudine
C. An associated myopathy, peripheral neuropathy and pancreatitis may occur as well
D. Most of the patients recover

18. All of the following are true regarding hepatitis B virus (HBV) infection in AIDS patients *except:*
A. Clinical and autopsy studies showed upto 90% seroprevalence of hepatitis B markers indicating past or present infection
B. There is an accelerated loss of naturally acquired anti-HBS even in those patients who remain HbsAg negative
C. Biochemical and histological liver disease is more severe
D. Vaccination appears to be ineffective, regardless of the stage of immunocompromised

19. All of the following are true regarding HBV and HDV infection in AIDS patients *except:*
A. In HBV infection after institution of HAART patients may develop an acute flare
B. Inclusion of Lamividine into HAART regimen may reduce the acute flare
C. All patient to receive HAART therapy should be screened for active or past HBV infection
D. HIV coinfection suppresses delta virus replication

20. All of the following are true regarding HCV (Hepatitis C virus infection) in AIDS patient *except:*
A. Assaying antibodies to hepatitis C virus alone without RNA may underestimated the true prevalence

B. Unlike hepatitis B virus, the clinical course of hepatitis C virus appears to worsen as HIV related immunocompromised advances
C. HCV causes progression of HIV disease
D. Coinfected patients also have a higher rate active cirrhosis on biopsy

21. **All of the following are true regarding liver involvement in AIDS patients *except:***
A. Cryptococcus typically found in the sinusoids of liver
B. Candida infection of liver is common
C. Kaposi's sarcoma has a predilection for periportal region of liver
D. Cell of origin of Kaposi's sarcoma is the lymphatic endothelial cells

22. **All are true regarding bacillary peliosis hepatitis *except:***
A. Caused by either bartonella henselae or bartonella quintana
B. Liver function tests are normal
C. Warthin starry stain or electron microscopy reveals clumps of organisms
D. Treatment is with either erythromycin, tetracycline, minocycline, or a cephalosporin

23. **All of the following are true regarding biliary tract involvement in AIDS patients *except:***
A. Jaundice is usual
B. The etiology in most cases of AIDS cholangiopathy is infectious because of cryptosporidium CMV or microsporidium
C. AIDS cholangiopathy is not associated with a shortened survival
D. Acalculous cholecystitis is most frequently caused by CMV

24. **All of the following are true regarding bleeding peptic ulcer disease *except:***
A. Responsible for nearly 50% of all cases of cute upper GI bleed
B. Corticosteroids alone increases the risk for peptic ulcer bleed
C. 5% of patients can have hematochezia
D. Endoscopic methods can control bleeding in nearly 90% of cases

25. **All of the following are true regarding perforation of peptic ulcer *except:***
A. No prior history of peptic ulcer symptoms seen in 10% to 25% of patients
B. Ulcer on posterior wall of duodenum perforate in most cases
C. In 10% of patients perforation is accompanied by hemorrhage
D. Plain X-ray abdomen reveals free air under diaphragm in 70% of cases

26. **All of the following are true regarding gastric outlet obstruction because of peptic ulcer *except:***
A. Succession splash is seen in 1/3rd of patients
B. Gastric aspirate volume of more 200 ml at 4 hours after a meal confirms delayed gastric emptying
C. In saline load test recovery of more than 300 ml after 30 minutes confirms delayed gastric emptying
D. Cab be managed with medical and endoscopic means in approximately 70% of cases

27. **All of the following are true regarding highly selective vagotomy a surgery for peptic ulcer *except:***
A. Also termed parietal cell vagotomy
B. Drainage procedure is not needed
C. Recurrence rates are seen in 5% to 20%
D. Indicated for pyloric and prepyloric gastric ulcers

28. **All of the following are true regarding surgeries for peptic ulcer disease:**
A. Ulcer recurrence rate is least with vagotomy and antrectomy
B. Mortality rate is more with vagotomy and antrectomy
C. Morbidity rate is least with highly selective vagotomy
D. Ulcer recurrence rates with vagotomy and pyloroplasty is 5%

29. **All of the following are true regarding development of cancers after peptic ulcer surgery *except:***
A. Post gastrectomy patients have a two-fold increase in gastric cancer risk 15 years after resection
B. Reflux of intestinal contents and bile into the gastric remnant leads formation of carcinogens
C. Risk of gastric cancer is low in patients who had gastrectomy rather than vagotomy and a drainage procedure
D. These patients have risk for development of pancreatic cancer

30. **All of the following are true regarding dumping syndrome *except:***
A. Early dumping syndrome occurs about 30 minutes after meals
B. Symptoms of later dumping syndrome occurs 1 to 2 after meals
C. Rich carbohydrate diet is advised
D. Octreotide is effective both in early and late dumping syndromes

Explanation

1. **Ans. (A)** Many patients with CD4 counts less than 100/ul who initially receive HAART experience during long term therapy an increase to more than 200/ul, the threshold for the development of most OIS.

(Sleisenger, 9th edition, Pp-523-524)

2. **Ans. (A)** Clinical signs and symptoms infrequently suggests a specific diagnosis.

(Sleisenger, 9th edition, P-524)

3. **Ans. (D)** Numerous antimicrobial agents have been tested most without significant effect. The agent that has shown the most efficacy, albeit modest, is paramomycin, an oral aminoglycoside. Other drugs which are effective are Nitatoxanide and Atithromycin.

(Sleisenger, 9th edition, Pp-526-527)

4. **Ans. (A)** Microsporidium typical symptoms include watery non bloody diarrhea of mild to moderate severity usually without associated crampy abdominal pain.

(Sleisenger, 9th edition, P-527)

5. **Ans. (A)** Although there is deficiency of cell mediated immunity in HIV patients, however, frequencies of E. histolytica and giardia are not increased.

(Sleisenger, 9th edition, Pp-526-529)

6. **Ans. (C)** Cultures for CMV are usually positive when inclusions are present, but they are less sensitive and specific than histopathologic identification.

(Sleisenger, 9th edition, P-528)

7. **Ans. (C)** The basis for mucosal atrophy in AIDS enteropathy is not established but has been proposed to results from diminished numbers of activated lymphocytes expressing the interleukin 2 receptor (CD25 cells), leading to a reduces mucosal responsiveness to this trophic lymphokine. Addition of protease inhibitor relief the patient.

(Sleisenger, 9th edition, P-529)

8. **Ans. (C)** Diarrhea due to clostridium difficile is common in AIDS patient, not because it is an OI but rather because antibiotic use is far greater and hospitalization more frequent in this population than in healthy hosts.

(Sleisenger, 9th edition, P-529)

9. **Ans. (C)** In AIDS patients with MAC infection response to antibiotic therapy is variable and depends in part on the extent of immunocompromised; however eradications is rarely achieved. As with other OIS, institution of HAART in these patients may improve immune function, hasten clinical resolution of the infection and prevent relapse.

(Sleisenger, 9th edition, Pp-526-530)

10. **Ans. (C)** In general the diarrhea is mild to moderate in severity and is not associated with weight loss.

(Sleisenger, 9th edition, P-530)

11. **Ans. (B)** In AIDS patient with diarrhea initial evaluations should include no less than three stools for ova and parasite examination, including acid fast smear, as well as culture for enteric bacterial pathogens.

(Sleisenger, 9th edition, Pp-526-530)

12. **Ans. (C)** In contrast with CMV esophagitis and idiopathic ulcer, Herpes simplex ulcers tend to be shallow: large, deep ulcers are rare.

(Sleisenger, 9th edition, Pp-524-525)

13. **Ans. (C)** The most common cause of pancreatitis in AIDS is drug induced disease, most frequently didanosine (DDL) or pentamidine.

(Sleisenger, 9th edition, Pp-530-531)

14. **Ans. (D)** Cytologic specimens of the anal canal, similar to PAP smears, are sensitive means to detect dysplasia.

(Sleisenger, 9th edition, P-531)

15. **Ans. (D)** MAC, microsporidia and cryptosporidium causes watery diarrhoea in AIDS patient.

(Sleisenger, 9th edition, Pp-531-532)

16. **Ans. (C)** In contrast to hepatotoxicity from sulfonamides, where liver biopsy typically shows evidence of granulomas containing eosinophils, the histologic findings of drug induced injury from newer antiretroviral agents, has not been well characterized.

(Sleisenger, 9th edition, P-532)

17. Ans. (D) Although reversal of this syndrome has occurred in some patients following drug withdrawal most patients have worsening disease and death. Liver transplantation is curative.

(Slesisenger, 9th edition, Pp-532-533)

18. Ans. (C) Although HIV infection leads to more prevalent chronic HBV carriage, it appears to attenuate the severity of biochemical and histologic liver disease is most but not all patients. In one study, the mean alanine aminotransferase (ALT) level correlated with CD4 lymphocyte count. The mechanism for reduced hepatitis B virus related liver injury following HIV infection is not certain but has been attributed to a diminution in lymphocyte-mediated hepatocellular injury as a result of HIV effects on lymphocytes.

(Sleisenger, 9th edition, P-533)

19. Ans. (D) In small series HIV coinfection was associated with enhanced delta virus replication without increased liver disease and in a single patient, reactivation of delta hepatitis was ascribed to acute HIV infection.

(Sleisenger, 9th edition, P-533)

20. Ans. (C) Like hepatitis B, hepatitis C virus does not cause progression of HIV disease.

(Sleisenger, 9th edition, P-533)

21. Ans. (B) Candida infection of the liver is rare, in contrast to its high prevalence in mucosal site.

(Sleisenger, 9th edition, P-534)

22. Ans. (B) Liver function test in bacillary peliosis hepatic usually show a disproportionate elevation of the alkaline phosphates.

(Sleisenger, 9th edition, P-534)

23. Ans. (A) Biliary tract involvement in AIDS may result in marked liver test abnormalities and right upper quadrant symptoms, jaundice is unusual. In AIDS cholangiopathy marked elevation of alkaline phosphates and minimal elevation of bilirubin, AST and ALT are seen.

(Sleisenger, 9th edition, P-534)

24. Ans. (B) Although corticosteroids use alone does not appear to increase the risk for bleeding ulcer substantially, the combined use of corticosteroids and NSAIDS may increase the risk of this complication by nearly 10-fold approximately 20% of patients with bleeding peptic ulcers present with melena and 30% present with hematemesis, whereas 50% have both melena and hematemesis on initial presentation.

(Sleisenger, 9th edition, P-878)

25. Ans. (B) Duodenal ulcers that perforate involve the anterior wall of the duodenal bulb in most cases. Perforated gastric ulcer usually involve the lesser curvature.

(Sleisenger, 9th edition, Pp-883-885)

26. Ans. (B) A gastric aspirate volume of more than > 400 ml at 4 hours after a meal or more than 200 ml after an overnight fast is evidence of delayed gastric emptying.

(Sleisenger, 9th edition, P-884)

27. Ans. (D) Highly selective vagotomy is contraindicated for pyloric and prepyloric gastric ulcers, with 30% of patients experiencing difficult gastric emptying or recurrent ulcer after operation.

(Sleisenger, 9th edition, P-952)

28. Ans. (D) Ulcer recurrence rate with vagotomy and pyloroplasty is 10-15%.

(Sleisenger, 9th edition, P-948)

29. Ans. (C) The overall risk of developing gastric carcinoma post peptic ulcer surgery is higher in patients who had gastric ulcer, in men and in patient who had gastrectomy rather than vagotomy and a drainage procedure.

(Sleisenger, 9th edition, P-891)

30. Ans. (C) It is advisable to place all gastric surgery patients on anti-dumping diets, which limit the size and increase the frequency of meals (six small feeding per day) restrict carbohydrate while increasing the protein content of meals replace simple sugars with starches, avoid milk products, and encourage intake of liquids between rather than during meals.

(Sleisenger, 9th edition, P-891)

Chapter 12

NUTRITION

1. **The Na^+ K^+-ATPase pump:**
   A. Establishes a high intracellular Na^+ concentration to drive transport
   B. Is electroneutral
   C. Is present in all intestinal epithelial cells
   D. Is dependent on calcium

2. **In addition to the regulatory mechanisms intrinsic to the epithelium itself, electrolyte transport is regulated by all of the following pathways *except*:**
   A. Endocrine and paracrine regulation
   B. ATP
   C. Enteric neural regulation
   D. Intestinal immune system

3. **Secretory mechanism throughout the gastro-intestinal tract largely center on the transcellular secretion of:**
   A. Sodium B. Potassium
   C. Hydrogen D. Chloride

4. **The absorption of hydrophobic compounds is reduced as a result of ineffective Micellar concentration in all of the following conditions *except*:**
   A. Menetrier disease
   B. Biliary obstruction
   C. Bacterial overgrowth
   D. Zollinger-Ellison

5. **Each of the following statements regarding intestinal fatty acid-binding proteins is true *except*:**
   A. They are abundant in enterocytes of the small intestine
   B. They facilitate the intracellular trafficking of fatty acids from the brush border endoplasmic reticulum
   C. They exported from the cell into the intestinal lumen
   D. They have been postulated to assist in the formation of chylomicrons and very-low-density lipoproteins for eventual secretion into the post circulation

6. **The colon is able to readily absorb each of the following *except*:**
   A. Monosaccharides B. Acetate
   C. Propionate D. Butyrate

7. **True statements regarding iron deficiency anemia include each of the following *except*:**
   A. Decreased acid production impairs the absorption of nonheme ferric iron
   B. The first stage of iron deficiency is the depletion of iron stores and is manifest by a low serum ferritin level
   C. The level of transferring saturation is less because the decrease in serum iron concentration is greater than the decrease in transferrin
   D. Dietary iron, in the form of heme iron, has a low bioavailability due to variable absorption

8. **Each of the following conditions may explain the presence of abnormal liver chemistries in patients receiving a total parenteral nutrition (TPN) *except*:**
   A. Hepatic steatosis
   B. Acalculous cholecystitis
   C. Calculous cholecystitis
   D. TPN-associated hemolysis

9. **Metabolic responses to illness and injury include all the following *except*:**
   A. Thermoregulatory setpoint of the body temperature increases by 1°C to 2°C
   B. Lipolysis increases
   C. Glucose production and insulin sensitivity increase
   D. Protein synthesis and breakdown increase

10. **True statements regarding vitamins and minerals include all of the following *except*:**
    A. Vitamin K is fat-soluble; therefore, there are large total body stores of this vitamin
    B. Iron and zinc inhibit copper absorption
    C. High doses of vitamin C can produce diarrhea
    D. Vitamin E acts as a antioxidant and free-radical scavenge

11. **Which of the following statements regarding glutamine metabolism by enterocytes is true?**
A. Enterocytes obtain glutamine from the intestinal lumen but not from the intestinal circulation
B. Enterocytes use glutamine primarily as an energy source, not as a substrate for protein synthesis
C. Glutamine is a poor source of ammonia for enterocytes
D. Glutamine enters the enterocyte primarily by passive diffusion

12. **Each of the following condition is a likely explanation for the diarrhea in short bowel syndrome *except*:**
A. Increased osmolarity of luminal contents
B. Increased secretions into the gut
C. Bacterial overgrowth
D. Steatorrhea

13. **In addition to total parenteral nutrition, the initial management of diarrhea in this patient should include each of the following *except*:**
A. H_2-receptor antagonist therapy
B. Pancreatic enzyme replacement
C. Anti-diarrheal agents (e.g. loperamide)
D. Oral nutrition

14. **This acute change in mental status is a patient with TPN therapy due to:**
A. Zinc deficiency
B. Magnesium deficiency
C. Folate deficiency
D. Vitamin B_{12} deficiency

15. **A 53-year-old man with short bowel syndrome present with severe right flank pain and hematuria. Which of the following is most likely to predispose the patient to these symptoms?**
A. Short bowel with an ileostomy
B. Short bowel with a subtotal colectomy
C. Short bowel requiring daily total parenteral nutrition and inability to tolerate oral feeding
D. Short bowel with an intact colon

16. **Which of the following is an absolute contra-indication for placement of a precautious endo-scopic gastrostomy?**
A. Ascites
B. Ventriculoperitoneal shunt
C. Morbid obesity
D. Peritoneal dialysis

17. **All of the following reduce lactase-phlorhizin hydrolase activity in adults *except*:**
A. Starvation
B. Infection with human immunodeficiency virus
C. Inflammatory bowel disease
D. Corticosteroid use

18. **All of the following statements regarding bile salts are true *except*:**
A. They are passively absorbed in the proximal small intestine
B. They are absorbed by active transport in the ileum
C. They are reabsorbed very efficiently in the small intestine
D. They result in the generation of short-chain fatty acids within the colon

19. **The gastric phase of protein digestion:**
A. Includes the secretion of pepsinogen by parietal cells
B. Is controlled by factors also involved in regulating acid secretion
C. Is a mandatory phase for intestinal protein assimilation
D. Is independent of the gastric pH

20. **All of the following statements regarding small intestine assimilation of protein are true *except*:**
A. It occurs exclusively by absorption of single amino acids
B. It can be used as an energy source by the small bowel epithelium
C. It involves a sodium-independent transporter
D. It results in the delivery of free amino acids into the portal circulation

21. **All of the following statements regarding iron absorption are true *except*:**
A. Iron absorption increases in response to iron deficiency
B. Unlike ferric iron (Fe), ferrous iron (Fe2) remains soluble across a broad pH range
C. Dietary substances such as sugars, amino acids and ascorbate promote iron absorption
D. Iron is absorbed at the brush-border membrane by passive effusion

22. **All of the following statements are true *except*:**
A. The recommended daily allowance is the minimum intake required to prevent a negative balance
B. Vegetable oils are rich sources of essential fatty acids
C. The intake of polyunsaturated fats should be increased
D. The average intake of fruit and vegetables on a western diet is less than 1 serving per day

23. Total parenteral nutrition is indicated for each of the following clinical situation *except*:

A. Elderly patients with decreased oral intake secondary to dysphagia
B. Severely malnourished patients requiring surgery
C. Severe, active Crohn's disease with malabsorption
D. During prolonged bowel rest resulting from the inability to tolerate oral feeding

24. Which of the following statements concerning the increased risk of serious medical complication associated with obesity is the most correct?

A. Although obesity is a risk factor for developing cardiovascular disease, the degree of obesity does not correlate with the extent of cardiovascular risk
B. The body mass include (BMI) can be used to assess the degree of an individual obesity and is calculated as height divided by body weight
C. For the same BMI, individuals with primarily upper body obesity are at higher risk for developing diabetes, hypertension and ischemic heart disease
D. Upper body obesity is more common in women than in men

25. Which of the following statements regarding food allergy or food hypersensitivity is true?

A. Most cases of immunologically mediated food allergy are IgE-mediated
B. The majority of cases presenting with 'food allergy' are immune-mediated
C. Most food allergens are of high molecular weight (greater than 150 kd) and are resistant to proteolysis
D. Skin tests of specific antigen are available for most common food allergens and are helpful in the diagnosis of food allergy in cases of life-threatening anaphylactic reaction

Explanation

1. **Ans. (C)** The Na^+ Ka^+-ATPase pump, in the presence of Mg2, catalyzes the efflux of three Na^+ ions out of the cell and the uptake of two K^+ ions into the cell. This action is electrogenic and acts to maintain a high extracellular concentration of Na^+. The gradient established by this pump is then used to drive many Na^+ dependent transporters. The pump is located on the basolateral membrane and exists in all intestinal epithelial cells.

(Sleisenger, 9th edition, P-1690)

2. **Ans. (B)** The interceullar regulatory mechanism of electrolyte transport include endocrine (Blood-borne hormones from distant sites), Paracrine (Local) ever endings within the enteric nervous system and resident and infiltrating immune and inflammatory cells types. The mediators released by these pathways generally are regulated by these pathways generally are regulated by Ca^{++} or cAMP, which act as second messengers.

(Sleisenger, 9th edition, Pp-1675-1694)

3. **Ans. (D)** Although bicarbonate secretion is important in selected regions of the gut (e.g., bile and pancreatic duct, duodenal mucosa), secretory mechanisms throughout the gastrointestinal tract largely centre on the active transcellular secretion of chloride into the lumen. Sodium, potassium and water follow passively through the tight junctions.

(Sleisenger, 9th edition, P-1679)

4. **Ans. (A)** A lack of bile salts at effective micellar concentrations may occur as a result of low intraluminal levels of bile salts (e.g., cholestasis), bacterial deconjugation (e.g., bacterial overgrowth), or abnormal acidic condition.

(Sleisenger, 9th edition, P-1701)

5. **Ans. (C)** Fatty acid-binding proteins (FABPs) are two cytosolic proteins that are independently regulated, with separate roles in the liver and the intestine. In the intestine FABPs are essential in the directed intracellular trafficking of absorbed long-chain fatty acids, retinylesters and probably cholesterol. By so directing the movement of lipids intracellularly and assisting in their uptake from the lumen, FABPs are ultimately involved in the disposition of cellular lipids into secretable forms such as chymicrons and very-low-density lipoprotein. FABPs are obligate intracellular peptides that are not exported out of the cells.

(Sleisenger, 9th edition, Pp-1701-1704)

6. **Ans. (A)** Monosaccharides are not readily absorbed by the colonic mucosa. Fermentation converts monosac-charides to short-chain fatty acids which are readily absorbed.

(Sleisenger, 9th edition, Pp-1706-1712)

7. **Ans. (D)** The two major sources of dietary iron are heme and nonheme iron. Meat, fish and poultry provide heme iron. These sources offer high bioavailability because the iron is absorbed intact within the porphyrin ring of hemoglobin and myoglobin. Nonheme iron is present in vegetables, grain and fruits. Absorption of non heme iron is highly variable and is affected by other meal components.

(Sleisenger, 9th edition, Pp-1723-1725)

8. **Ans. (D)** There is no increased risk of hemolysis in patients receiving total parenteral nutrition. Elevated liver chemistries in patients receiving total parenteral nutrition are likely to be multifactorial, including hepatic steatosis and calculous as well as acalculous cholecystitis.

(Sleisenger, 9th edition, Pp-85-87)

9. **Ans. (C)** Hypermetabolism negative nitrogen balance, insulin resistance leading to hyperglycemia and increased mobilization of adipose tissue triglycerides characterize the metabolic response to illness and injury.

(Sleisenger, 9th edition, Pp-69-70)

10. **Ans. (A)** Vitamin K is passively absorbed in the small intestine a process that requires bile-salt micelles and pancreatic enzymes. Unlike the other fat-soluble vitamin. These are consistently taken up from the circulation by the small intestine mucosa.

(Sleisenger, 9th edition, P-1722)

11. **Ans. (B)** Glutamine and glutamic acid are major energy sources for enterocytes and are the only amino acids

that are consistently taken up from the circulation by the small intestine mucosa.

(Sleisenger, 9th edition, Pp-1782-1783)

12. **Ans. (C)** Malabsorption (leading to osmotic diarrhea), increased luminal secretion and fat malabsorption all occur in short bowel syndrome. Bacterial overgrowth is not commonly encountered in patients with short bowel syndrome.

(Sleisenger, 9th edition, Pp-1780-1792)

13. **Ans. (D)** The first phase of short bowel syndrome is characterized by severe diarrhea during oral nutrition, with the development of dehydration and electrolyte abnormalities. The diarrhea is caused by decreased transit time secondary to physical shortening of the small intestine and motility disturbances. Incomplete digestion and absorption of carbohydrates increases the osmotic load, drawing more water into the lumen. Gastric hypersecretion occurs, as does steatorrhea. Bacterial overgrowth can contribute to the diarrhea by increasing the osmotic load of the gut but is less likely to be problem in the early postoperative period. Generally, at least 30 to 50 cm of healthy small intestine and an intact colon are necessary for the patients to be maintained without parenteral nutrition. Although functional pancreatic enzyme insufficiency can occur, pancreatic enzyme insufficiency can occur, pancreatic enzyme replacements are not needed in most patients. Oral nutrition should be encouraged to stimulated intestinal mucosal adaptation. Anti-diarrheal agents may provide symptom relief. H_2-receptor antagonists may reduce diarrhea by decreasing gastric secretory component of the stool output.

(Sleisenger, 9th edition, Pp-1785-1795)

14. **Ans. (D)** This patient has signs of Vitamin B_{12} and/or thiamine deficiency. Glucose administration prior to thiamine supplementation in deficient patients can lead to an acute clinical deterioration. Because the body has such large stores of vitamin B_{12}. It may take individuals consuming a diet deficient in Vitamin B_{12} as long as 1 to 3 years to develop evidence of deficiency. Most patients with Vitamin B_{12} deficiency will also be lacking in the other B vitamins.

(Sleisenger, 9th edition, Pp-1790-1791)

15. **Ans. (D)** Short bowel syndrome predisposes the patient to hyperoxaluria and oxalate kidney stones. Normally, dietary oxalates are bound by dietary calcium to form insoluble calcium oxalate. In patients with steatorrhea, fatty acids compete for dietary calcium oxalate, and free oxalate is available for absorption, especially in the colon. In addition, malabsorption of bile salts and free fatty acids alters the permeability of the colonic mucosa, which further increases the absorption of oxalate. For this sequence of events to occur, the colon must be intact.

(Sleisenger, 9th edition, P-1790)

16. **Ans. (A)** Contraindication to PEG replacements are gastric varices, severe obesity, major gastric resection, ascites and coagulopathy.

(Sleisenger, 9th edition, Pp-90-91)

17. **Ans. (A)** Although starvation in adults leads to a reduction of many saccharidases, lactase-phlorhizin hydrolase activity is not reduced. Human immunodeficiency virus infection, corticosteroids and inflammatory conditions are all associated with reduced enzyme activity.

(Sleisenger, 9th edition, Pp-1754-1755)

18. **Ans. (D)** During fatty acid absorption, conjugated bile salts are passively absorbed by enterocytes in the upper small intestine. In addition sodium-coupled active transport retrieves bile salts in the ileum. Together, these absorptive processes are very efficient with a nearly 95% recovery of bile acids in the bloodstream. A small percentage of circulating bile salts enter the colon, where they are deconjugated and dehydroxylated by colonic bacteria and passed in the stool, short-chain fatty acid are generated by the colonic metabolism of unabsorbed dietary carbohydrates.

(Sleisenger, 9th edition, Pp-1701-1702)

19. **Ans. (B)** Pepsinogens are secreted by chief cells in response to gastrin, histamine and vagal stimulation the same factors that regulate acid secretion. Activation of pepsinogens to pepsins I and II is extremely pH-dependent and will not ocular above a pH of 4.5. Patients who are achlorhydric or who have had a gastrectomy do not show evidence of protein maldigestion because of the extensive contribution of pancreatic proteases and intestinal brush-border enzymes to the digestion of protein, indicating that intestinal events are more significant than gastric factors for protein digestion.

(Sleisenger, 9th edition, Pp-1712-1713)

20. **Ans. (A)** Intestinal epithelial cells can assimilate dipeptides and tripeptides as well as single amino acids. This has been shown in congenital diseases such as Hartnup disease and cystinuria, wherein defects in basic amino acid transporters occur in the small intestine and renal epithelium. In these conditions, measurable levels of the excluded amino acids are absorbed as a

result of the intracellular processing of absorbed dipeptides and tripeptides.

(Sleisenger, 9th edition, Pp-1716-1717)

21. **Ans. (D)** Iron absorption involves carrier-medicated translocation across the intestinal brush-border.

(Sleisenger, 9th edition, Pp-1723-1725)

22. **Ans. (A)** The recommended daily allowance is the level judged to be high enough to ensure an adequate intake for the majority of the normal population.

(Sleisenger, 9th edition, Pp-47-58)

23. **Ans. (A)** Whenever possible, oral feeding should be used to meet the patient's nutritional requirement rather than total parenteral nutrition. Malnourished preoperative patients, those with severe Crohn's disease, and patients with pancreatic pseudocyts have been shown to benefit from total parenteral nutrition. Elderly patients who cannot swallow are better managed by enteral feedings provided through a feeding tube.

(Sleisenger, 9th edition, Pp-85-87)

24. **Ans. (C)** In general, the degree of obesity is directly correlated with comorbidity risk. The body mass index is a useful measure of obesity, but is calculated as the weight in kilograms divided by the square of the height in meter. Upper body fat is more of a risk factor for diabetes, hypertension and ischemic heart disease than lower body fat. Men more commonly have upper body obesity compared to women.

(Sleisenger, 9th edition, Pp-103-110)

25. **Ans. (A)** Only a minority of cases of "food allergy" are immune-mediated. Many are the result of food intolerance from a variety of nonimmunologically medicated causes. Most cases of immunologic food allergy are IgE-mediated, causes an immediate-type hypersensitivity as a result of the degranulation of mass cell. Most food allergens are small (<70 kd) and are heat and acid-stable. Skin testing or food challenges in patients with severe anaphylactic reactions can be dangerous. In vitro tests for antigen specific IgE may be helpful in these cases.

(Sleisenger, 9th edition, Pp-139-142)

Chapter 13

LIVER BIOPSY

1. **The original description of liver biopsy in 1883 was done by:**
   A. Ehrlich
   B. Paul Lining
   C. Schiff
   D. G. Mehghini
   E. Vim Silverman
2. **Needle biopsy of the liver is preferred even during laparotomy because:**
   A. There is preponderance of the Glissen's capsule.
   B. Wider portal tracts in the sub capsular area
   C. Frequent but inconsequential surgically induced hepatitis
   D. All of the above
   E. None of the above
3. **The following are examples of suction needle used for liver biopsy *except*:**
   A. Menghini's needle
   B. Klatskin
   C. Jamshide
   D. Vim Silverman
4. **In a liver biopsy specimen preferential deposits of iron in Kupffer cells is associated with iron overload due to:**
   A. Multiple transfusions
   B. Hereditary haemochromatosis
   C. Chronic hepatitis C infection
   D. Alcoholic liver disease
5. **An independent predictor of sustained response in initial liver biopsy of the liver in HC:**
   A. Absence of bridging fibrosis/cirrhosis
   B. Iron overload
   C. Fatty change
   D. α_1 antitrypsin inclusion
6. **Liver biopsy specimens in patients with hereditary haemochromatosis show HIC (Hepatic iron concentration) of:**
   A. >3000 microgam/gm of dry weight
   B. <1500 micorgam/gm of dry weight
   C. <300 nitrogen of dry weight
   D. >1000 nitrogen of dry weight
7. **Hypokalemia precipitates hepatic encephalopathy by the following mechanism:**
   A. Increase in intestinal production of ammonia
   B. Increase in renal production of ammonia and favour cellular uptake of ammonia
   C. Decrease in conversion to urea
   D. Unknown mechanism
8. **Increase is the ratio of plasma aromatic ammonia acids to branched chain amino acids precipitate the hepatic encephalopathy by:**
   A. Increase in ammonia production
   B. Decrease in ammonia degradation
   C. Increase in production of false neutrotransmitters
   D. Stimulation of GABA receptor complex
9. **In the following statements which is true?**
   A. Arterial ammonia levels always correlate with severity of hepatic encephalopathy
   B. Normal ammonia levels can occur in hepatic encephalopathy
   C. Normal ammonia levels cannot occur in hepatic encephalopathy
   D. Venous ammonia always correlates with hepatic coma
10. **In the partosystemic encephalopathy index, which of the following measurement not included?**
    A. Clinical assessment of mental stat.
    B. Asterixis
    C. Arterial ammonia
    D. EEG
    E. MRI spectroscopy
11. **Lactitol is synthetic disaccharide otherwise called:**
    A. 1,4 galactosido fructose
    B. Beta galactosido sorbitol
    C. 1,4 galactosido sorbitol
    D. Beta galactosido fructose
12. **Lactitol has the following advantages over lactulose *except*:**
    A. Less sweet
    B. Quicker action
    C. Less flatulence
    D. More diarrhea

13. **Therapy with flumazenil should be limited to the following situations in hepatic encephalopathy:**
 A. Reversing the effects of exogenous benzodiazepines
 B. Aiding in the establishment of a diagnosis of encephalopathy
 C. Providing information about prognosis and optimizing brain function in hepatic encephalopathy
 D. When hepatic coma is complicated by bleeding tendency

14. **Common precipitating factor for hepatic encephalopathy is:**
 A. Azotemia B. Sedatives
 C. GI bleed D. Constipation

15. **Asterixis can be elicitied in the following region *except*:**
 A. Head B. Extremities
 C. Tongue D. Trunk

16. **TI weighted MRI scan in hepatic encephalopathy commonly shown lesion in:**
 A. Globus pallidus
 B. Thalamus
 C. Putamen
 D. Mesencephalon

17. **Globus pallidal hyper intensity in MRI scan in hepatic encephalopathy is due to deposition of:**
 A. Zinc
 B. Ammonia
 C. Manganese
 D. False neurotransmitters

18. **L-ornithine L-aspirate in hepatic encephalo-pathy decrease the ammonia by:**
 A. Stimulation of urea genesis in the peripheral organs
 B. Stimulation of urea genesis in the perivenular hepatocytes
 C. Decrease the absorption of urea from intestine
 D. Decrease the production of ammonia from intestine

19. **Spuriously low level of aminotransferases values can be seen in:**
 A. Myocardial infarction
 B. Skeletal diseases
 C. Uraemia
 D. Cholestatic

20. **AST is present in many tissues *except*:**
 A. Liver B. Heart
 C. Bone D. Kidney

21. **AST/ALT> 1 is seen in following conditions:**
 A. Alcoholic hepatitis
 B. Fatty liver of pregnancy
 C. Acute Wilson's disease
 D. CBD obstruction

22. **All clotting factors are synthesised in liver *except*:**
 A. VIII B. IX
 C. V D. VII

23. **Half life of factor VII is:**
 A. 24 hours B. 6 hours
 C. 12 hours D. 48 hours

24. **The time interval that requires normalization of prothrombin time after injection:**
 A. Within 48-72 hours
 B. Within 24-48 hours
 C. Within 4 hours
 D. 3-4 days

25. **In hepatic encephalopathy after treatment, ammonia levels usually return to normal level:**
 A. Immediately with improvement of neurological status
 B. Within 24 hours improvement of neurological status
 C. Within 48-72 hours improvement of neurological status
 D. Within 3-4 days improvement of neurological status

26. **Increased serum alkaline phosphatase and normal Gamma GTP is usually seen in *except*:**
 A. BRIC B. Byler's disease
 C. Bone disease D. CBD obstruction

27. **Increased GGTP and normal alkaline phosphatase is usually seen in:**
 A. Alcohol and drug B. Viral hepatitis
 C. Cholangitis D. CBD stricture

28. **Approximately how much of albumin synthesed and secreted by liver each day:**
 A. 10 gm/day B. 15 gm/day
 C. 6 gm/day D. 5.5 gm/day

29. **Unconjugated hyperbilirubinaemia is called when unconjugated bilirubin is:**
 A. Just more than conjugated bilirubin
 B. >85% of total bilirubin
 C. >60% of total bilirubin
 D. >70% of total bilirubin

30. **Following histological changes can be seen in chronic hepatitis C *except*:**

A. Steatosis
B. Lymphoid aggregates
C. Bile duct damage
D. Ground glass cells

31. **Marked elevation (1000 u/l) of ALT can be seen in following conditions *except*:**
A. Alcoholic hepatitis
B. Toxic hepatitis
C. Viral hepatitis
D. Ischemic hepatitis

32. **Increased ALT and increased LDH is usually seen in:**
A. Alcoholic hepatitis
B. Toxic hepatitis
C. Viral hepatitis
D. Ischemic hepatitis

33. **Sustained LDH elevation, with elevation of alkaline phosphatase level suggests:**
A. Ischemic hepatitis
B. Malignant infiltration of the liver
C. CBD obstruction
D. Viral hepatitis

34. **Prothrombin time prolonged in following conditions *except*:**
A. Liver failure
B. Consumptive coagulopathy
C. Prolonged antibiotics
D. von Willebrand's disease

Explanation

1. **Ans. (A)** Needle biopsy of the liver was first performed by Paul Ehrlich in 1883.

(Sherlock, 12th edition, P-36)

2. **Ans. (D)** Liver biopsy can be done during laparotomy because of wider portal tract in subcapsular area. Although hepatitis is frequent, but is mild and self-limiting.

(Sherlock, 12th edition, Pp-36-37)

3. **Ans. (D)** Menghin Klatskin and Jamshide needle obtain specimen by aspiration, while Vim Silverman uses a cutting technique.

(Sherlock, 12th edition, Pp-37-38)

4. **Ans. (A)** Kupffer cell sparing (Iron deposition) occurs in hereditary hemochromatosis, but in secondary iron over load (due to multiple blood transfusion iron deposition occurs predominately in Kupffer cell and reticuloendothelial cell.

(Sleisenger, 9th edition, Pp-1239-1246)

5. **Ans. (A)** Absence of bridging fibrosis and cirrhosis in pretreatment liver biopsy specimen is a future predictor of maintaining rapid virological response (RVR), early virological response (EVR) and sustained virological response (SUR).

(Sleisenger, 9th edition, Pp-1322-1323)

6. **Ans. (A)** Typically patient with HFE-related hereditary hemochromatosis has a HIC grade of 10,000 microgram/gram of liver weight (Normal<1500 microgram/gm of liver tissue.

(Sleisenger, 9th edition, P-1244)

7. **Ans. (B)** Hypokalemia increases renal production of ammonia and favors cellular uptake of ammonia precipitating hepatic encephalopathy.

(Sleisenger, 9th edition, Pp-1543-1546)

8. **Ans. (C)** Increased amount of aromatic aminoacid intake increases false neurotransmitter in brain precipitating hepatic encephalopathy.

(Sleisenger, 9th edition, Pp-1543-1547)

9. Serum ammonia level has no correlation with severity of hepatic encephalopathy and may be normal in patient with hepatic encephalopathy.

(Sleisenger, 9th edition, P-1544)

10. **Ans. (E)** In addition to clinical assessment, asterixis, arterial ammonia level, electroencephalography are used for calculating encephalopathy index.

(Sherlock, 12th edition, Pp-124-127)

11. **Ans. (B)** Lactitol is a beta galactosidosorbitol is a second generation disaccharide is efficacious with quicker onset of action and better tolerated with fewer side effects.

(Sherlock, 12th edition, P-142)

12. **Ans. (D)** For explanation see Ans. No.11.

(Sherlock, 12th edition, P-142)

13. **Ans. (A)** Flumazenil induce transient, variable short term improvement in hepatic encephalopathy, so not recommended routinely use limited reversing the effects of exogenous benzodiazepine.

(Sherlock, 12th edition, Pp-143-144)

14. **Ans. (C)** Gastrointestinal bleed is the most common precipitating factor for hepatic encephalopathy.

(Sleisenger, 9th edition, Pp-1543-1545)

15. **Ans. (C)** Asterixis elicited in arms, neck jaw, closed eyelid, trunk and extremities.

(Sherlock, 12th edition, P-122)

16. **Ans. (A)** T1-weighted MRI scan commonly show lesion in globus pallidus.

(Sherlock, 12th edition, P-127)

17. **Ans. (C)** Globus pallidal hyperintesity in MRI in hepatic encephalopathy is due to deposition of manganese.

(Sherlock, 12th edition, Pp-127-128)

18. **Ans. (A)** L-ornithine–L-asparate (LOLA) treatment promotes removal of ammonia by stimulating residual hepatic urea cycle activity and promoting glutamine synthesis particularly in skeletal muscle.

(Sherlock, 12th edition, P-143)

19. **Ans. (C)** Low serum aminotransferase level in chronic kidney disease patient on hemodialysis due to Vit-B6 deficiency.

(Sleisenger, 9th edition, P-1230)

20. **Ans. (C)** AST found in cytosol and mitochondria in the following organs. Liver > heart > skeletal muscle > brain > kidney > pancreas > lung > RBC > leucocytes.

(Sleisenger, 9th edition, P-1229)

21. **Ans. (A)** AST/ALT >1-seen in alcoholic hepatitis.

(Sleisenger, 9th edition, P-1230)

22. **Ans. (A)** All clotting factors produced in the liver with the exception of factor VIII, which is produced by vascular endothelial cell.

(Sleisenger, 9th edition, P-1234)

23. **Ans. (B)** Factor VII has the shortest half life of all clotting factor (of six hours).

(Sleisenger, 9th edition, P-1234)

24. **Ans. (A)** After Vit-K injection-normalization of prothrombin time occurs after 48-72 hours.

(Sleisenger, 9th edition, P-1234)

25. In hepatic encephalopathy, following treatment, ammonia level usually return to normal within 48-72 hours in improvement of neurological status.

(Sherlock, 12th edition, Pp-140-150)

26. **Ans. (C)** GGTP not elevated in bone diseases. Byler's disease there is elevation of GGTP.

(Sleisenger, 9th edition, P-1232)

27. **Ans. (A)** GGTP elevated in patients taking phenytoin, barbiturates, some drugs like highly active antiretroviral therapy.

(Sleisenger, 9th edition, P-1232)

28. **Ans. (A)** Daily synthesis of albumin 0.15 gm/kg body weight.

(Sleisenger, 9th edition, P-437)

29. **Ans. (B)** Conjugated bilirubinemia is defined as >15% of total bilirubin is conjugated.

(Sleisenger, 9th edition, P-1228)

30. **Ans. (C)** Bile duct damage is not the usual features of chronic hepatitis C, it occurs more in the setting of chronic rejection following liver transplant.

(Sleisenger, 9th edition, Pp-1322-1324)

31. **Ans. (A)** Marked elevation of ALT occurs in acute viral hepatitis, ischemic hepatitis, acute Budd-Chiari syndrome, acute bile duct obstruction.

(Sleisenger, 9th edition, P-1230)

32. **Ans. (D)** Increased ALT and LDH is usually seen in ischemic hepatitis.

(Sleisenger, 9th edition, P-1230)

33. **Ans. (B)** Sustained LDH elevation with elevated ALP may be found in malignant infiltration of liver such as lymphoma.

(Sleisenger, 9th edition, P-1235)

34. **Ans. (D)** In von-Willebrand's disease, there is prolongation of APTT, but no prolongation of prothrombin.

(Sleisenger, 9th edition, P-1234)

Chapter 14

Miscellaneous

1. **Motilin receptors are stimulated by:**
   A. Ampicillin
   B. Tetracycline
   C. Erythromycin
   D. Cephalosporins

2. **Metabolite measured in quantitative liver function test–MEG-X is:**
   A. Indocyanine green B. Aminopyrine
   C. Lignocaine D. Antipyrine

3. **Amount of fluid presented to the small intestine per day is:**
   A. 2-4 I B. 4-6 I
   C. 6-8 I D. 8-10 I

4. **Fecal leucocytes are present in all *except*:**
   A. Cholera
   B. Amoebic colitis
   C. Infective colitis
   D. Enteroinvasive E. coli

5. **One of the statement is wrong regarding omeprazole:**
   A. Prodrug
   B. Acts on parietal cells
   C. Reversible enzyme inhibition
   D. Proton pump blocker

6. **Cholera is treated by:**
   A. Tetracycline B. Ampicillin
   C. Erythromycin D. Chloramphenicol

7. **For replication of HBV highly sensitive test is:**
   A. HbeAg B. HbsAg
   C. HBV DNA D. HbcAg

8. **Hepatic adenomas are caused by:**
   A. Androgens B. Amiodarone
   C. Azathioprine D. Acetaminophen

9. **Gene for Wilson's disease is on chromosome:**
   A. 9
   B. 13
   C. 18
   D. 22

10. **Fibrolamellar carcinoma differs from hepatoma by:**
    A. Occurs in young
    B. No previous history of chronic liver disease
    C. Normal AFP
    D. All the above

11. **In MEN1 most common involvement is:**
    A. Gastrinoma
    B. Insulinoma
    C. Hyperparathyroidism
    D. Parathyroid adenoma

12. **Most common site of involvement in gastrinoma is:**
    A. Head of pancreas B. Body of pancreas
    C. Stomach D. Duodenum

13. **One of the following is not found in somatostatinoma:**
    A. Diabetes B. Gall stones
    C. Steatorrhea D. Hypokalemia

14. **H. pylori most commonly implicated in:**
    A. Duodenal ulcer B. Gastric ulcer
    C. Gastric carcinoma D. Gastritis

15. **Patients with gluten enteropathy are fed with:**
    A. Wheat B. Rye
    C. Barley D. Maize

16. **Most common cause of variceal bleed in children is:**
    A. Cirrhosis of liver
    B. EHPVO
    C. NCPF
    D. Budd-Chiari syndrome

17. **Taenia coli is formed by:**
    A. Mucosa
    B. Submucosa
    C. Muscularis mucosa
    D. Worm infestation

18. **Highest concentration of hepatitis E is seen in:**
    A. Stool B. Bile
    C. Intestinal juice D. Serum

19. Which is not seen in Menetrier's disease?
A. Hypoproteinemia and oedema
B. Hypertrophied folds
C. Proteinuria
D. Increased incidence of carcinoma

20. Which is not seen in hypertrophic pyloric stenosis?
A. Palpable stomach
B. Diagnosis by ultrasound abdomen
C. Visible peristalsis
D. Increased length of the pyloric muscle

21. All cause macrovesicular fatty liver *except*:
A. Obesity
B. Jejunoileal bypass
C. Alcohol
D. Reye's syndrome

22. Primary gastrointestinal lymphoma involves:
A. Small intestine B. Lymph nodes
C. Liver and spleen D. All the above

23. Brunner's glands develop by:
A. 14 weeks B. 20 weeks
C. 24 weeks D. 28 weeks

24. In oesophagus, stratified squamous epithelium develops by:
A. 16 weeks B. 20 weeks
C. 22 weeks D. 36 weeks

25. In glycolysis the number of ATP produced is:
A. 2 B. 4
C. 6 D. 8

26. Pancreas fully develops by:
A. 16 weeks B. 19 weeks
C. 24 weeks D. 28 weeks

27. In diffuse oesophageal spasm manometry shows:
A. Normal UES and high mid and lower oesophageal pressure
B. Normal UES with high lower oesophageal sphincter pressure
C. High UES pressure with normal mid and lower oesophagus
D. High pressure in both UES and LES

28. Absent peristalsis with hypotensive LES is seen in:
A. Achalasia
B. Scleroderma
C. Diffuse esophageal spasm
D. Pregnancy

29. Pancreatic rests show all *except*:
A. Malignant transformation
B. Pancreatitis
C. Gastric outlet obstruction
D. None of the above

30. All are tests for oesophageal motility disorder *except*:
A. Ergonovine test B. Pyridostigmine test
C. Bernstein test D. Manometry

31. False regarding early gastric malignancy:
A. Involves only mucosa
B. Involves mucosa and submucosa
C. Involves lymph nodes
D. Does not involve liver and spleen

32. Abnormality not seen in bacterial overgrowth is:
A. Folate malabsorption
B. B_{12} malabsorption
C. Positive D-xylose test
D. Abnormal xylose breath test

33. Pancreatic pseudocyst is commonly seen in the:
A. Head of pancreas B. Body of pancreas
C. Tail of pancreas D. Lesser sac

34. Hypergastrinaemia is seen in all *except*:
A. ZE syndrome
B. Antral G cell hyperplasia
C. Carcinoid syndrome
D. Small intestinal resection

35. Correct statement regarding ZE syndrome:
A. Two-third are malignant
B. Most common site is pancreas
C. Secretin stimulation test is positive in 75% of cases
D. Chemotherapy is treatment of choice

36. Most common bleeding site of diverticulosis is:
A. Ascending colon B. Transverse colon
C. Descending colon D. Rectosigmoid

37. Best test for gastric emptying is:
A. Barium meal follow through
B. Radioisotope scan
C. 24-hour pH monitoring
D. Hydrogen breath test

38. Protein losing enteropathy is seen in:
A. Intestinal tuberculosis
B. Lactose malabsorption
C. Chronic pancreatitis
D. Periampullary carcinoma

39. Most common indication of liver transplantation in children is:
A. Biliary atresia
B. Alpha 1 antitrypsin
C. Wilson's disease
D. Glycogen storage disease

40. Bacterial count in small intestine (ileum) is:
A. 104 B. 106
C. 108 D. 1012

41. All the following cause a similar type of skin rash *except*:
A. Acrodermatitis B. Zn deficiency
C. Amyloidosis D. Glucagonoma

42. The number of crypts surrounding each villous in jejunum is:
A. 2 B. 4
C. 6 D. 8

43. M cells are located in:
A. Duodenum B. Jejunum
C. Ileum D. Colon

44. In pregnancy all are seen *except*:
A. Gallbladder contractions are increased
B. Increased gastric emptying
C. Colonic transit time is increased
D. LES pressure is decreased

45. Treatment of choice for microscopic colitis is:
A. Bismuth B. Corticosteroids
C. Salazopyrine D. Azathioprine

46. All act at intestinal basolateral membrane *except*:
A. H-K-ATPase B. Na-K-ATPase
C. C1– transport D. None of the above

47. Most specific test for celiac disease is:
A. Anti-gliadin antibodies
B. Anti-endomyseal antibodies
C. Villous atrophy
D. Villous atrophy which responds to gluten free diet1

48. Patients with gluten enteropathy are fed with:
A. Wheat B. Rye
C. Barley D. Oat

49. In food hypersensitivity which is not a feature?
A. Anaphylactic shock
B. Pruritus ani
C. Arthritis
D. Macrocytic anemia

50. Prevalence of hepatitis B virus in India is:
A. 0.5% B. 1%
C. 2% D. 4%

51. Fulminant colitis is treated by:
A. 4ASA B. 5ASA
C. Corticosteroids D. Sulphapyridine

52. Most accepted theory for the cause of ulcerative colitis:
A. Infective theory
B. Immunological theory
C. Psychological
D. Heat shock protein

53. Candida is associated with all *except*:
A. Old age B. Steroid
C. Diabetes D. GERD

54. Acute pancreatitis is caused by:
A. Scorpion sting
B. Organophosphorus poisoning
C. Methyl dopa
D. High fatty meal

55. True statement regarding peptic stricture:
A. Always occurs in the lower end of esophagus
B. Many present with hematemesis
C. Causes long strictures
D. Always have history of heartburn

56. Primary biliary cirrhosis is associated with all *except*:
A. Renal tubular acidosis
B. Medullary sponge kidney
C. Renal stones
D. Sjögren's syndrome

57. Calcium absorption is altered by all *except*:
A. Phosphates B. Phytates
C. Lactose D. Cellulose

58. One of the following is incorrect regarding cystic fibrosis:
A. Inborn error of metabolism
B. Most common cause of pancreatic insufficiency in children
C. Most of the patients have respiratory complaints
D. In majority it presents with rectal prolapse

59. Sweat chloride levels are increased in all *except*:
A. Cystic fibrosis
B. Hyperparathyroidism
C. Hypothyroidism
D. Malnutrition

60. Hyperamylasaemia is seen in all *except*:
A. Burns B. Hypothyroidism
C. Macroamylasaemia D. Renal failure

Explanation

1. **Ans. (C)** Motilin receptor is stimulated by erythromycin. So they are effective in gastroparesis as it increases gastric emptying.

(Sleisenger, 9th edition, P-812)

2. **Ans. (C)** Metabolite of lignocaine is MEGX. Lignocaine is used for assessment of quantitative liver function.

(Sleisenger, 9th edition, P-1235)

3. **Ans. (D)** Total 8.5 liter of fluid is presented to small intestine, out of which 7 liters absorbed.

(Sleisenger, 9th edition, P-1676)

4. **Ans. (A)** Cholera is characterized by watery diarrhea. So, No evidence of fecal leucocytes in choleral stool.

(Sleisenger, 9th edition, P-185)

5. **Ans. (C)** Omeprazole is a prodrug, it act on parietal cell H^+-K^+-ATPase, is a proton pump inhibitors, they irreversible inhibits the H^+-K^+-ATPase.

(Sleisenger, 9th edition, Pp-722-723)

6. **Ans. (A)** Cholera is treated by tetracycline.

(Sleisenger, 9th edition, Pp-1851-1852)

7. **Ans. (C)** Serum HBV DNA level is the quantitative of hepatitis B virus replication phase.

(Sleisenger, 9th edition, P-1299)

8. **Ans. (A)** Hepatic adenoma is caused by ocps, androgens and synthetic steroids.

(Sleisenger, 9th edition, Pp-1584-1585)

9. **Ans. (B)** Gene for Wilson's disease lies in chromosome B.

(Sleisenger, 9th edition, P-1384)

10. **Ans. (D)** Fibrolamellar carcinoma no previous history of chronic liver disease usually occurs in young persons. The prognosis is usually better than classic hepatocellular carcinoma.

(Sleisenger, 9th edition, P-1575)

11. **Ans. (C)** In MEN1—Most common involvement is hyper-parathyroidism due to parathyroid adenoma and parathyroid hyperplasia.

(Sleisenger, 9th edition, Pp-499-501)

12. **Ans. (D)** Most common site of involvement of gastrinoma triangle, which is formed by junction of pancreatic body and neck medially junction of cystic and (BD posteriorly and junction of 2nd and 3rd part of duodenum laterally.

(Sleisenger, 9th edition, P-499)

13. **Ans. (D)** Hypokalemia most commonly found in vipoma but not in somatostatinoma.

(Sleisenger, 9th edition, Pp-511-512)

14. H. pylori commonly implicated in duodenal ulcer.

(Sleisenger, 9th edition, Pp-838-840)

15. **Ans. (D)** In gluten enteropathy rye, barley and wheat are contraindicated.

(Sleisenger, 9th edition, Pp-1813-1814)

16. **Ans. (B)** EHPVO (Extrahepatic portal vein obstruction) is the most common cause of variceal bleeding in children.

(Sleisenger, 9th edition, Pp-1499-1500)

17. **Ans. (C)** Taenia coli present in large intestine and derived from longitudinal muscle fibers.

(Sleisenger, 9th edition, P-1616)

18. **Ans. (A)** Highest concentration of HEV found in stool.

(Sleisenger, 9th edition, Pp-1337-1338)

19. **Ans. (C)** Protein losing enteropathy seen in menetrier's disease but not proteinuria. There is 15% risk of gastric carcinoma in menetrier's disease. Due to protein losing enteropathy, there is associated hypoproteinemia and odema.

(Sleisenger, 9th edition, P-400)

20. **Ans. (A)** In idiopathic hypertophic pyloric stenosis, there is palpable pylorous. In addition USG is useful to establish the diagnosis.

(Sleisenger, 9th edition, Pp-783-784)

21. **Ans. (D)** Reye syndrome, acute fatty liver of pregnancy, Jamaican vomiting sickness syndrome, and drugs like sodium valproate and tetracycline all are causes of microvesicular steatosis.

(Sleisenger, 9th edition, P-1414)

22. **Ans. (A)** Primary gastrointestinal lymphoma commonly involves stomach and followed by small intestine.

(Sleisenger, 9th edition, P-446)

23. **Ans. (B)** Brunner's gland develops by 20th week of gestation.

(Sleisenger, 9th edition, P-1352)

24. **Ans. (A)** In oesophagus, stratified squamous epithelium develops by 16 weeks of gestation.

(Sleisenger, 9th edition, P-668)

25. **Ans. (A)** In glycolysis total 2ATPS are produced.

(Sleisenger, 9th edition, P-1217)

26. **Ans. (B)** Pancreas fully developed by 20th week of gestation.

(Sleisenger, 9th edition, Pp-915-916)

27. **Ans. (A)** In distal oesophageal spasm, there is normal UES pressure, but high mid and lower oesophageal pressure with CFV-8 cm/second.

(Sleisenger, 9th edition, P-699)

28. **Ans. (B)** Absent peristalsis with hypotensive LES seen in scleroderma.

(Sleisenger, 9th edition, Pp-678-682)

29. **Ans. (D)** Pancreatic rest contains pancreatic tissue, most commonly located in the stomach, they may undergo complication like pancreatitis, gastric outlet obstruction and malignant change.

(Sleisenger, 9th edition, P-918)

30. **Ans. (C)** Bernstein test used for detecting oesophageal hypersensitivity. Rest others documented to detect the motility disorder.

(Sleisenger, 9th edition, Pp-698-702)

31. **Ans. (B)** Early gastric cancer is defined as it involves mucosa and submucosa irrespective of lymph node status.

(Sleisenger, 9th edition, P-900)

32. **Ans. (C)** In small intestinal bacterial overgrowth syndrome, there is increased folate and vit-K level, due to synthesis by bacteria.

(Sleisenger, 9th edition, Pp-1772-1773)

33. **Ans. (B)** Pancreatic pseudocyst most commonly occurs in body of pancreas.

(Sleisenger, 9th edition, Pp-980-981)

34. **Ans. (C)** Carcinoid syndrome is not associated with hypergastrinemia. However hypergastrinemia occurs following small bowel resection, PPI therapy, ZE syndrome.

(Sleisenger, 9th edition, Pp-498-500)

35. **Ans. (A)** ZES syndrome 50%-80% are malignant commonly occurs in duodenal triangle secretion stimulation are positive in 96% of cases. PPI are treatment of choice.

(Sleisenger, 9th edition, Pp-498-501)

36. **Ans. (A)** Most common site for bleeding in diverticulosis is from right sided colon.

(Sleisenger, 9th edition, Pp-2085-2087)

37. **Ans. (B)** Test meals labeled with radioisotopes are available to assess the gastric emptying in 4 hours emptying test if retention is more than > 10% is considered to have deployed gastric emptying.

(Sleisenger, 9th edition, P-803)

38. **Ans. (A)** Fecal estimation of $á_1$-antitrypsin level best correlates with protein losing enteropathy.

(Sleisenger, 9th edition, Pp-437-440)

39. **Ans. (A)** Most common indication for liver transplantation in children is extra hepatic biliary atresia.

(Sleisenger, 9th edition, Pp-1054-1055)

40. **Ans. (C)** Normal bacterial count in ileum is 10^8/gram of stool.

(Sleisenger, 9th edition, P-1770)

41. **Ans. (C)** Characteristic rash in glucagonoma is similar to rash seen in zinc deficiency and acrodermatitis.

(Sleisenger, 9th edition, Pp-505-509)

42. **Ans. (B)** Each crypt is surrounded by 4-5 villi in jejunum.

(Sleisenger, 9th edition, P-1784)

43. **Ans. (C)** M-cells are located most commonly in ileum.

(Sleisenger, 9th edition, P-25)

44. **Ans. (A)** In pregnancy, there is hypomotility of gallbladder leading to gallbladder stasis and cholelithiasis small intestine and large intestine transit time increased.

(Sleisenger, 9th edition, Pp-625-628)

45. **Ans. (B)** Corticosteroid is the treatment of choice for microscopic colitis.

(Sleisenger, 9th edition, Pp-2239-2243)

46. **Ans. (A)** H+ -K+ -ATPase located in a pilal membrane. Rest all located in basolateral membrane.

(Sleisenger, 9th edition, P-821)

47. Ans. (D) Most specific histologic finding in celiac disease is villous atrophy which respond to gluten-free diet.

(Sleisenger, 9th edition, Pp-1799-1803)

48. Ans. (D) Oat can be taken safely in celiac disease. rye, barley and wheat contraindicated in celiac disease.

(Sleisenger, 9th edition, Pp-1799-1808)

49. Ans. (D) In food hypersensitivity microcytic anemia is usually seen however macrocytic anemia is uncommon. Rheumatoid like arthritis can be manifestation of food hypersensitivity.

(Sleisenger, 9th edition, Pp-142-145)

50. Ans. (D) 3%-5% of population of India are hepatitis B carrier in contrast to 3% of general patient are having hepatitis C virus infection.

(Sleisenger, 9th edition, P-1287)

51. Ans. (C) Fulminant colitis are treated by parental steroids and immune suppressants.

(Sleisenger, 9th edition, Pp-1995-2001)

52. Ans. (B) Immunological theory is the most accepted theory for pathogenesis of ulcerative colitis.

(Sleisenger, 9th edition, Pp-1989-2000)

53. Ans. (D) Oesophageal candidiasis is associated with older age, long term steroid use, achalasia, scleroderma, use of immunosuppressants etc.

(Sleisenger, 9th edition, Pp-741-742)

54. Ans. (C) Acute pancreatitis can be caused by organophosphorous poisoning, scorpion bite high fatty meal etc.

(Sleisenger, 9th edition, P-969)

55. Ans. (B) Peptic stricture due to reflux may occur in 7%-25% of cases, are usually small size stricture. 80% of cases associated with pain sometimes it may present with hematemesis.

(Sleisenger, 9th edition, P-714)

56. Ans. (B) Primary biliary cirrhosis is associated with Sjögren syndrome, RTA, diabetes mellitus, hypothyroidism gallstones.

(Sleisenger, 9th edition, P-1480)

57. Ans. (C) Calcium absorption is decreased by phosphate, phytate and cellulose.

(Sleisenger, 9th edition, P-1705)

58. Ans. (B) Sweat chloride test increased in the following conditions:

Cystic fibrosis	Ectodermal dysplasia
GSD-type-I	Adrenal insufficiency
Familial hyperparathyroidism	Pitressin resistant
Fucoidosis	Diabetic insidious
Mucopolysaccharidosis syndrome	Familial cholestasis
Environmental deprivation syndrome	Acute respiratory disorders
Chronic respiratory disorder	

(Sleisenger, 9th edition, P-944)

59. Ans. (D) Only 20% of cases of cystic fibrosis patient presented with rectal prolapse.

(Sleisenger, 9th edition, P-945)

60. Ans. (B) Hyperamylasemia not seen in hypothyroidism.

(Sleisenger, 9th edition, P-946)